Contemporary Neuroimmunology

Contemporary Neuroimmunology

Editor: Lane Thompson

AMERICAN
MEDICAL PUBLISHERS
www.americanmedicalpublishers.com

AMERICAN
MEDICAL PUBLISHERS
www.americanmedicalpublishers.com

Cataloging-in-Publication Data

Contemporary neuroimmunology / edited by Lane Thompson.
p. cm.
Includes bibliographical references and index.
ISBN 978-1-63927-642-4
1. Neuroimmunology. 2. Nervous system--Diseases--Immunological aspects.
3. Immunology. 4. Neurosciences. I. Thompson, Lane.
QP356.47 .C66 2023
616.079--dc23

American Medical Publishers,
41 Flatbush Avenue,
1st Floor, New York,
NY 11217, USA

ISBN 978-1-63927-642-4 (Hardback)

Contents

Preface

I am honored to present to you this unique book which encompasses the most up-to-date data in the field. I was extremely pleased to get this opportunity of editing the work of experts from across the globe. I have also written papers in this field and researched the various aspects revolving around the progress of the discipline. I have tried to unify my knowledge along with that of stalwarts from every corner of the world, to produce a text which not only benefits the readers but also facilitates the growth of the field.

Neuroimmunology is a discipline of medical science that deals with the study of nervous system, neuroscience and immunology. It aims to understand the complex interplay of nervous system and immune system during development, homeostasis and injuries. The main aim of this discipline is to develop treatment, prevention methods for neurological diseases, which do not have apparent etiology. Symptoms of neuroimmunological disorders include considerably decreased capability to do regular activities, inability to talk, stand or sit straight, excessive sensitivity to light, sleep problems, and thinking and memory problems. Other common symptoms are night sweats, sore throat and muscle or joint pain. There is no treatment for these diseases but symptoms may be managed. This book unravels the recent studies in the field of neuroimmunology. It will also provide interesting topics for research which interested readers can take up. Through it, we attempt to further enlighten the readers about the new concepts in this field.

Finally, I would like to thank all the contributing authors for their valuable time and contributions. This book would not have been possible without their efforts. I would also like to thank my friends and family for their constant support.

Editor

1

Overview of Traumatic Brain Injury: An Immunological Context

Damir Nizamutdinov [1,2] and Lee A. Shapiro [1,2,*]

1 Department of Surgery, Texas A & M University Health Science Center, College of Medicine, Temple, TX 76504, USA; dnizamutdinov@medicine.tamhsc.edu
2 Department of Neurosurgery, Neuroscience Research Institute, Baylor Scott & White Health, Temple, TX 76504, USA
* Correspondence: lshapiro@medicine.tamhsc.edu

Academic Editor: Donna Gruol

Abstract: Traumatic brain injury (TBI) afflicts people of all ages and genders, and the severity of injury ranges from concussion/mild TBI to severe TBI. Across all spectrums, TBI has wide-ranging, and variable symptomology and outcomes. Treatment options are lacking for the early neuropathology associated with TBIs and for the chronic neuropathological and neurobehavioral deficits. Inflammation and neuroinflammation appear to be major mediators of TBI outcomes. These systems are being intensively studies using animal models and human translational studies, in the hopes of understanding the mechanisms of TBI, and developing therapeutic strategies to improve the outcomes of the millions of people impacted by TBIs each year. This manuscript provides an overview of the epidemiology and outcomes of TBI, and presents data obtained from animal and human studies focusing on an inflammatory and immunological context. Such a context is timely, as recent studies blur the traditional understanding of an "immune-privileged" central nervous system. In presenting the evidence for specific, adaptive immune response after TBI, it is hoped that future studies will be interpreted using a broader perspective that includes the contributions of the peripheral immune system, to central nervous system disorders, notably TBI and post-traumatic syndromes.

Keywords: traumatic brain injury; neuroimmunity; neuroinflammation

---

1. Types of Traumatic Brain Injuries in Humans

1.1. Epidemiology of TBI in the United States

A traumatic brain injury (TBI) is an injury that disrupts the normal function of the brain and can be caused by a bump, blow or jolt to the head, rapid acceleration and deceleration of the calvarium, or a penetrating head injury [1]. In 2010, the Centers for Disease Control and Prevention estimated that TBIs accounted for approximately 2.5 million emergency department (ED) visits in the United States. Of these, approximately 87% (2,213,826) were treated and released, 11% (283,630) were hospitalized and discharged, and approximately 2% (52,844) died [2]. The leading causes of non-fatal TBI in the U.S. are falls (35%), motor vehicle-associated accidents (17%) and strikes or blows to the head from/against objects, including sport injuries (17%) [3]. The leading causes of TBI-related deaths are motor vehicle crashes, suicides and falls. In the United States, children aged 0–4 years, adolescents aged 15–19 years, and older adults aged >75 years have the highest rates of TBI-related hospitalizations and deaths among all age groups [3]. Approximately 145,000 children/adolescent (aged 0–19 years) and 775,000 older adults (>75 years) are estimated to be living with substantial and long-lasting limitations in social, behavioral, physical and/or cognitive functioning following a TBI [4]. In every age group, TBI-related ED visit rates are higher for males than for females, which were 800.4 vs. 633.7 cases per 100,000, respectively [2]. Males aged 0–4 years have the highest rates for TBI-related emergency department visits, hospitalizations and deaths combined. Regarding the military, Department of Defense data revealed that from 2000–2011, 235,046 service members (4.2% of the 5,603,720 who served in the Army, Air Force, Navy and Marine Corps) were diagnosed with a TBI [5]. Thus, TBI afflicts millions of people each year, including civilian and military populations. It is pertinent to note that these statistics do not account for those people suffering from concussion/mild TBI who did not receive medical care or had outpatient/office-based visits, estimated by some to be hundreds of thousands, if not millions of people each year [3].

1.2. Classification of TBI

The severity of TBIs is typically categorized using the Glasgow Coma Scale and can range from: (a) mild; (b) moderate; to (c) severe [6]. TBI outcomes are often determined by using the Glasgow Outcome Scale, which categorizes gross neurobehavioral ranges of recovery: (a) dead; (b) vegetative state; (c) severe disability; (d) moderate disability; (e) good recovery [7]. An alternative prognosis, using Russell and Smith's classification, is divided as severe or very severe [8]. Considering that detailed classification helps to determine the severity of injury, informs treatment options and is used to assess prognosis and functional recovery, recent suggestions have indicated that better diagnostic and assessment criteria are needed in the TBI field [9,10].

1.3. TBI Prognosis

The effects of TBI can adversely affect quality of life, including cognitive, behavioral, emotional and physical deficiencies. Any one or more of these can negatively impact interpersonal, social and occupational functioning, as well as families, communities and the economy in general [11,12]. Impairment of cognitive function can lead to difficulties with memory, attention, learning, coordination and sleep disturbances [12] and can persist for days, months or even years following the initial injury. Other long-term deficiencies include: language and communication problems (19%), dysarthria (30%), dysphagia (17%) [13], mood disorders [14,15] and cognitive impairment, even six months after mild TBI [16]. Another post-traumatic syndrome that can have a relatively delayed onset is post-traumatic epilepsy [14,15,17]. While all epilepsies are seizure disorders, not all seizures are epilepsy. As such, the incidence of early post-traumatic seizures (seizures immediately following, up to the first few days after the TBI) is higher than the incidence of post-traumatic epilepsy. Notably, about 25% of brain contusion patients and 32%–53% of patients with penetrating TBI develop different degrees of early post-traumatic seizures. Post-traumatic seizures also seem to be more prevalent following severe TBIs, although mild and moderate TBIs can also result in seizures [18]. Considering the negative impact of these numerous disorders associated with post-traumatic deficiencies, as well as the significant numbers of people suffering from the chronic effects of TBIs, research efforts are underway in the hopes of better understanding the pathogenic progression, and developing successful treatments of and diagnostic criterion for TBI.

2. A Brief Review of Experimental TBI Animal Models

In view of the heterogeneous clinical nature of TBI, numerous animal models have been developed for experimentation. Although larger animals are closer in size and physiology to humans, rodents are a valuable and commonly-used model in TBI research. Their modest cost, biological similarities, more manageable size and standardized outcome measurements are all advantageous. Such models have been incorporated for studies aimed at improving our understanding of the detrimental, complex molecular cascades that are initiated by head trauma, as well as the long-term neurological and behavioral consequences. Therefore, unless otherwise indicated, this review focuses on data from animal models (primarily rodents) of TBI. Among them, several models are widely used in research: fluid percussion injury (FPI) [19–22], cortical impact injury (CCI) [23–25], penetrating ballistic-like brain injury [26], weight drop/impact acceleration injury [27] and blast TBI injury [28,29]. Although we will highlight the two most highly-cited animal models, FPI and CCI, it is important to note that many similarities with regard to the general neuroinflammatory responses are observed across rodent models of TBI, despite the different methods and modalities of the injuries.

2.1. Percussion Injury Animal Models

In percussive injury models, there are two devices that are most commonly incorporated into experiments. In the FPI model, the insult is inflicted by a pendulum striking the piston of a reservoir of fluid, and this generates a fluid pressure pulse that is delivered to the intact dura, via a syringe secured over an opened midline or lateral craniotomy [30,31]. In the second percussive TBI, an injury is delivered by a piston that is controlled either pneumatically or via a piezoelectric mechanism [32–34]. The percussion produces brief displacement and deformation of brain tissue, and the severity of injury depends on the strength of the pressure pulse [31], as well as the location of the craniotomy/injury. FPI models replicate clinical TBI without skull fracture [35] and, despite the craniotomy, are considered a closed head injury model [36]. The FPI model is often considered to be of mild to moderate severity, rather than severe [30]. A number of studies have shown that FPI can reliably reproduce intracranial hemorrhage [30,31], swelling [31,37], neuroinflammation [37–39] and gray matter damage [19,30], all of which are pathophysiological changes observed in human TBIs [40]. Based on the position of the craniotomy, FPI models can be divided into midline (centered on the sagittal suture), parasagittal (<3.5 mm lateral to midline) and lateral models (>3.5 mm lateral to midline; LFPI) [31,41–43]. The midline FPI model of TBI was first developed for use in cats and rabbits [37,44], secondly adapted for rats [30] and subsequently modified for use in mice [19,31]. FPI has also been used for studying TBI pathophysiology and pharmacology in other species [37,45,46], although the volume of literature pales in comparison to that for rodents.

In rodents, FPI produces a rapid combination of focal cortical contusion and diffuse subcortical (such as hippocampus and thalamus) neuronal injury. These can occur within minutes of the impact, progress to a loss of neurons by 12 h and are accompanied by a rapid neuroinflammatory response that is initially focused in the peri-injury region [38,39]. Neuronal death and neuroinflammatory signaling seem to peak at around three days after FPI and in many other models [38]. This inflammation persists, albeit at levels lower than the peak, well into chronic time points (≥1 month). In the days and months following the injury, progressive degenerative cascades that include chronic inflammation continue to be observed in a variety of brain regions implicated in higher cognitive functions. These include the hippocampus, thalamus, medial septum, striatum and amygdala [35,47,48]. It is often deduced that the neuropathology in these regions underlies the observed neurobehavioral and cognitive deficits that are commonly seen in the FPI model [36,49,50]. Of significance is the fact that analogous symptoms are often seen in patients with TBI-related injuries to corresponding brain regions [36,49].

2.2. Controlled Cortical Impact Injury Animal Model

The CCI model uses a pneumatic or electromagnetic impact device to drive a rigid impactor onto the exposed intact dura and mimics cortical tissue loss, acute subdural hematoma, axonal injury, concussion, blood-brain barrier (BBB) dysfunction and even coma [23–25]. It has been applied to a number of animals, such as ferrets [24], swine and monkeys [51] and, most prominently, rodents [23,25]. CCI is delivered to the intact dura through a craniotomy and results in deformation of the underlying cortex [23]. The damage created is highly reproducible and includes a rapid and sometimes widespread neuropathological damage. This damage is most prominent in the peri-injury area, includes neurodegenerative and neuroinflammatory responses [52], and can also encompass cortical, hippocampal and thalamic degeneration [53]. The histopathological severity of CCI rises with increasing cortical deformation, as does the cognitive impairment that is likely related to the extent of damage [54–59]. Similar to the FPI model, the neuropathology and associated cognitive and behavioral deficits after CCI persist chronically, and diffuse neuropathology is evident [60,61].

Similarly, the neuroinflammatory response appears to play a major role in both the early and chronic deficiencies observed following TBI.

3. Mechanisms of Neuropathology Following TBI

It is now widely acknowledged that TBI is a complex multimodal disease process, not a single pathophysiological event [62]. It causes structural and functional damage, which lead to deficits resulting from both primary and secondary injury mechanisms [63]. The primary injury is the result of the immediate mechanical damage from direct contact and/or inertial forces to the brain that occurs at the moment of the traumatic impact. This damage can include direct neuronal, glial and other cellular damage, contusion, damage to blood vessels (hemorrhage) and axonal shearing [64,65]. Secondary injury evolves over minutes, to days, to months, to years after the primary injury and is the result of cascades of metabolic, cellular and molecular events. These occur concurrently with, and contribute to, alterations of endogenous neurochemical, inflammatory and neuroinflammatory mechanisms. Such mechanisms ultimately lead to brain cell death or rescue, plasticity, tissue damage and atrophy [35,66,67]. Many biochemical alterations responsible for secondary injury have also been identified. These include, perturbation of cellular calcium homeostasis, glutamate excitotoxicity, mitochondrial dysfunction, increased free radical generation, inflammation, neuroinflammation, increased lipid peroxidation, apoptosis and diffuse axonal injury (DAI) [68]. Interestingly, all of these alterations can be linked either directly or indirectly to neuroinflammation, and such inflammation has been implicated in the early and chronic components of TBI-induced neuropathology [69–71].

4. Inflammation Following TBI: An Immunological Perspective

4.1. Innate, Non-Specific Immune Response to TBI

At present, the prevailing viewpoint in the TBI field has been that most, if not all of the inflammation that follows a TBI can be considered components of the innate immune response [72–74]. However, accumulating evidence using updated technology suggests that specific adaptive immune mechanisms are also at play. Thus, a working operational definition is needed to define immune specificity after TBI, and few authors have adequately separated innate from adaptive immune components after a TBI. The early neuroinflammatory response across injuries and injury models occurs in a relatively stereotypical manner and can largely be considered to consist mainly of innate immune mechanisms. When damage to the brain takes place during TBI, it triggers the release and production of cytokines and chemokines, which activate receptors, and results in local and systemic immune responses [72,75,76]. The net effect of these innate inflammatory mediators is aimed at limiting the spread of the injury and restoring homeostatic balance [77].

4.2. Cytokines in TBI

Cytokines are categorized by structural and functional components, can be either pro- and/or anti-inflammatory and, in a classical immunological sense, are mediators of the cellular immune response, as well as of antibody synthesis and release. Cytokines can be synthesized and/or released by a wide variety of cells, including microglia, macrophages, T and B lymphocytes, endothelial and mast cells [78,79]. Although a full discussion of cytokine changes and functions after TBI is beyond the scope of this review, several reports indicate that interleukin (IL) IL1-β, IL18 and tumor necrosis factor alpha (TNFα) are involved in the onset and development of the inflammatory cascade after TBI in rodents and humans [72–74]. IL1-β binds to IL1-receptors, primarily localized on microglia and astrocytes in the brain, but also to other cell types, including infiltrating immune cells [80,81]. Activation of the neuroglial and immune cell IL1-receptors initiates the production and release of inflammatory cytokines, including increased production of IL1-β and IL18 [82]. This results in a self-perpetuating, pro-inflammatory environment, which may be damaging to the CNS parenchyma [75,76,83,84].

The damaging effects of IL1-β can also be related to activation of other pro-inflammatory pathways, such as, TNFα [85] and IL18 [72].

Several studies support the evidence of rapid and sustained induction of TNFα in damaged brain tissue, within one hour after TBI in rodent models [75,76,86]. TNFα triggers the production of other cytokines (IL1-β, IL6), chemokines [75] and nuclear factor kappa B (NF-κB) family (p50, p52 and p65) of transcription factors. Thus, TNFα is an important modulator of inflammation, at the transcriptional and translational levels, in the nervous system and in non-neural tissues [87,88]. IL18 also appears to play an important inflammatory role after TBI. IL18 has been shown to be elevated following a number of CNS inflammatory insults [89–91], including TBI [72]. In humans and rodents, the IL18 pathway can contribute to delayed neuronal injury, up to 14 days following TBI [72]. Activated neuroglial and immune cells in the area of injury secrete IL18, which binds to the IL18 receptor. Activation of the IL18 receptor initiates inflammatory signaling cascades [92]. Thus, cytokines, some of which have been mentioned here, are major contributors to the inflammatory and neuroinflammatory response.

4.3. Chemokines in TBI

Chemokines (CCL) are chemotactic inflammatory proteins that mediate interactions among inflammatory cells and target cells. In general, chemokines are typically 10 KDa or smaller. CCLs are synthesized and/or released along with other mediator molecules by a variety of cell types that include: astrocytes, microglia, macrophages, eosinophils, neutrophils, dendritic cells, mast cells and natural killer cells (NK cells) [93–95]. Release of chemokines serves to chemotactically guide receptor-sensitive cells, primarily through activation of G protein-coupled receptors [96]. Similar to cytokines, chemokines can be either pro- and/or anti-inflammatory. After a TBI, chemokines contribute to the attraction of a wide range of immune cells to the site of damage [97,98]. The specific activities of classes of chemokines have been elucidated following TBIs [99–101]. Although a full discussion is beyond the scope of this review, one example, CXC chemokines, activates the migration of neutrophils to the site of the lesion [96]. Alternatively, chemokines CCL2, CCL3, CCL5, CCL7, CCL8, CCL13, CCL17 and CCL22 attract monocytes and macrophages [102–104]. Other chemokines, such as, CCL1, CCL2, CCL17 and CCL22, are involved in the recruitment of T-lymphocytes [103].

Another important role of cytokine and chemokine release is to activate pattern recognition receptors (PRRs). PRRs are proteins of the innate immune system and identify danger-associated molecular patterns (DAMPs) of cellular stress. This identification, and the ensuing response, helps defend against cell and/or tissue damage [105,106]. The PRRs are divided into several subgroups, depending on cell localization, type and function. One such group is the nucleotide-binding domain leucine-rich repeats (NLRs) [107], which are also called the nucleotide oligomerization domain (NOD)-like receptors. These receptors are located in the cytoplasm and help to regulate the host inflammatory, apoptotic and innate immune responses [108,109]. The NLR family of proteins can be activated by multiple types of cell/tissue damage that are seen in TBI and can form multi-protein complexes called "inflammasomes" [110]. The unique compositions of these inflammasomes depend on the extent and type of cell and tissue damage. Some reports suggested the specific contributions of NLR family proteins (NLRP3-inflammasome) after TBI [110,111]. The NLRP3-inflammasome has been detected in neurons, astrocytes and microglia in the cortex after TBI [110], and the NLRP3-inflammasome complex is associated with increases in the aforementioned IL1-β and IL18 [108,110,112]. Interestingly, the NLRP3-inflammasome has also been demonstrated to associate with other CNS inflammatory disorders, including Alzheimer's disease (AD) [113], which is an increased risk factor following TBI.

Thus, the overall contributions of the cytokines and chemokines released after TBI are mediated by the release, and subsequent recruitment of immune cells to the site of injury, and to coordinate the ensuing activity of these cells. These immune cells are an essential part of the innate immune response and also the putative transition to the adaptive immune response and will be discussed below.

4.4. Cellular Immune Response to TBI

Several reports show that TBI and the associated neuroinflammation lead to local deposition of specific immune cells at the peri-injury area and beyond [97,114,115]. In addition, peripheral inflammation can also influence TBI outcomes [116]. There appears to be a rapid expansion and activation of peripheral immune cells after experimental TBI, as well as a significant extravasation of immune cells from the spleen, resulting in splenic hypotrophy following TBI [117,118]. It is also known that some of these immune cells that exit the spleen can contribute to the innate immune response, and some may also contribute to an ensuing adaptive immune response following a TBI [116,119,120]. Similarly, it is also known that some of these immune cells will infiltrate the CNS [121–123]. Immune cells involved in coordinating the innate immune response include: (1) monocytes, which develop into macrophages; (2) mast cells; (3) granulocytes (basophils, eosinophils and neutrophils); (4) dendritic cells (DC); and (5) natural killer cells.

Neutrophils and macrophages strongly infiltrate the brain in the early phase of TBI [121,123,124]. Neutrophils appear to be the most numerous type of granulocytes and possess high phagocytic potential. These cells are highly migratory and were reported to be involved in phagocytosing damaged elements within the brain parenchyma following a TBI [115,122]. The processes whereby neutrophils function are by: (1) secreting lysosomal enzymes; (2) releasing free radicals; (3) decreasing blood flow by direct physical microvascular occlusion; (4) increasing vascular permeability [125–127]. Interestingly, neutrophils can be found in the microvasculature lining the peri-injury region by as early as 2 h after injury and in brain parenchyma shortly thereafter [115,122]. Thus, neutrophils can contribute to the development of BBB breakdown and subsequent brain edema formation [122,128]. It is possible that neutrophils contribute to the secondary damage seen after TBI. Consistent with this notion, blocking neutrophil migration and adhesion decreases the total area of neuronal damage after a TBI in rabbits [129].

It has been hypothesized that accumulation of DCs at the site of damaged brain parenchyma can negatively contribute to brain tissue damage after the onset of TBI [122,130]. Infiltrating DCs may be activated by contact with the damaged cells at the site of injury. Antigen materials get processed by DCs, which can than travel to distant lymph nodes, present antigen and generate a local immune response. Once this response is initiated, antigen-specific T cells may migrate into CNS parenchyma and cause extended, chronic damage to the brain [131,132]. T cell accumulation at the site of injury, concurrent with DC accumulation, has also been indicated to negatively influence TBI outcomes [115].

Activated macrophages and/or microglia also contribute to neuronal damage [122,133]. It has been reported that different molecules released after TBI contribute to microglia/macrophage phenotype shifts [134,135]. Although the utility of classifying the M1/M2 phenotype in vivo has come into question [136,137], it is still useful to review the potential impact of the different phenotypes. For example, damaged endothelial cells can mediate microglia/macrophage polarization through secretion of cytokines [138], such as TNF-α, IL-6, IL-25, transforming growth factor beta (TGF-β), interferon-gamma (IFN-gamma), including substance-P and lipocalin-2 [139–141]. Additionally, infiltrating peripheral immune cells (T lymphocytes specifically) can induce macrophage/microglial phenotype transformation [142]. Recent studies suggest that such phenotype changes can alter neurogenesis after TBI, such that macrophage polarization from M2 toward M1 stimulates the release of soluble factors that impair basal neurogenesis [138], and this may impair functional recovery [134,143]. Thus, macrophages and/or microglial cells can be acted upon by a number of factors that ultimately determine the functional consequences of these cell types.

Macrophages, including both resident (microglia) and infiltrating (peripheral macrophages), are observed in relatively high numbers following TBIs [133]. Macrophages appeared to be abundant between 12 and 72 h and predominate in damaged cortical regions [122,144]. These cells accumulate near the area of injury [144], and this accumulation is a result of at least two mechanisms. One is through attractions by locally-secreted chemo- and cytokines released at the site of injury, as previously discussed. The other mechanism appears to occur via the T-cell activation. Once in the damaged area, the T cells get activated by direct contact with antigen presentation on DCs, macrophages and microglia [145,146]. It is this latter activation which is the hallmark of a transition from a non-specific innate immune response, to a specific adaptive immune response; e.g. T cell recognition of presented antigen.

T lymphocytes play an important role in the development and maintenance of secondary brain injury after TBI, through engagement of different cell types and mechanisms. Steady increases in the number and composition of T cells at the site of injury are highly suggestive of a transition to an adaptive immune response following a TBI. The peak of brain tissue infiltration by T cells after TBI, seems to occur within a range of 1–5 days, although the data on this topic are inconsistent [147,148]. Despite these inconsistencies, it appears that gamma delta T cells ($\gamma\delta$ T cells), which are a distinct class of T cells largely developed in thymus and express $\gamma\delta$ receptors, rather than $\alpha\beta$ T-cell receptor (TCR) on their surface, are early responders to the site of brain injury [149]. Combined with CD8+ T lymphocytes and CD4+ T-helper 1 (TH1) cells, these cells may worsen damage by cytotoxic and pro-inflammatory actions [150,151]. However, some suggest that the infiltration of immune cells into the CNS after TBI can also be neuroprotective [120,152,153]. This hypothesis is substantiated by the supposition that antigen-activated T cells provide protection, maintenance of neurological integrity and repair of tissue after a TBI [154]. Reports indicate that CD4+ T-helper 2 (TH2) cells specific for myelin basic protein (MBP) and CD4+ T cells may play such role of protection in neuronal survival [155,156]. Despite the pathogenic potential of anti-MBP T cells, they were also found in human immune system of healthy individuals [157,158]. It seems that regulatory T cells (CD4+ CD25+ Foxp3+) might also play important role in protection by suppressing autoimmune activity [159,160]. They derive from naive CD4 cells and are known for their immunosuppressive action, which downregulate the induction and proliferation of effector T cells [159,160].

Thus, it is possible that after TBI, the inflammatory sequelae result in antigen processing and presentation, as well as an eventual transition to an adaptive immune response. The implications of a transition to an adaptive immune response after a TBI are poorly understood and may have a positive and/or negative impact on the CNS. Here, we will summarize the existing data supporting an adaptive immune response after TBI, and we will provide a novel hypothesis to generate a foundation from which ensuing studies can occur in the context of adaptive immunity and TBI.

4.5. Adaptive Immune Response to TBI

Although scant, following TBI, some studies have provided strong evidence for a switch from a non-specific innate immune response, to a specific, adaptive immune response. As such, a paradigm shift in thinking may be necessary to fully understand and appreciate the sequelae that occur in the early and chronic stages after a TBI. A switch to an adaptive immune response has occurred, once antigen is processed and presented by professional antigen-presenting cells (APCs), and T cells recognize the presented antigen. The evidence supporting the transition to an adaptive immune response following TBI has been observed following retinal crush studies [161,162], fluid percussion injury in mice [116] and in human TBI patients [163]. The cellular components of the adaptive immune response may entail resident brain cells and/or infiltrating immune cells, as described above. In the case of infiltrating immune cells, they can gain access to the CNS via the compromised BBB, as well as the aforementioned chemotactic signaling. The humoral component of the adaptive immunity can be initially mediated by B cells and subsequently by T cells, which produce antigen-specific antibodies. Although the evidence is lacking for a direct connection between antibody production by T cells and neurodegeneration, accumulating evidence supports a role in the adaptive immune response in neurodegeneration. Once a transition from an adaptive immune response occurs, the possible outcomes have the potential to profoundly influence the outcomes for TBI.

In the case of most TBIs, the injuries are non-penetrating; thus, it would seem, if an adaptive immune response is occurring, then the antibody response is likely to be against self-antigen. Indeed, in human patients, evidence for this is found in the fact that antibodies to glial fibrillary acidic protein (GFAP)-fragments have been observed in the cerebral spinal fluid (CSF), at various time points after a TBI [164]. Moreover, proteolytic fragments of MBP, neuron specific enolase and to ubiquitin D-terminal hydrolase-L-1 (UCH-L1), which is a highly specific protein to neurons and an essential component of the ubiquitin proteasome system, have also been observed in humans and animal models of TBI [165–168]. Moreover, auto-reactive T cell responses to MBP have been documented in humans after TBI [169], further supporting a switch to an adaptive immune response. Considering that white matter loss has been reported after TBI in humans and animals, the observation of antibodies and T cells to MBP could have a tremendous implication on the loss of white matter and axonal degeneration that is observed at chronic time points after a TBI. A potential consequence of antibody production and the implied transition to an adaptive immune response is that memory immune cells are formed. It is possible that reactivation of the memory T cells, by another injury or perhaps by other neuroinflammatory stimulus, such as bacterial or viral infections [170], might re-open the BBB and expose the memory immune cells to self-antigens, such as GFAP, UCH-L1 or MBP. In this scenario, the subsequent appearance of post-traumatic syndromes may only appear after appropriate spatial and temporal stimuli, hence explaining the wide variation in when, why and what types of post-traumatic syndromes appear. Therefore, the development of post-TBI auto-antibody response might be highly pathogenic and contribute to chronic neuropathology that persists for a relatively long duration (days, week, months, years) after injury, and there is evidence in support of this notion from a wide swath of neurological and immunological studies [171–174].

Resident brain immune cells, such as microglial cells, infiltrate the CNS very early during development [175,176] and do not seem as likely a candidate to present self-antigen, despite the fact that these resident microglial cells are highly competent, professional APCs, and they can also express major histocompatibility complex class II molecules (MHCII). Considering that resident microglial cells in the brain are continuously exposed to GFAP, UCH-L1 and MBP and there does not seem to be any auto-reactivity in normal conditions, one alternative scenario is that infiltrating immune cells are responding to the antigenic peptide fragments of GFAP, UCH-L1 and MBP [165–167,177–180].

Another important factor to consider in the context of an adaptive immune response after TBI is the recent reports of two distinct lymphatic portals that directly service the brain. First, sitting subjacent to the superior sagittal sinus is a lymphatic area that has recently been shown to have white blood cells that dip in and out of the CNS, even in normal conditions [181,182]. Immune signals from the CNS have been shown to directly signal through this lymphatic portal and to initiate a global immune response that can exacerbate the severity of an injury [147,183,184]. Second is the "glymphatic" system, which allows for clearance of CNS waste products and soluble proteins. This system also has been shown to provide a substrate for the signaling of CNS components to the more classically-defined peripheral lymphatic system [184–187]. In either of these two CNS "lymphatic compartments", there can be a rapid communication between the CNS and the periphery, and this signaling can exacerbate injuries, such as stroke or TBI [184,188]. In the stroke literature, removing the spleen (splenectomy) and, therefore, reducing the number of B and T cells capable of responding to the TBI results in a significant improvement in lesion size and functional outcome measures. However, the data were inconsistent between humans and rodent models [189–191]; thus, the true functional implications require further examination. Interestingly, other studies that have blocked the expansion and activation of B and T cells in the spleen after a TBI have demonstrated significant neuroprotection [116]. Thus, the role of peripheral immune cells after TBI might provide novel targets for the development of therapeutic options to treat TBIs and post-traumatic syndromes.

5. Conclusions

TBI remains a complex, multi-system pathology, with a wide-ranging potential for short- and long-term detrimental outcomes. Using the existing and newly-developed animal models, as well as clinical and translational studies, research continues to unravel the complex interactions between the brain, the periphery and the immune system. New understanding of these interactions will lead to novel therapeutic targets, with the hope of improving the outcomes for millions of people each year.

Acknowledgments: This work was supported by a Department of Defense (DOD) research grant.

Author Contributions: Conception and design of the research: Damir Nizamutdinov, Lee A. Shapiro. Drafted the manuscript: Damir Nizamutdinov, Lee A. Shapiro. Edited and revised the manuscript: Damir Nizamutdinov, Lee A. Shapiro. Approved the final version of the manuscript: Damir Nizamutdinov, Lee A. Shapiro.

References

1. Marr, A.L.; Coronado, V.G. *Central Nervous System Injury Surveillance Data Submission Standards—2002*; Department of Health and Human Services: Washington, DC, USA, 2004.
2. Centers for Disease Control and Prevention (CDC). Traumatic Brain Injury in the United States: Fact Sheet. Available online: https://www.cdc.gov/traumaticbraininjury/get_the_facts.html (accessed on 15 September 2016).
3. Faul, M.X.; Xu, L.; Wald, M.M.; Coronad, V.G. Traumatic Brain Injury in the United States: Emergency Department Visits, Hospitalizations and Deaths 2002–2006. Available online: https://www.cdc.gov/traumaticbraininjury/pdf/blue_book.pdf (accessed on 15 September 2016).
4. Zaloshnja, E.; Miller, T.; Langlois, J.A.; Selassie, A.W. Prevalence of long-term disability from traumatic brain injury in the civilian population of the United States, 2005. *J. Head Trauma Rehabil.* **2008**, *23*, 394–400. [CrossRef] [PubMed]
5. Centers for Disease Control and Prevention (CDC); United States Department of Defense (DOD); VA Leadership Panel. Report to Congress on Traumatic Brain Injury in the United States: Understanding the Public Health Problem among Current and Former Military Personnel. Available online: https://www.cdc.gov/traumaticbraininjury/pdf/report_to_congress_on_traumatic_brain_injury_2013-a.pdf (accessed on 15 September 2016).
6. Teasdale, G.; Jennett, B. Assessment of coma and impaired consciousness. A practical scale. *Lancet* **1974**, *2*, 81–84. [CrossRef]
7. Jennett, B.; Bond, M. Assessment of outcome after severe brain damage. *Lancet* **1975**, *1*, 480–484. [CrossRef]
8. Nakase-Richardson, R.; Sherer, M.; Seel, R.T.; Hart, T.; Hanks, R.; Arango-Lasprilla, J.C.; Yablon, S.A.; Sander, A.M.; Barnett, S.D.; Walker, W.C.; et al. Utility of post-traumatic amnesia in predicting 1-year productivity following traumatic brain injury: Comparison of the Russell and Mississippi PTA classification intervals. *J. Neurol. Neurosurg. Psychiatry* **2011**, *82*, 494–499. [CrossRef] [PubMed]
9. Brenner, L.A.; Vanderploeg, R.D.; Terrio, H. Assessment and diagnosis of mild traumatic brain injury, posttraumatic stress disorder, and other polytrauma conditions: Burden of adversity hypothesis. *Rehabil. Psychol.* **2009**, *54*, 239–246. [CrossRef] [PubMed]
10. Turan, N.; Miller, B.A.; Heider, R.A.; Nadeem, M.; Sayeed, I.; Stein, D.G.; Pradilla, G. Neurobehavioral testing in subarachnoid hemorrhage: A review of methods and current findings in rodents. *J. Cereb. Blood Flow Metab.* **2016**. [CrossRef] [PubMed]
11. Riggio, S.; Wong, M. Neurobehavioral sequelae of traumatic brain injury. *Mt. Sinai J. Med.* **2009**, *76*, 163–172. [CrossRef] [PubMed]
12. Walker, W.C.; Pickett, T.C. Motor impairment after severe traumatic brain injury: A longitudinal multicenter study. *J. Rehabil. Res. Dev.* **2007**, *44*, 975–982. [CrossRef] [PubMed]
13. Safaz, I.; Alaca, R.; Yasar, E.; Tok, F.; Yilmaz, B. Medical complications, physical function and communication skills in patients with traumatic brain injury: A single centre 5-year experience. *Brain Inj.* **2008**, *22*, 733–739. [CrossRef] [PubMed]
14. Rosenthal, M.; Christensen, B.K.; Ross, T.P. Depression following traumatic brain injury. *Arch. Phys. Med. Rehabil.* **1998**, *79*, 90–103. [CrossRef]
15. Hart, T.; Brenner, L.; Clark, A.N.; Bogner, J.A.; Novack, T.A.; Chervoneva, I.; Nakase-Richardson, R.; Arango-Lasprilla, J.C. Major and minor depression after traumatic brain injury. *Arch. Phys. Med. Rehabil.* **2011**, *92*, 1211–1219. [CrossRef] [PubMed]

16. Stulemeijer, M.; Vos, P.E.; Bleijenberg, G.; van der Werf, S.P. Cognitive complaints after mild traumatic brain injury: Things are not always what they seem. *J. Psychosom. Res.* **2007**, *63*, 637–645. [CrossRef] [PubMed]
17. Agrawal, A.; Timothy, J.; Pandit, L.; Manju, M. Post-traumatic epilepsy: An overview. *Clin. Neurol. Neurosurg.* **2006**, *108*, 433–439. [CrossRef] [PubMed]
18. Bazarian, J.J.; Cernak, I.; Noble-Haeusslein, L.; Potolicchio, S.; Temkin, N. Long-term neurologic outcomes after traumatic brain injury. *J. Head Trauma Rehabil.* **2009**, *24*, 439–451. [CrossRef] [PubMed]
19. Carbonell, W.S.; Maris, D.O.; McCall, T.; Grady, M.S. Adaptation of the fluid percussion injury model to the mouse. *J. Neurotrauma* **1998**, *15*, 217–229. [CrossRef] [PubMed]
20. Dixon, C.E.; Lighthall, J.W.; Anderson, T.E. Physiologic, histopathologic, and cineradiographic characterization of a new fluid-percussion model of experimental brain injury in the rat. *J. Neurotrauma* **1988**, *5*, 91–104. [CrossRef] [PubMed]
21. Dixon, C.E.; Lyeth, B.G.; Povlishock, J.T.; Findling, R.L.; Hamm, R.J.; Marmarou, A.; Young, H.F.; Hayes, R.L. A fluid percussion model of experimental brain injury in the rat. *J. Neurosurg.* **1987**, *67*, 110–119. [CrossRef] [PubMed]
22. Mukherjee, S.; Zeitouni, S.; Cavarsan, C.F.; Shapiro, L.A. Increased seizure susceptibility in mice 30 days after fluid percussion injury. *Front. Neurol.* **2013**, *4*, 28. [CrossRef] [PubMed]
23. Dixon, C.E.; Clifton, G.L.; Lighthall, J.W.; Yaghmai, A.A.; Hayes, R.L. A controlled cortical impact model of traumatic brain injury in the rat. *J. Neurosci. Methods* **1991**, *39*, 253–262. [CrossRef]
24. Lighthall, J.W. Controlled cortical impact: A new experimental brain injury model. *J. Neurotrauma* **1988**, *5*, 1–15. [CrossRef] [PubMed]
25. Smith, D.H.; Soares, H.D.; Pierce, J.S.; Perlman, K.G.; Saatman, K.E.; Meaney, D.F.; Dixon, C.E.; McIntosh, T.K. A model of parasagittal controlled cortical impact in the mouse: Cognitive and histopathologic effects. *J. Neurotrauma* **1995**, *12*, 169–178. [CrossRef] [PubMed]
26. Williams, A.J.; Hartings, J.A.; Lu, X.C.; Rolli, M.L.; Dave, J.R.; Tortella, F.C. Characterization of a new rat model of penetrating ballistic brain injury. *J. Neurotrauma* **2005**, *22*, 313–331. [CrossRef] [PubMed]
27. Marmarou, A.; Foda, M.A.; van den Brink, W.; Campbell, J.; Kita, H.; Demetriadou, K. A new model of diffuse brain injury in rats. Part I: Pathophysiology and biomechanics. *J. Neurosurg.* **1994**, *80*, 291–300. [CrossRef] [PubMed]
28. Cernak, I.; Savic, J.; Malicevic, Z.; Zunic, G.; Radosevic, P.; Ivanovic, I.; Davidovic, L. Involvement of the central nervous system in the general response to pulmonary blast injury. *J. Trauma* **1996**, *40*, S100–S104. [CrossRef] [PubMed]
29. Warden, D. Military tbi during the iraq and afghanistan wars. *J. Head Trauma Rehabil.* **2006**, *21*, 398–402. [CrossRef] [PubMed]
30. McIntosh, T.K.; Noble, L.; Andrews, B.; Faden, A.I. Traumatic brain injury in the rat: Characterization of a midline fluid-percussion model. *Cent. Nerv. Syst. Trauma* **1987**, *4*, 119–134. [CrossRef] [PubMed]
31. McIntosh, T.K.; Vink, R.; Noble, L.; Yamakami, I.; Fernyak, S.; Soares, H.; Faden, A.L. Traumatic brain injury in the rat: Characterization of a lateral fluid-percussion model. *Neuroscience* **1989**, *28*, 233–244. [CrossRef]
32. Kabadi, S.V.; Hilton, G.D.; Stoica, B.A.; Zapple, D.N.; Faden, A.I. Fluid-percussion-induced traumatic brain injury model in rats. *Nat. Protoc.* **2010**, *5*, 1552–1563. [CrossRef] [PubMed]
33. Walter, B.; Bauer, R.; Fritz, H.; Jochum, T.; Wunder, L.; Zwiener, U. Evaluation of micro tip pressure transducers for the measurement of intracerebral pressure transients induced by fluid percussion. *Exp. Toxicol. Pathol.* **1999**, *51*, 124–129. [CrossRef]
34. Alder, J.; Fujioka, W.; Lifshitz, J.; Crockett, D.P.; Thakker-Varia, S. Lateral fluid percussion: Model of traumatic brain injury in mice. *J. Vis. Exp.* **2011**, *54*, e3063. [CrossRef] [PubMed]
35. Thompson, H.J.; Lifshitz, J.; Marklund, N.; Grady, M.S.; Graham, D.I.; Hovda, D.A.; McIntosh, T.K. Lateral fluid percussion brain injury: A 15-year review and evaluation. *J. Neurotrauma* **2005**, *22*, 42–75. [CrossRef] [PubMed]
36. Morales, D.M.; Marklund, N.; Lebold, D.; Thompson, H.J.; Pitkanen, A.; Maxwell, W.L.; Longhi, L.; Laurer, H.; Maegele, M.; Neugebauer, E.; et al. Experimental models of traumatic brain injury: Do we really need to build a better mousetrap? *Neuroscience* **2005**, *136*, 971–989. [CrossRef] [PubMed]
37. Hartl, R.; Medary, M.; Ruge, M.; Arfors, K.E.; Ghajar, J. Blood-brain barrier breakdown occurs early after traumatic brain injury and is not related to white blood cell adherence. *Acta Neurochir. Suppl.* **1997**, *70*, 240–242. [PubMed]

38. Das, M.; Leonardo, C.C.; Rangooni, S.; Pennypacker, K.R.; Mohapatra, S.; Mohapatra, S.S. Lateral fluid percussion injury of the brain induces CCL20 inflammatory chemokine expression in rats. *J. Neuroinflamm.* **2011**, *8*, 148. [CrossRef] [PubMed]
39. Xiong, Y.; Mahmood, A.; Chopp, M. Animal models of traumatic brain injury. *Nat. Rev. Neurosci.* **2013**, *14*, 128–142. [CrossRef] [PubMed]
40. Graham, D.I.; McIntosh, T.K.; Maxwell, W.L.; Nicoll, J.A. Recent advances in neurotrauma. *J. Neuropathol. Exp. Neurol.* **2000**, *59*, 641–651. [CrossRef] [PubMed]
41. Sanders, M.J.; Dietrich, W.D.; Green, E.J. Cognitive function following traumatic brain injury: Effects of injury severity and recovery period in a parasagittal fluid-percussive injury model. *J. Neurotrauma* **1999**, *16*, 915–925. [CrossRef] [PubMed]
42. Vink, R.; Mullins, P.G.; Temple, M.D.; Bao, W.; Faden, A.I. Small shifts in craniotomy position in the lateral fluid percussion injury model are associated with differential lesion development. *J. Neurotrauma* **2001**, *18*, 839–847. [CrossRef] [PubMed]
43. Floyd, C.L.; Golden, K.M.; Black, R.T.; Hamm, R.J.; Lyeth, B.G. Craniectomy position affects morris water maze performance and hippocampal cell loss after parasagittal fluid percussion. *J. Neurotrauma* **2002**, *19*, 303–316. [CrossRef] [PubMed]
44. Hayes, R.L.; Stalhammar, D.; Povlishock, J.T.; Allen, A.M.; Galinat, B.J.; Becker, D.P.; Stonnington, H.H. A new model of concussive brain injury in the cat produced by extradural fluid volume loading: II. Physiological and neuropathological observations. *Brain Inj.* **1987**, *1*, 93–112. [CrossRef] [PubMed]
45. Millen, J.E.; Glauser, F.L.; Fairman, R.P. A comparison of physiological responses to percussive brain trauma in dogs and sheep. *J. Neurosurg.* **1985**, *62*, 587–591. [CrossRef] [PubMed]
46. Pfenninger, E.G.; Reith, A.; Breitig, D.; Grunert, A.; Ahnefeld, F.W. Early changes of intracranial pressure, perfusion pressure, and blood flow after acute head injury. Part 1: An experimental study of the underlying pathophysiology. *J. Neurosurg.* **1989**, *70*, 774–779. [CrossRef] [PubMed]
47. Hicks, R.; Soares, H.; Smith, D.; McIntosh, T. Temporal and spatial characterization of neuronal injury following lateral fluid-percussion brain injury in the rat. *Acta Neuropathol.* **1996**, *91*, 236–246. [CrossRef] [PubMed]
48. Liu, Y.R.; Cardamone, L.; Hogan, R.E.; Gregoire, M.C.; Williams, J.P.; Hicks, R.J.; Binns, D.; Koe, A.; Jones, N.C.; Myers, D.E.; et al. Progressive metabolic and structural cerebral perturbations after traumatic brain injury: An in vivo imaging study in the rat. *J. Nucl. Med.* **2010**, *51*, 1788–1795. [CrossRef] [PubMed]
49. Hamm, R.J. Neurobehavioral assessment of outcome following traumatic brain injury in rats: An evaluation of selected measures. *J. Neurotrauma* **2001**, *18*, 1207–1216. [CrossRef] [PubMed]
50. Pierce, J.E.; Smith, D.H.; Trojanowski, J.Q.; McIntosh, T.K. Enduring cognitive, neurobehavioral and histopathological changes persist for up to one year following severe experimental brain injury in rats. *Neuroscience* **1998**, *87*, 359–369. [CrossRef]
51. King, C.; Robinson, T.; Dixon, C.E.; Rao, G.R.; Larnard, D.; Nemoto, C.E. Brain temperature profiles during epidural cooling with the chillerpad in a monkey model of traumatic brain injury. *J. Neurotrauma* **2010**, *27*, 1895–1903. [CrossRef] [PubMed]
52. Acosta, S.A.; Tajiri, N.; Shinozuka, K.; Ishikawa, H.; Grimmig, B.; Diamond, D.M.; Sanberg, P.R.; Bickford, P.C.; Kaneko, Y.; Borlongan, C.V. Long-term upregulation of inflammation and suppression of cell proliferation in the brain of adult rats exposed to traumatic brain injury using the controlled cortical impact model. *PLoS ONE* **2013**, *8*, e53376. [CrossRef]
53. Hall, E.D.; Sullivan, P.G.; Gibson, T.R.; Pavel, K.M.; Thompson, B.M.; Scheff, S.W. Spatial and temporal characteristics of neurodegeneration after controlled cortical impact in mice: More than a focal brain injury. *J. Neurotrauma* **2005**, *22*, 252–265. [CrossRef] [PubMed]
54. Goodman, J.C.; Cherian, L.; Bryan, R.M., Jr.; Robertson, C.S. Lateral cortical impact injury in rats: Pathologic effects of varying cortical compression and impact velocity. *J. Neurotrauma* **1994**, *11*, 587–597. [CrossRef] [PubMed]
55. Saatman, K.E.; Feeko, K.J.; Pape, R.L.; Raghupathi, R. Differential behavioral and histopathological responses to graded cortical impact injury in mice. *J. Neurotrauma* **2006**, *23*, 1241–1253. [CrossRef] [PubMed]

56. Petraglia, A.L.; Plog, B.A.; Dayawansa, S.; Chen, M.; Dashnaw, M.L.; Czerniecka, K.; Walker, C.T.; Viterise, T.; Hyrien, O.; Iliff, J.J.; et al. The spectrum of neurobehavioral sequelae after repetitive mild traumatic brain injury: A novel mouse model of chronic traumatic encephalopathy. *J. Neurotrauma* **2014**, *31*, 1211–1224. [CrossRef] [PubMed]
57. Fox, G.B.; Fan, L.; Levasseur, R.A.; Faden, A.I. Sustained sensory/motor and cognitive deficits with neuronal apoptosis following controlled cortical impact brain injury in the mouse. *J. Neurotrauma* **1998**, *15*, 599–614. [CrossRef] [PubMed]
58. Washington, P.M.; Forcelli, P.A.; Wilkins, T.; Zapple, D.N.; Parsadanian, M.; Burns, M.P. The effect of injury severity on behavior: A phenotypic study of cognitive and emotional deficits after mild, moderate, and severe controlled cortical impact injury in mice. *J. Neurotrauma* **2012**, *29*, 2283–2296. [CrossRef] [PubMed]
59. Marklund, N.; Hillered, L. Animal modelling of traumatic brain injury in preclinical drug development: Where do we go from here? *Br. J. Pharmacol.* **2011**, *164*, 1207–1229. [CrossRef] [PubMed]
60. Dixon, C.E.; Kraus, M.F.; Kline, A.E.; Ma, X.; Yan, H.Q.; Griffith, R.G.; Wolfson, B.M.; Marion, D.W. Amantadine improves water maze performance without affecting motor behavior following traumatic brain injury in rats. *Restor. Neurol. Neurosci.* **1999**, *14*, 285–294. [PubMed]
61. Dixon, C.E.; Kochanek, P.M.; Yan, H.Q.; Schiding, J.K.; Griffith, R.G.; Baum, E.; Marion, D.W.; DeKosky, S.T. One-year study of spatial memory performance, brain morphology, and cholinergic markers after moderate controlled cortical impact in rats. *J. Neurotrauma* **1999**, *16*, 109–122. [CrossRef] [PubMed]
62. Masel, B.E.; DeWitt, D.S. Traumatic brain injury: A disease process, not an event. *J. Neurotrauma* **2010**, *27*, 1529–1540. [CrossRef] [PubMed]
63. Davis, A.E. Mechanisms of traumatic brain injury: Biomechanical, structural and cellular considerations. *Crit. Care Nurs. Q.* **2000**, *23*, 1–13. [CrossRef] [PubMed]
64. Gaetz, M. The neurophysiology of brain injury. *Clin. Neurophysiol.* **2004**, *115*, 4–18. [CrossRef]
65. Cernak, I. Animal models of head trauma. *NeuroRx* **2005**, *2*, 410–422. [CrossRef] [PubMed]
66. Bramlett, H.M.; Dietrich, W.D. Progressive damage after brain and spinal cord injury: Pathomechanisms and treatment strategies. *Prog. Brain Res.* **2007**, *161*, 125–141. [PubMed]
67. Marklund, N.; Bakshi, A.; Castelbuono, D.J.; Conte, V.; McIntosh, T.K. Evaluation of pharmacological treatment strategies in traumatic brain injury. *Curr. Pharm. Des.* **2006**, *12*, 1645–1680. [CrossRef] [PubMed]
68. Povlishock, J.T.; Christman, C.W. The pathobiology of traumatically induced axonal injury in animals and humans: A review of current thoughts. *J. Neurotrauma* **1995**, *12*, 555–564. [CrossRef] [PubMed]
69. Arvin, B.; Neville, L.F.; Barone, F.C.; Feuerstein, G.Z. Brain injury and inflammation. A putative role of TNF alpha. *Ann. N. Y. Acad. Sci.* **1995**, *765*, 62–71. [CrossRef] [PubMed]
70. Isaksson, J.; Lewen, A.; Hillered, L.; Olsson, Y. Up-regulation of intercellular adhesion molecule 1 in cerebral microvessels after cortical contusion trauma in a rat model. *Acta Neuropathol.* **1997**, *94*, 16–20. [CrossRef] [PubMed]
71. Yang, K.; Mu, X.S.; Xue, J.J.; Whitson, J.; Salminen, A.; dixon, C.E.; Liu, P.K.; Hayes, R.L. Increased expression of c-fos mRNA and AP-1 transcription factors after cortical impact injury in rats. *Brain Res.* **1994**, *664*, 141–147. [CrossRef]
72. Yatsiv, I.; Morganti-Kossmann, M.C.; Perez, D.; Dinarello, C.A.; Novick, D.; Rubinstein, M.; Otto, V.I.; Rancan, M.; Kossmann, T.; Redaelli, C.A.; et al. Elevated intracranial IL-18 in humans and mice after traumatic brain injury and evidence of neuroprotective effects of IL-18-binding protein after experimental closed head injury. *J. Cereb. Blood Flow Metab.* **2002**, *22*, 971–978. [CrossRef] [PubMed]
73. Hutchinson, P.J.; O'Connell, M.T.; Rothwell, N.J.; Hopkins, S.J.; Nortje, J.; Carpenter, K.L.; Timofeev, I.; Al-Rawi, P.G.; Menon, D.K.; Pickard, J.D. Inflammation in human brain injury: Intracerebral concentrations of IL-1alpha, IL-1beta, and their endogenous inhibitor IL-1ra. *J. Neurotrauma* **2007**, *24*, 1545–1557. [CrossRef] [PubMed]
74. Utagawa, A.; Truettner, J.S.; Dietrich, W.D.; Bramlett, H.M. Systemic inflammation exacerbates behavioral and histopathological consequences of isolated traumatic brain injury in rats. *Exp. Neurol.* **2008**, *211*, 283–291. [CrossRef] [PubMed]
75. Minami, M.; Kuraishi, Y.; Satoh, M. Effects of kainic acid on messenger RNA levels of IL-1 beta, IL-6, TNF alpha and lif in the rat brain. *Biochem. Biophys. Res. Commun.* **1991**, *176*, 593–598. [CrossRef]
76. Liu, T.; Clark, R.K.; McDonnell, P.C.; Young, P.R.; White, R.F.; Barone, F.C.; Feuerstein, G.Z. Tumor necrosis factor-alpha expression in ischemic neurons. *Stroke* **1994**, *25*, 1481–1488. [CrossRef] [PubMed]

77. Chizzolini, C.; Dayer, J.M.; Miossec, P. Cytokines in chronic rheumatic diseases: Is everything lack of homeostatic balance? *Arthritis Res. Ther.* **2009**, *11*, 246. [CrossRef] [PubMed]
78. Iwasaki, A.; Medzhitov, R. Regulation of adaptive immunity by the innate immune system. *Science* **2010**, *327*, 291–295. [CrossRef] [PubMed]
79. Zhang, J.M.; An, J. Cytokines, inflammation, and pain. *Int. Anesthesiol. Clin.* **2007**, *45*, 27–37. [CrossRef] [PubMed]
80. Dinarello, C.A. Immunological and inflammatory functions of the interleukin-1 family. *Annu. Rev. Immunol.* **2009**, *27*, 519–550. [CrossRef] [PubMed]
81. Garlanda, C.; Dinarello, C.A.; Mantovani, A. The interleukin-1 family: Back to the future. *Immunity* **2013**, *39*, 1003–1018. [CrossRef] [PubMed]
82. Pearson, V.L.; Rothwell, N.J.; Toulmond, S. Excitotoxic brain damage in the rat induces interleukin-1beta protein in microglia and astrocytes: Correlation with the progression of cell death. *Glia* **1999**, *25*, 311–323. [CrossRef]
83. Dinarello, C.A. Blocking IL-1 in systemic inflammation. *J. Exp. Med.* **2005**, *201*, 1355–1359. [CrossRef] [PubMed]
84. Dinarello, C.A. Interleukin 1 and interleukin 18 as mediators of inflammation and the aging process. *Am. J. Clin. Nutr.* **2006**, *83*, 447S–455S. [PubMed]
85. Lu, K.T.; Wang, Y.W.; Wo, Y.Y.; Yang, Y.L. Extracellular signal-regulated kinase-mediated IL-1-induced cortical neuron damage during traumatic brain injury. *Neurosci. Lett.* **2005**, *386*, 40–45. [CrossRef] [PubMed]
86. Liu, T.; Young, P.R.; McDonnell, P.C.; White, R.F.; Barone, F.C.; Feuerstein, G.Z. Cytokine-induced neutrophil chemoattractant mRNA expressed in cerebral ischemia. *Neurosci. Lett.* **1993**, *164*, 125–128. [CrossRef]
87. Grilli, M.; Memo, M. Nuclear factor-kappaB/Rel proteins: A point of convergence of signalling pathways relevant in neuronal function and dysfunction. *Biochem. Pharmacol.* **1999**, *57*, 1–7. [CrossRef]
88. Baeuerle, P.A.; Baltimore, D. NF-kappa B: Ten years after. *Cell* **1996**, *87*, 13–20. [CrossRef]
89. Jander, S.; Stoll, G. Differential induction of interleukin-12, interleukin-18, and interleukin-1beta converting enzyme mRNA in experimental autoimmune encephalomyelitis of the lewis rat. *J. Neuroimmunol.* **1998**, *91*, 93–99. [CrossRef]
90. Losy, J.; Niezgoda, A. IL-18 in patients with multiple sclerosis. *Acta Neurol. Scand.* **2001**, *104*, 171–173. [CrossRef] [PubMed]
91. Fassbender, K.; Mielke, O.; Bertsch, T.; Muehlhauser, F.; Hennerici, M.; Kurimoto, M.; Rossol, S. Interferon-gamma-inducing factor (IL-18) and interferon-gamma in inflammatory CNS diseases. *Neurology* **1999**, *53*, 1104–1106. [CrossRef] [PubMed]
92. Sims, J.E.; Smith, D.E. The IL-1 family: Regulators of immunity. *Nat. Rev. Immunol.* **2010**, *10*, 89–102. [CrossRef] [PubMed]
93. Kremlev, S.G.; Roberts, R.L.; Palmer, C. Differential expression of chemokines and chemokine receptors during microglial activation and inhibition. *J. Neuroimmunol.* **2004**, *149*, 1–9. [CrossRef] [PubMed]
94. Gyoneva, S.; Ransohoff, R.M. Inflammatory reaction after traumatic brain injury: Therapeutic potential of targeting cell-cell communication by chemokines. *Trends Pharmacol. Sci.* **2015**, *36*, 471–480. [CrossRef] [PubMed]
95. Choi, S.S.; Lee, H.J.; Lim, I.; Satoh, J.; Kim, S.U. Human astrocytes: Secretome profiles of cytokines and chemokines. *PLoS ONE* **2014**, *9*, e92325. [CrossRef] [PubMed]
96. Ono, S.J.; Nakamura, T.; Miyazaki, D.; Ohbayashi, M.; Dawson, M.; Toda, M. Chemokines: Roles in leukocyte development, trafficking, and effector function. *J. Allergy Clin. Immunol.* **2003**, *111*, 1185–1199. [CrossRef] [PubMed]
97. Helmy, A.; Carpenter, K.L.; Menon, D.K.; Pickard, J.D.; Hutchinson, P.J. The cytokine response to human traumatic brain injury: Temporal profiles and evidence for cerebral parenchymal production. *J. Cereb. Blood Flow Metab.* **2011**, *31*, 658–670. [CrossRef] [PubMed]
98. Helmy, A.; Antoniades, C.A.; Guilfoyle, M.R.; Carpenter, K.L.; Hutchinson, P.J. Principal component analysis of the cytokine and chemokine response to human traumatic brain injury. *PLoS ONE* **2012**, *7*, e39677. [CrossRef] [PubMed]
99. Glabinski, A.R.; Tani, M.; Aras, S.; Stoler, M.H.; Tuohy, V.K.; Ransohoff, R.M. Regulation and function of central nervous system chemokines. *Int. J. Dev. Neurosci.* **1995**, *13*, 153–165. [CrossRef]

100. Ghirnikar, R.S.; Lee, Y.L.; Eng, L.F. Inflammation in traumatic brain injury: Role of cytokines and chemokines. *Neurochem. Res.* **1998**, *23*, 329–340. [CrossRef] [PubMed]
101. Cartier, L.; Hartley, O.; Dubois-Dauphin, M.; Krause, K.H. Chemokine receptors in the central nervous system: Role in brain inflammation and neurodegenerative diseases. *Brain Res. Brain Res. Rev.* **2005**, *48*, 16–42. [CrossRef] [PubMed]
102. Proudfoot, A.E.; Handel, T.M.; Johnson, Z.; Lau, E.K.; LiWang, P.; Clark-Lewis, I.; Borlat, F.; Wells, T.N.; Kosco-Vilbois, M.H. Glycosaminoglycan binding and oligomerization are essential for the in vivo activity of certain chemokines. *Proc. Natl. Acad. Sci. USA* **2003**, *100*, 1885–1890. [CrossRef] [PubMed]
103. Mantovani, A.; Sica, A.; Sozzani, S.; Allavena, P.; Vecchi, A.; Locati, M. The chemokine system in diverse forms of macrophage activation and polarization. *Trends Immunol.* **2004**, *25*, 677–686. [CrossRef] [PubMed]
104. Shi, C.; Pamer, E.G. Monocyte recruitment during infection and inflammation. *Nat. Rev. Immunol.* **2011**, *11*, 762–774. [CrossRef] [PubMed]
105. Tang, D.; Kang, R.; Coyne, C.B.; Zeh, H.J.; Lotze, M.T. PAMPs and DAMPs: Signal 0s that spur autophagy and immunity. *Immunol. Rev.* **2012**, *249*, 158–175. [CrossRef] [PubMed]
106. Sansonetti, P.J. The innate signaling of dangers and the dangers of innate signaling. *Nat. Immunol.* **2006**, *7*, 1237–1242. [CrossRef] [PubMed]
107. Trinchieri, G.; Sher, A. Cooperation of toll-like receptor signals in innate immune defence. *Nat. Rev. Immunol.* **2007**, *7*, 179–190. [CrossRef] [PubMed]
108. Ting, J.P.; Lovering, R.C.; Alnemri, E.S.; Bertin, J.; Boss, J.M.; Davis, B.K.; Flavell, R.A.; Girardin, S.E.; Godzik, A.; Harton, J.A.; et al. The NLR gene family: A standard nomenclature. *Immunity* **2008**, *28*, 285–287. [CrossRef] [PubMed]
109. Strober, W.; Murray, P.J.; Kitani, A.; Watanabe, T. Signalling pathways and molecular interactions of NOD1 and NOD2. *Nat. Rev. Immunol.* **2006**, *6*, 9–20. [CrossRef] [PubMed]
110. Liu, H.D.; Li, W.; Chen, Z.R.; Hu, Y.C.; Zhang, D.D.; Shen, W.; Zhou, M.L.; Zhu, L.; Hang, C.H. Expression of the NLRP3 inflammasome in cerebral cortex after traumatic brain injury in a rat model. *Neurochem. Res.* **2013**, *38*, 2072–2083. [CrossRef] [PubMed]
111. Needham, E.; Zandi, M.S. Recent advances in the neuroimmunology of cell-surface CNS autoantibody syndromes, Alzheimer's disease, traumatic brain injury and schizophrenia. *J. Neurol.* **2014**, *261*, 2037–2042. [CrossRef] [PubMed]
112. Martinon, F.; Burns, K.; Tschopp, J. The inflammasome: A molecular platform triggering activation of inflammatory caspases and processing of proil-beta. *Mol. Cell* **2002**, *10*, 417–426. [CrossRef]
113. Halle, A.; Hornung, V.; Petzold, G.C.; Stewart, C.R.; Monks, B.G.; Reinheckel, T.; Fitzgerald, K.A.; Latz, E.; Moore, K.J.; Golenbock, D.T. The NALP3 inflammasome is involved in the innate immune response to amyloid-beta. *Nat. Immunol.* **2008**, *9*, 857–865. [CrossRef] [PubMed]
114. Trahanas, D.M.; Cuda, C.M.; Perlman, H.; Schwulst, S.J. Differential activation of infiltrating monocyte-derived cells after mild and severe traumatic brain injury. *Shock* **2015**, *43*, 255–260. [CrossRef] [PubMed]
115. Rhodes, J. Peripheral immune cells in the pathology of traumatic brain injury? *Curr. Opin. Crit. Care* **2011**, *17*, 122–130. [CrossRef] [PubMed]
116. Tobin, R.P.; Mukherjee, S.; Kain, J.M.; Rogers, S.K.; Henderson, S.K.; Motal, H.L.; Newell Rogers, M.K.; Shapiro, L.A. Traumatic brain injury causes selective, CD74-dependent peripheral lymphocyte activation that exacerbates neurodegeneration. *Acta Neuropathol. Commun.* **2014**, *2*, 143. [CrossRef] [PubMed]
117. Schwulst, S.J.; Trahanas, D.M.; Saber, R.; Perlman, H. Traumatic brain injury-induced alterations in peripheral immunity. *J. Trauma Acute Care Surg.* **2013**, *75*, 780–788. [CrossRef] [PubMed]
118. Rasouli, J.; Lekhraj, R.; Ozbalik, M.; Lalezari, P.; Casper, D. Brain-spleen inflammatory coupling: A literature review. *Einstein J. Biol. Med.* **2011**, *27*, 74–77. [CrossRef] [PubMed]
119. Schwartz, M.; Deczkowska, A. Neurological disease as a failure of brain-immune crosstalk: The multiple faces of neuroinflammation. *Trends Immunol.* **2016**, *37*, 668–679. [CrossRef] [PubMed]
120. Schwartz, M. Helping the body to cure itself: Immune modulation by therapeutic vaccination for spinal cord injury. *J. Spinal Cord Med.* **2003**, *26*, S6–S10. [CrossRef] [PubMed]
121. Foley, L.M.; Hitchens, T.K.; Ho, C.; Janesko-Feldman, K.L.; Melick, J.A.; Bayir, H.; Kochanek, P.M. Magnetic resonance imaging assessment of macrophage accumulation in mouse brain after experimental traumatic brain injury. *J. Neurotrauma* **2009**, *26*, 1509–1519. [CrossRef] [PubMed]

122. Soares, H.D.; Hicks, R.R.; Smith, D.; McIntosh, T.K. Inflammatory leukocytic recruitment and diffuse neuronal degeneration are separate pathological processes resulting from traumatic brain injury. *J. Neurosci.* **1995**, *15*, 8223–8233. [PubMed]
123. Kenne, E.; Erlandsson, A.; Lindbom, L.; Hillered, L.; Clausen, F. Neutrophil depletion reduces edema formation and tissue loss following traumatic brain injury in mice. *J. Neuroinflamm.* **2012**, *9*, 17. [CrossRef] [PubMed]
124. Clark, R.S.; Schiding, J.K.; Kaczorowski, S.L.; Marion, D.W.; Kochanek, P.M. Neutrophil accumulation after traumatic brain injury in rats: Comparison of weight drop and controlled cortical impact models. *J. Neurotrauma* **1994**, *11*, 499–506. [CrossRef] [PubMed]
125. Harlan, J.M. Leukocyte-endothelial interactions. *Blood* **1985**, *65*, 513–525. [PubMed]
126. Kochanek, P.M.; Hallenbeck, J.M. Polymorphonuclear leukocytes and monocytes/macrophages in the pathogenesis of cerebral ischemia and stroke. *Stroke* **1992**, *23*, 1367–1379. [CrossRef] [PubMed]
127. Lucchesi, B.R.; Mullane, K.M. Leukocytes and ischemia-induced myocardial injury. *Annu. Rev. Pharmacol. Toxicol.* **1986**, *26*, 201–224. [CrossRef] [PubMed]
128. Burke-Gaffney, A.; Keenan, A.K. Modulation of human endothelial cell permeability by combinations of the cytokines interleukin-1 alpha/beta, tumor necrosis factor-alpha and interferon-gamma. *Immunopharmacology* **1993**, *25*, 1–9. [CrossRef]
129. Clark, W.M.; Madden, K.P.; Rothlein, R.; Zivin, J.A. Reduction of central nervous system ischemic injury in rabbits using leukocyte adhesion antibody treatment. *Stroke* **1991**, *22*, 877–883. [CrossRef] [PubMed]
130. Schwartz, M.; Yoles, E. Macrophages and dendritic cells treatment of spinal cord injury: From the bench to the clinic. *Acta Neurochir. Suppl.* **2005**, *93*, 147–150. [PubMed]
131. Zindler, E.; Zipp, F. Neuronal injury in chronic CNS inflammation. *Best Pract. Res. Clin. Anaesthesiol.* **2010**, *24*, 551–562. [CrossRef] [PubMed]
132. Herz, J.; Zipp, F.; Siffrin, V. Neurodegeneration in autoimmune CNS inflammation. *Exp. Neurol.* **2010**, *225*, 9–17. [CrossRef] [PubMed]
133. Jin, X.; Ishii, H.; Bai, Z.; Itokazu, T.; Yamashita, T. Temporal changes in cell marker expression and cellular infiltration in a controlled cortical impact model in adult male C57BL/6 mice. *PLoS ONE* **2012**, *7*, e41892. [CrossRef] [PubMed]
134. Hu, X.; Li, P.; Guo, Y.; Wang, H.; Leak, R.K.; Chen, S.; Gao, Y.; Chen, J. Microglia/macrophage polarization dynamics reveal novel mechanism of injury expansion after focal cerebral ischemia. *Stroke* **2012**, *43*, 3063–3070. [CrossRef] [PubMed]
135. Rolls, A.; Shechter, R.; London, A.; Segev, Y.; Jacob-Hirsch, J.; Amariglio, N.; Rechavi, G.; Schwartz, M. Two faces of chondroitin sulfate proteoglycan in spinal cord repair: A role in microglia/macrophage activation. *PLoS Med.* **2008**, *5*, e171. [CrossRef] [PubMed]
136. Heppner, F.L.; Ransohoff, R.M.; Becher, B. Immune attack: The role of inflammation in alzheimer disease. *Nat. Rev. Neurosci.* **2015**, *16*, 358–372. [CrossRef] [PubMed]
137. Martinez, F.O.; Gordon, S. The M1 and M2 paradigm of macrophage activation: Time for reassessment. *F1000Prime Rep.* **2014**, *6*, 13. [CrossRef] [PubMed]
138. Verma, S.; Nakaoke, R.; Dohgu, S.; Banks, W.A. Release of cytokines by brain endothelial cells: A polarized response to lipopolysaccharide. *Brain Behav. Immun.* **2006**, *20*, 449–455. [CrossRef] [PubMed]
139. Jang, E.; Lee, S.; Kim, J.H.; Kim, J.H.; Seo, J.W.; Lee, W.H.; Mori, K.; Nakao, K.; Suk, K. Secreted protein lipocalin-2 promotes microglial M1 polarization. *FASEB J.* **2013**, *27*, 1176–1190. [CrossRef] [PubMed]
140. Starossom, S.C.; Mascanfroni, I.D.; Imitola, J.; Cao, L.; Raddassi, K.; Hernandez, S.F.; Bassil, R.; Croci, D.O.; Cerliani, J.P.; Delacour, D.; et al. Galectin-1 deactivates classically activated microglia and protects from inflammation-induced neurodegeneration. *Immunity* **2012**, *37*, 249–263. [CrossRef] [PubMed]
141. Rocher, C.; Singla, D.K. SMAD-PI3K-Akt-mTOR pathway mediates BMP-7 polarization of monocytes into M2 macrophages. *PLoS ONE* **2013**, *8*, e84009. [CrossRef] [PubMed]
142. Biswas, S.K.; Mantovani, A. Macrophage plasticity and interaction with lymphocyte subsets: Cancer as a paradigm. *Nat. Immunol.* **2010**, *11*, 889–896. [CrossRef] [PubMed]
143. Roughton, K.; Andreasson, U.; Blomgren, K.; Kalm, M. Lipopolysaccharide-induced inflammation aggravates irradiation-induced injury to the young mouse brain. *Dev. Neurosci.* **2013**, *35*, 406–415. [CrossRef] [PubMed]

144. Mukherjee, S.; Katki, K.; Arisi, G.M.; Foresti, M.L.; Shapiro, L.A. Early tbi-induced cytokine alterations are similarly detected by two distinct methods of multiplex assay. *Front. Mol. Neurosci.* **2011**, *4*, 21. [CrossRef] [PubMed]
145. Ni, K.; O'Neill, H.C. The role of dendritic cells in T cell activation. *Immunol. Cell Biol.* **1997**, *75*, 223–230. [CrossRef] [PubMed]
146. Pozzi, L.A.; Maciaszek, J.W.; Rock, K.L. Both dendritic cells and macrophages can stimulate naive CD8 T cells in vivo to proliferate, develop effector function, and differentiate into memory cells. *J. Immunol.* **2005**, *175*, 2071–2081. [CrossRef] [PubMed]
147. Kelso, M.L.; Gendelman, H.E. Bridge between neuroimmunity and traumatic brain injury. *Curr. Pharm. Des.* **2014**, *20*, 4284–4298. [CrossRef] [PubMed]
148. Gyoneva, S.; Kim, D.; Katsumoto, A.; Kokiko-Cochran, O.N.; Lamb, B.T.; Ransohoff, R.M. *Ccr2* deletion dissociates cavity size and tau pathology after mild traumatic brain injury. *J. Neuroinflamm.* **2015**, *12*, 228. [CrossRef] [PubMed]
149. Gelderblom, M.; Arunachalam, P.; Magnus, T. Gammadelta T cells as early sensors of tissue damage and mediators of secondary neurodegeneration. *Front. Cell Neurosci.* **2014**, *8*, 368. [CrossRef] [PubMed]
150. Sobottka, B.; Harrer, M.D.; Ziegler, U.; Fischer, K.; Wiendl, H.; Hunig, T.; Becher, B.; Goebels, N. Collateral bystander damage by myelin-directed CD8+ T cells causes axonal loss. *Am. J. Pathol.* **2009**, *175*, 1160–1166. [CrossRef] [PubMed]
151. Melzer, N.; Meuth, S.G.; Wiendl, H. CD8+ T cells and neuronal damage: Direct and collateral mechanisms of cytotoxicity and impaired electrical excitability. *FASEB J.* **2009**, *23*, 3659–3673. [CrossRef] [PubMed]
152. Serpe, C.J.; Coers, S.; Sanders, V.M.; Jones, K.J. CD4+ T, but not CD8+ or B, lymphocytes mediate facial motoneuron survival after facial nerve transection. *Brain Behav. Immun.* **2003**, *17*, 393–402. [CrossRef]
153. Schwartz, M.; Shechter, R. Systemic inflammatory cells fight off neurodegenerative disease. *Nat. Rev. Neurol.* **2010**, *6*, 405–410. [CrossRef] [PubMed]
154. Cohen, I.R. The cognitive paradigm and the immunological homunculus. *Immunol. Today* **1992**, *13*, 490–494. [CrossRef]
155. Moalem, G.; Leibowitz-Amit, R.; Yoles, E.; Mor, F.; Cohen, I.R.; Schwartz, M. Autoimmune T cells protect neurons from secondary degeneration after central nervous system axotomy. *Nat. Med.* **1999**, *5*, 49–55. [PubMed]
156. Bradl, M.; Bauer, J.; Flugel, A.; Wekerle, H.; Lassmann, H. Complementary contribution of CD4 and CD8 T lymphocytes to T-cell infiltration of the intact and the degenerative spinal cord. *Am. J. Pathol.* **2005**, *166*, 1441–1450. [CrossRef]
157. Burns, J.; Rosenzweig, A.; Zweiman, B.; Lisak, R.P. Isolation of myelin basic protein-reactive T-cell lines from normal human blood. *Cell. Immunol.* **1983**, *81*, 435–440. [CrossRef]
158. Martin, R.; Jaraquemada, D.; Flerlage, M.; Richert, J.; Whitaker, J.; Long, E.O.; McFarlin, D.E.; McFarland, H.F. Fine specificity and HLA restriction of myelin basic protein-specific cytotoxic T cell lines from multiple sclerosis patients and healthy individuals. *J. Immunol.* **1990**, *145*, 540–548. [PubMed]
159. Sakaguchi, S. Naturally arising Foxp3-expressing $CD25^+CD4^+$ regulatory T cells in immunological tolerance to self and non-self. *Nat. Immunol.* **2005**, *6*, 345–352. [CrossRef] [PubMed]
160. Fontenot, J.D.; Gavin, M.A.; Rudensky, A.Y. Foxp3 programs the development and function of CD4+CD25+ regulatory T cells. *Nat. Immunol.* **2003**, *4*, 330–336. [CrossRef] [PubMed]
161. Ben Simon, G.J.; Hovda, D.A.; Harris, N.G.; Gomez-Pinilla, F.; Goldberg, R.A. Traumatic brain injury induced neuroprotection of retinal ganglion cells to optic nerve crush. *J. Neurotrauma* **2006**, *23*, 1072–1082. [CrossRef] [PubMed]
162. Fisher, J.; Levkovitch-Verbin, H.; Schori, H.; Yoles, E.; Butovsky, O.; Kaye, J.F.; Ben-Nun, A.; Schwartz, M. Vaccination for neuroprotection in the mouse optic nerve: Implications for optic neuropathies. *J. Neurosci.* **2001**, *21*, 136–142. [PubMed]
163. Hazeldine, J.; Lord, J.M.; Belli, A. Traumatic brain injury and peripheral immune suppression: Primer and prospectus. *Front. Neurol.* **2015**, *6*, 235. [CrossRef] [PubMed]
164. Jesse, S.; Steinacker, P.; Cepek, L.; von Arnim, C.A.; Tumani, H.; Lehnert, S.; Kretzschmar, H.A.; Baier, M.; Otto, M. Glial fibrillary acidic protein and protein s-100b: Different concentration pattern of glial proteins in cerebrospinal fluid of patients with alzheimer's disease and creutzfeldt-jakob disease. *J. Alzheimers Dis.* **2009**, *17*, 541–551. [CrossRef] [PubMed]

165. Posti, J.P.; Takala, R.S.; Runtti, H.; Newcombe, V.F.; Outtrim, J.; Katila, A.J.; Frantzen, J.; Ala-Seppala, H.; Coles, J.P.; Hossain, M.I.; et al. The levels of glial fibrillary acidic protein and ubiquitin c-terminal hydrolase-l1 during the first week after a traumatic brain injury: Correlations with clinical and imaging findings. *Neurosurgery* **2016**, *79*, 456–464. [PubMed]
166. Mondello, S.; Kobeissy, F.; Vestri, A.; Hayes, R.L.; Kochanek, P.M.; Berger, R.P. Serum concentrations of ubiquitin c-terminal hydrolase-l1 and glial fibrillary acidic protein after pediatric traumatic brain injury. *Sci. Rep.* **2016**, *6*, 28203. [CrossRef] [PubMed]
167. Yan, E.B.; Satgunaseelan, L.; Paul, E.; Bye, N.; Nguyen, P.; Agyapomaa, D.; Kossmann, T.; Rosenfeld, J.V.; Morganti-Kossmann, M.C. Post-traumatic hypoxia is associated with prolonged cerebral cytokine production, higher serum biomarker levels, and poor outcome in patients with severe traumatic brain injury. *J. Neurotrauma* **2014**, *31*, 618–629. [CrossRef] [PubMed]
168. Ottens, A.K.; Golden, E.C.; Bustamante, L.; Hayes, R.L.; Denslow, N.D.; Wang, K.K. Proteolysis of multiple myelin basic protein isoforms after neurotrauma: Characterization by mass spectrometry. *J. Neurochem.* **2008**, *104*, 1401–1414. [CrossRef] [PubMed]
169. Cox, A.L.; Coles, A.J.; Nortje, J.; Bradley, P.G.; Chatfield, D.A.; Thompson, S.J.; Menon, D.K. An investigation of auto-reactivity after head injury. *J. Neuroimmunol.* **2006**, *174*, 180–186. [CrossRef] [PubMed]
170. Kalia, V.; Sarkar, S.; Ahmed, R. Cd8 t-cell memory differentiation during acute and chronic viral infections. *Adv. Exp. Med. Biol.* **2010**, *684*, 79–95. [PubMed]
171. Goverman, J. Autoimmune t cell responses in the central nervous system. *Nat. Rev. Immunol.* **2009**, *9*, 393–407. [CrossRef] [PubMed]
172. McFarland, H.F.; Martin, R. Multiple sclerosis: A complicated picture of autoimmunity. *Nat. Immunol.* **2007**, *8*, 913–919. [CrossRef] [PubMed]
173. Lucchinetti, C.; Bruck, W.; Parisi, J.; Scheithauer, B.; Rodriguez, M.; Lassmann, H. Heterogeneity of multiple sclerosis lesions: Implications for the pathogenesis of demyelination. *Ann. Neurol.* **2000**, *47*, 707–717. [CrossRef]
174. Ransohoff, R.M.; Kivisakk, P.; Kidd, G. Three or more routes for leukocyte migration into the central nervous system. *Nat. Rev. Immunol.* **2003**, *3*, 569–581. [CrossRef] [PubMed]
175. Ginhoux, F.; Lim, S.; Hoeffel, G.; Low, D.; Huber, T. Origin and differentiation of microglia. *Front. Cell Neurosci.* **2013**, *7*, 45. [CrossRef] [PubMed]
176. Harry, G.J. Microglia during development and aging. *Pharmacol. Ther.* **2013**, *139*, 313–326. [CrossRef] [PubMed]
177. Papa, L.; Brophy, G.M.; Welch, R.D.; Lewis, L.M.; Braga, C.F.; Tan, C.N.; Ameli, N.J.; Lopez, M.A.; Haeussler, C.A.; Mendez Giordano, D.I.; et al. Time course and diagnostic accuracy of glial and neuronal blood biomarkers gfap and uch-l1 in a large cohort of trauma patients with and without mild traumatic brain injury. *JAMA Neurol.* **2016**, *73*, 551–560. [CrossRef] [PubMed]
178. Zoltewicz, J.S.; Scharf, D.; Yang, B.; Chawla, A.; Newsom, K.J.; Fang, L. Characterization of antibodies that detect human gfap after traumatic brain injury. *Biomark. Insights* **2012**, *7*, 71–79. [CrossRef] [PubMed]
179. Bogoslovsky, T.; Wilson, D.; Chen, Y.; Hanlon, D.; Gill, J.; Jeromin, A.; Song, L.; Moore, C.; Gong, Y.; Kenney, K.; et al. Increases of plasma levels of glial fibrillary acidic protein, tau, and amyloid beta up to 90 days after traumatic brain injury. *J. Neurotrauma* **2017**, *34*, 66–73. [CrossRef] [PubMed]
180. Su, E.; Bell, M.J.; Kochanek, P.M.; Wisniewski, S.R.; Bayir, H.; Clark, R.S.; Adelson, P.D.; Tyler-Kabara, E.C.; Janesko-Feldman, K.L.; Berger, R.P. Increased csf concentrations of myelin basic protein after tbi in infants and children: Absence of significant effect of therapeutic hypothermia. *Neurocrit. Care* **2012**, *17*, 401–407. [CrossRef] [PubMed]
181. Raper, D.; Louveau, A.; Kipnis, J. How do meningeal lymphatic vessels drain the cns? *Trends Neurosci.* **2016**, *39*, 581–586. [CrossRef] [PubMed]
182. Louveau, A.; Da Mesquita, S.; Kipnis, J. Lymphatics in neurological disorders: A neuro-lympho-vascular component of multiple sclerosis and alzheimer's disease? *Neuron* **2016**, *91*, 957–973. [CrossRef] [PubMed]
183. Brait, V.H.; Arumugam, T.V.; Drummond, G.R.; Sobey, C.G. Importance of t lymphocytes in brain injury, immunodeficiency, and recovery after cerebral ischemia. *J. Cereb. Blood Flow Metab.* **2012**, *32*, 598–611. [CrossRef] [PubMed]

184. Louveau, A.; Smirnov, I.; Keyes, T.J.; Eccles, J.D.; Rouhani, S.J.; Peske, J.D.; Derecki, N.C.; Castle, D.; Mandell, J.W.; Lee, K.S.; et al. Structural and functional features of central nervous system lymphatic vessels. *Nature* **2015**, *523*, 337–341. [CrossRef] [PubMed]
185. Yang, L.; Kress, B.T.; Weber, H.J.; Thiyagarajan, M.; Wang, B.; Deane, R.; Benveniste, H.; Iliff, J.J.; Nedergaard, M. Evaluating glymphatic pathway function utilizing clinically relevant intrathecal infusion of csf tracer. *J. Transl. Med.* **2013**, *11*, 107. [CrossRef] [PubMed]
186. Iliff, J.J.; Lee, H.; Yu, M.; Feng, T.; Logan, J.; Nedergaard, M.; Benveniste, H. Brain-wide pathway for waste clearance captured by contrast-enhanced mri. *J. Clin. Invest.* **2013**, *123*, 1299–1309. [CrossRef] [PubMed]
187. Xie, L.; Kang, H.; Xu, Q.; Chen, M.J.; Liao, Y.; Thiyagarajan, M.; O'Donnell, J.; Christensen, D.J.; Nicholson, C.; Iliff, J.J.; et al. Sleep drives metabolite clearance from the adult brain. *Science* **2013**, *342*, 373–377. [CrossRef] [PubMed]
188. Aspelund, A.; Antila, S.; Proulx, S.T.; Karlsen, T.V.; Karaman, S.; Detmar, M.; Wiig, H.; Alitalo, K. A dural lymphatic vascular system that drains brain interstitial fluid and macromolecules. *J. Exp. Med.* **2015**, *212*, 991–999. [CrossRef] [PubMed]
189. Li, M.; Li, F.; Luo, C.; Shan, Y.; Zhang, L.; Qian, Z.; Zhu, G.; Lin, J.; Feng, H. Immediate splenectomy decreases mortality and improves cognitive function of rats after severe traumatic brain injury. *J. Trauma* **2011**, *71*, 141–147. [CrossRef] [PubMed]
190. Chu, W.; Li, M.; Li, F.; Hu, R.; Chen, Z.; Lin, J.; Feng, H. Immediate splenectomy down-regulates the mapk-nf-kappab signaling pathway in rat brain after severe traumatic brain injury. *J. Trauma Acute Care Surg.* **2013**, *74*, 1446–1453. [CrossRef] [PubMed]
191. Teixeira, P.G.; Karamanos, E.; Okoye, O.T.; Talving, P.; Inaba, K.; Lam, L.; Demetriades, D. Splenectomy in patients with traumatic brain injury: Protective or harmful? A national trauma data bank analysis. *J. Trauma Acute Care Surg.* **2013**, *75*, 596–601. [CrossRef] [PubMed]

2

Neuroimmunology Research: A Report from the Cuban Network of Neuroimmunology

María de los Angeles Robinson-Agramonte [1,*], Lourdes Lorigados Pedre [1] and Orlando Ramón Serrano-Barrera [2]

[1] Neuroimmunology Laboratory, Immunochemical Department, International Center for Neurological Restoration, Ave 25 # 15805 b/w 158 and 160, Playa, Havana 11300, Cuba; lourdesl@neuro.ciren.cu

[2] Las Tunas General Hospital, Post Office Box 27, Las Tunas 75100, Cuba; orlandosb@infomed.sld.cu

* Correspondence: maria.robinson@infomed.sld.cu

Abstract: Neuroimmunology can be traced back to the XIX century through the descriptions of some of the disease's models (e.g., multiple sclerosis and Guillain Barret syndrome, amongst others). The diagnostic tools are based in the cerebrospinal fluid (CSF) analysis developed by Quincke or in the development of neuroimmunotherapy with the earlier expression in Pasteur's vaccine for rabies. Nevertheless, this field, which began to become delineated as an independent research area in the 1940s, has evolved as an innovative and integrative field at the shared edges of neurosciences, immunology, and related clinical and research areas, which are currently becoming a major concern for neuroscience and indeed for all of the scientific community linked to it. The workshop focused on several topics: (1) the molecular mechanisms of immunoregulation in health and neurological diseases, (like multiple sclerosis, autism, ataxias, epilepsy, Alzheimer and Parkinson's disease); (2) the use of animal models for neurodegenerative diseases (ataxia, fronto-temporal dementia/amyotrophic lateral sclerosis, ataxia-telangiectasia); (3) the results of new interventional technologies in neurology, with a special interest in the implementation of surgical techniques and the management of drug-resistant temporal lobe epilepsy; (4) the use of non-invasive brain stimulation in neurodevelopmental disorders; as well as (5) the efficacy of neuroprotective molecules in neurodegenerative diseases. This paper summarizes the highlights of the symposium.

Keywords: neuroimmunology; neurodevelopmental disorders; neurodegenerative disorders; non-invasive brain stimulation; Alzheimer disease's; Parkinson's disease; autism; demyelinating disease; neuropsychology; ataxy

---

1. Introduction

Neuroimmunology has arisen as an innovative and integrative field in the shared edges of neurosciences, immunology, as well as related areas. The current research was carried out in order to get insight into the current development of neuroimmunology, in terms of scientists, events and literature shaping and reflecting its main achievements: the delineation and evolution of a central paradigm. A first topic addressed was to review some events on the history of neuroimmunology. This talk fixed the roots of neuroimmunology in the 19th century, with the descriptions of some of the model diseases (e.g., multiple sclerosis, neuromyelitisoptica, Guillain-Barré syndrome), the diagnostic examination of cerebrospinal fluid (CSF) by Quincke or the development of neuroimmunotherapy with the vaccine for rabies by Pasteur, and it showed that the field began to become delineated as an independent research area in the 1940s, after Medawar's statements on the peculiarities of the brain in antigenic tolerance and the findings by Waksman and Adams on experimental allergic (later coined as autoimmune) encephalomyelitis. Reviewed aspects of neuroimmunology were shown to have evolved from neurological infections and immunopathological conditions to the conformation of a supracontrol system integrating neural and immune mechanisms toward a better adaptation of the organism in an ever-changing environment, and this allowed for a definition of the purpose of the work and its significance in this field [1,2].

This meeting was the fourth edition of the International Workshop of Neuroimmunology and the first of the Cuban Network of Neuroimmunology "CUBANNI", going from the 10 to 14 June 2017. The first session chaired by Professor Von Wee Yong and Professor Maria Robinson opened with an atypical but very interesting talk from Prof. Orlando Serrano from Tunas University, Cuba. This talk offered an overview on the history of neuroimmunology. After that, some very experienced speakers in this field showed some advances in this field and discussed current topics relative to how the immune reaction occurs in the context of the neurological disorders, as well as discussing, in some cases, ways to restore functions or to modulate aberrant mechanisms to get beneficial effects that are disease related. Several diseases were revised, such as multiple sclerosis (MS), Alzheimer's disease, epilepsy, strock, autism, Parkinson disease, as well as others. Interesting lectures served as guides to offer a better understanding of the molecular processes underlying neuroimmune pathology in neurodegenerative, neurodevelopmental, and neurovascular diseases, as well as to understand some vulnerabilities and comorbidities occurring in these disorders. Relevant to this topic was the lecture of Prof. Jack Antel on a new approach in microRNA in MS vulnerabilities [1].

The papers that referred to new therapeutic approaches for interventions in neuroimmunology were presented by experts: Prof. Diogo O Souza from UFRGS, Brazil; Prof. Von Wee Yong from the University of Calgary, Canada, Prof. Luis Velazquez from the Center for the Research and Rehabilitation of Hereditary Ataxias (CIRAH), Holguín, Cuba, Prof. Lázaro Gómez from the International Center for Neurological Restoration (CIREN), Havana, Cuba, and Prof. Miriam Marañón Cardonne from the Applied Electromagnetism Center, Santiago de Cuba, Cuba. An experiment in the use of protector molecules in neurological diseases was also presented by Prof. Yanier Núñez-Figueredo from the Center for Drugs Research and Development (CIDEM), Havana City, Cuba.

2. Lecture Highlights

Manfred Schedlowski, from the Institute of Medical Psychology and Behavioral Immunobiology, University Clinic Essen, Germany, delivered his lecture entitled "Learned immune responses—mechanisms and potential clinical application".

This speaker introduced experimental data in rodent and humans demonstrating that peripheral humoral and cellular immune functions can be modulated by associative learning processes. In a taste-immune learning paradigm in rats employing the immunosuppressive drug cyclosporine A as an unconditioned stimulus, the behaviorally conditioned suppressive effects on IL-2 and IFN-γ mRNA expression, cytokine production and T cell activity were shown to be centrally mediated via the insular cortex and amygdala, and peripherally via the sympathetic innervation of lymphatic organs and the beta-adrenoreceptor-dependent inhibition of the calcineurin activity. This learned immunosuppression is of biological relevance, since behavioral conditioning significantly attenuated allergic responses and symptom severity in chronic inflammatory autoimmune diseases. Moreover, behaviorally conditioned immunosuppression has also been demonstrated in healthy humans and in diseases. The presented data provided proof of the principle that learning strategies can be implemented in a immunopharmacological regimen, the aim being to reduce the amount of drugs, thereby minimizing unwanted toxic drug side effects while maximizing the therapeutic benefit for patients [3,4].

Professor Wekerle from the Max Planx Institute, Germany entitled his lecture: "Nature and Nurture-Gut Microbiota and Multiple Sclerosis". This very experienced investigator commented on his work group's extensive experience, spanning multiple years, in using a spontaneous variant of relapsing-remitting experimental autoimmune encephalomyelitis (EAE) to study the triggering events of brain autoimmunity. Single transgenic JL/J mice expressing a myelin oligodendrocyte glycoprotein (MOG) showed autoreactive T cell receptor in about 70% of their CD4+ T cell repertoire. He showed how the disease risk is modulated by the modification of the microbiota, for instance by antibiotic treatments or by dietary interventions, as well as showing how they currently explore the effect of microbial samples from people with MS on initiation of EAE in the RR-mouse model. Prof. Wekerle's pioneering work in this field also exposed the previous results observed in a rodent model with spontaneous EAE, establishing the relevance of gut flora in disease-triggering demyelination [5–8]: gut-associated lymphoid tissue, gut microbes and the susceptibility to experimental autoimmune encephalomyelitis [9].

The human gut commensal microbiota forms a complex population of microorganisms that survive by maintaining a symbiotic relationship with the host. Amongst the metabolic benefits, it plays an important role in the formation of an adaptive immune system and in the maintenance of its homeostasis, and it is crucial in the induction, training, and function of the host immune system. An optimal immune system-microbiota alliance allows the induction of protective responses to pathogens and the maintenance of regulatory pathways to the tolerance to innocuous antigens. Nevertheless, a mutual impact of the gastrointestinal tract (GIT) and central nervous system (CNS) functions was recognized since the mid-twentieth century, and it has been accepted that the so-called gut-brain axis provides a two-way homeostatic communication, through immunological, hormonal and neuronal signals [10,11].

The GIT might represent a vulnerable area through which pathogens influence all aspects of physiology, even inducing CNS neuro-inflammation. A dysfunction of this axis has been associated with the pathogenesis of some diseases outside the GIT that have shown an increase in incidence over the last decades. Some papers had looked at how the commensal gut microbiota influences a systemic immune response in some neurological disorders, highlighting its impact cognition in multiple sclerosis, Guillain-Barrè syndrome, neurodevelopmental and behavioral disorders and Alzheimer's disease [12]. Nevertheless there no full comprehension on the implication of the potential microbiota-gut-brain dialogue in neurodegenerative diseases that might provide an insight on the pathogenesis and therapeutic strategies of these disorders.

The discussion of this talk focused on the fact that genes identified as having a susceptibility to MS do not satisfy the risk that argued for MS development. It was emphasized that many environmental risk factors to MS are described [13,14], but a growing number of studies demonstrate that gut microbes could directly play a role in the onset or progression of MS. A study led by researchers at the Max Planck Institute in Germany and co-authored by Cekanaviciute and Baranzini was referred to, in which it was found that microbiome transplants from MS patients could exacerbate symptoms in mice with a genetic model of the disease and which identified that specific species of bacteria more common in people with MS—*Akkermansia muciniphila* and *Acinetobacter calcoaceticus*—triggered the cells to become pro-inflammatory responses in human peripheral blood mononuclear cells and in monocolonized mice, while a species of bacteria found at lever that were lower than usual in MS patients—*Parabacteroides distasonis*—triggered immune-regulatory responses, stimulating anti-inflammatory IL-10-expressing human $CD4^+CD25^+$ T cells and $IL\text{-}10^+FoxP3^+$ Tregs in mice [13,14].

Finally, the experiment with microbiota transplants from MS patients to germ-free mice resulted in more severe symptoms of experimental autoimmune encephalomyelitis and reduced proportions of IL-10+ Tregs compared with mice that were "humanized" with microbiota from healthy controls. This study identified specific human gut bacteria that regulate adaptive autoimmune responses, suggesting a therapeutic targeting of the microbiota as a treatment for MS at time that provided evidence that MS-derived microbiota contain factors that precipitate an MS-like autoimmune disease in a transgenic mouse model.

Microbial colonization of the infant gastrointestinal tract (GIT) begins at birth, is shaped by the maternal microbiota, and is profoundly altered by antibiotictreatment [15,16]. Antibiotictreatment of mothers during pregnancy influences the colonization of the GIT microbiota of their infants [15]. The role of the GIT microbiota in regulating the adaptive immune function against systemic viral infections during infancy remains undefined. Nevertheless, an undisturbed colonization and progression of the GIT microbiota during infancy are necessary to promote robust adaptive immune responses. The topic of symbiotic and antibiotic interactions between gut commensal microbiota and the host immune system was discussed, regarding the integral elements of commensal microbiota that stimulate responses of different parts of the immune system and lead to health or disease, as well as on the conditions and factors that contribute to gut commensal microbiota's transformation from a symbiotic to an antibiotic relationship with humans [16]. The authors suggested to continue research efforts to better understand the host-microbiota interactions in physiological and disease settings, which might lead to the development of rational-based treatments.

For decades, the brain was considered an autonomous tissue that performs best without any assistance from the immune system. It is now widely accepted, largely through our work, that circulating monocytes and CD4+ T cells are needed for supporting brain reparation and functional plasticity. It was demonstrated that leukocytes could gain access to the brain's territory through a unique interface, the epithelial layer that forms the blood-CSF-barrier, the choroid plexus (CP) [5,8]. Michal Schwartz and Aleksandra Deczkowska, from The Weizmann Institute of Science, Rehovot, Israel, exposed these considerations in their lecture entitled "Reversing age-related dementia and Alzheimer's disease by restoring the brain-immune axis". Evidences from a Robust RNAseq analysis demonstrated that, in aging, the function of this interface is suppressed due to a systemic loss of interferon-gamma (IFN-γ), and due to a local elevation of type I interferon (type 1-IFN), which not only interferes with the activity of the CP but also negatively affects microglial activity. The intracerebral administration of anti-IFN-β receptor antibodies restored CP activity, reversed the microglial cognitive-impairing phenotype, and improved the overall cognitive ability in aged mice [17–20].

In an animal model of Alzheimer's disease, the CP was found to be dysfunctional, mainly due to low IFN-γ availability, which results from systemic immune suppression/exhaustion. Transiently reducing the systemic immunosuppression via the depletion of Foxp3+ regulatory T cells, or via the blocking of the inhibitory PD-1/PD-L1 immune checkpoint pathways, led to an increase of the activation of the CP to express trafficking molecules, which in turn led to the recruitment of immune regulatory cells to sites of brain pathology. Treatments with anti-PD-1 antibodies were found to be effective in several mouse models of AD in reversing cognitive loss, the removal of plaques, and in restoring brain homeostasis as determined by the inflammatory molecular profile. Such an approach is not meant to be against any single disease-escalating factor in AD, but rather empowers the individual's immune system to drive the process of repair. By directly targeting the immune system, rather than a single disease risk factor in the brain, this approach provides a comprehensive therapy that addresses numerous factors that become detrimental in the AD brain [21].

The role of the S100B protein, in neuroinflammation and Alzheimer's disease, was presented by Prof. Carlos-Alberto Gonçalves from the Federal University of Rio Grande do Sul, Puerto Alegre, Brazil. Alzheimer's disease (AD) is characterized by two main neuropathological brain patterns: the senile plaques formed by deposits of the β-amyloid protein (Aβ) at cholinergic terminals and the neurofibrillary tangles produced by tau protein hyper-phosphorilation. This evidence points to the fact that AD is not restricted to neurons; that neuroinflammation precedes AD pathogenesis; and that glial activation occurs early on in AD, even before cognitive deficit and amyloid deposition. Like microglia, astrocytes recognize danger-associated and pathogen-associated molecular patterns and release inflammatory mediators, as well as supporting and modulating neuronal activity. S100B is a calcium-binding protein mainly expressed in astrocytes in brain tissue, and experimental evidence indicates its involvement in neuroinflammation and degenerative disorders, including AD. This protein has many putative intracellular targets; it is secreted and has autocrine and paracrine effects on glia, neurons and microglia, while showing a toxic effect at a high concentration [22]. Some proposed intracellular targets of S100B include proteins of the cytoskeleton (e.g., GFAP), modulators of the cell cycle (e.g., p53 and Ndr kinase), the protein kinase C and phosphatase 2B (calcineurin). The extracellular effect of S100B, observed in neural cultures, depends on its concentration, since it is neurotrophic at pico and nanomolar levels and apoptotic at micromolar levels. The activation of RAGE and signaling pathways such as ERK, NF-κB and NFAT, following the effects of S100B observed in culture were discussed by Prof. Gonçalves, along with its role in the inflammatory response and its putative use as a biomarker in the three stages of AD [23–27].

The results of a novel study on the participation of neuroinflammatory processes in neurological pathologies such as epilepsy were shown. In this field, Dr. Lourdes Lorigados and collaborators presented clinical evidence of the involvement of inflammatory processes both centrally and peripherally in drug-resistant epilepsy with their work entitled: Two year follow-up of IL-1, IL-6 in temporal lobe drug-resistant epilepsy patient treated surgically [28,29].

Autism spectrum disorders are neurodevelopmental disorders which involve moderately to severely disrupted functioning in regard to social skills and socialization, expressive and receptive communication, and repetitive or stereotyped behaviors and interests [30]. "How Neuropsychology informs Neuroimmunology—Understanding the Cognitive and Behavioral Vulnerabilities in Autism Spectrum Disorders", was the lecture delivered by Prof. Scott Hunter of Chicago University, USA. This presentation addressed the current understanding of the neuropsychology of autism spectrum disorders (ASD), in association with ongoing research on neuroimmunological factors that contribute to higher risks of neurodevelopmental disorders. The spectrum of challenges experienced by children with ASD and the multiple levels of influence that occur neurodevelopmentally, both prenatally and postnatally, were reviewed [31]. A proposal for an integrated collaboration between researchers and clinicians was also offered, to guide considerations regarding etiology and treatment in this disorder.

"From clinical to molecular in autism: A pending task to the science", delivered by Prof. Maria Robinson Agramonte from the International Center for Neurological Restoration, Havana, Cuba, was based on a study involving clinical and molecular analysis. It showed how necessary it became to perform multidisciplinary studies in autism in order to advance the understanding of the disease pathology toward better clinical management and toward the implementation of novel therapies in development. Referring to the contribution of inflammatory markers to vulnerabilities in autism, this paper showed the potentialities of EEG findings in aiding information on clinical decision making for children with autism spectrum disorders [32].

Dalina Laffita from Florida Atlantic University, delivered a talk entitled "Suppressing Igf-1 signaling pathway rescues neuronal overgrowth of Pten+/- mice". Macrocephaly is associated with ASD. The alteration of mTOR signaling pathways has been shown to be involved in 14% of ASD individuals [33]. The research supports divergent trajectories of brain growth in the regressive vs. non-regressive phenotype of ASD; however, the degree to which the cellular mechanisms underlying these profiles differ is not clear [34]. PTEN is a gene associated with ASD, the macrocephaly is observed in the heterozygous mutation in PTEN (PTEN+/-), which leads to a negative regulation in PI3K/Akt/mTOR signaling pathways; it is a great model for studying ASD, as these mice show social behavioral deficits that are observed in humans. During this study, there was evidence that Pten is a regulator of β-catenin. An increase was seen in the β-catenin signal, but the manner in how both of these are associated is not well understood. Measurements of the soma cell size of the fifth layer of the cerebral cortex in a Pten+/- mouse were taken. There was a decrease in the sizes of the neurons; thus, the ultimate goal was to recover the original size after birth, by upregulating the PI3K/Akt/mTOR signaling pathway. The inhibition of the insulin-like growth factor receptor 1 (IGF1R), which is found upstream of this pathway, led to a significant decrease in soma cell size in Pten+/-/Igf-1r+/- mice. The authors considered this a very promising result because it opens the door for a new pharmacological agent that could recover the damage done by this mutation. The pathway being targeted is a cellular pathway, so this brings up the challenge that the pharmacological agent must be able to cross the blood brain barrier and be able to only influence this cellular pathway within the brain to prevent side effects.

Georg Auburger from Goethe University Hospital Frankfurt, Germany, delivered a lecture on Ataxin-2 as a translation factor with a specificity for mitochondrial precursors. Prof. Auburger introduced his lecture by referencing the Ataxin-2 (ATXN2) gene family characterization, saying that, via yeast, it extends from man to plants and that it appears to be so important for all forms of eukaryotic life that several gene copies exist in most vertebrates, as well as in plants and fungi. Mammalian Ataxin-2 is transcriptionally induced during starvation; he said and continued saying that in periods of nutrient depletion, oxidative stress or infection, its subcellular localization changes from the ribosomal translation apparatus to stress granules, where RNA quality control and RNA repair occur [35].

Ataxin-2 is a key element of the stress granules component. Over the last two years, it was shown in yeast, worms and mammals that Ataxin-2 represses global mRNA translation via diminished mTORC1 signaling, a pathway where several drugs are already available. Importantly however, the abundance of selected factors requires Ataxin-2 expression. One example is the PAS domain containing the factor period. The PAS domains are signal modules that are widely distributed in proteins across all kingdoms of life. They are common in photoreceptors and transcriptional regulators of eukaryotic circadian clocks and mainly possess protein-protein interaction and light-sensing functions [36], which triggers rest and the decline of metabolic activity during nighttime. Another example is the mitochondrial matrix enzyme Iso-Valeryl-Dehydrogenase, which is responsible for leucine degradation and thus reduces mTORC1 activity. Further examples are branched chain amino acid enzymes in the mitochondrial matrix, which are responsible for fatty acid degradation. Additionally, mitochondrial matrix enzymes in the tricarboxylic acid (TCA) cycle of glycolysis are enhanced by Ataxin-2 expression. When Ataxin-2 is not absent, fat accumulates subcutaneously and in liver lipid droplets, parallel to glycogen granules. Thus, the recruitment of stored alternative fuels in times of glucose depletion or of excessive bioenergetic demands is dependent on Ataxin-2. Given that cellular lipid uptake via the endocytosis of trophic receptors is impaired by Ataxin-2, cells are more dependent on their own nutrient reserves, and autophagy would probably increase. Interestingly, Ataxin-2 expression also enhances the abundance of PINK1, an autophagy-regulator that is responsible for the quality control and repair of mitochondria. A conclusion of this lecture was that these cellular roles seem essential for neurodegenerative diseases, given that ATXN2 depletion is surprisingly effective in protecting motor neurons and cerebellar neurons in ALS and in Spinocerebellar Ataxias (SCAs), as demonstrated in mouse models and flies.

Spinocerebellar Ataxias (SCA) are neurodegenerative disorders characterized by the degeneration of the cerebellum and its afferent and efferent connections, brainstem, spinal cord and peripheral nerves. In the past 20 years, clinical trials have been carried out in SCAs to slow down or stop disease progression and disability. However, the main findings were often negative due to the fact that the included patients had a severe degeneration of the nervous system. The best moment to start with clinical trials is before ataxia onset, where the neurodegeneration is beginning. Recently, two phases before ataxia onset were defined: the asymptomatic and the preclinical stages in SCAs. The asymptomatic phase is characterized by an absence of neurological abnormalities. However, in the preclinical phase, there are several clinical and paraclinical complaints in SCAs. "Spinocerebellar Ataxias: Early diagnosis and ethical dilemmas during preclinical trials", was presented by Prof. Luis Velázquez-Pérez from the Center for Research and Rehabilitation of Hereditary Ataxias, Holguin, Cuba. In this talk, he commented on how the first studies of the preclinical stage were carried out in a Cuban SCA2 population. The dorsal lemniscal system, saccades movements, visual motor performance, REM sleep, and autonomic nervous system were evaluated. 35% of the preclinical subjects have cerebellar alterations such as abnormal tandem gait, mild incoordination deficit and nistagmus. The non-cerebellar manifestations were muscle cramps, sensory symptoms and sleep disorders. Clinical examination showed hyperreflexia, saccade slowing and cognitive dysfunction. The early clinical trials raise ethical dilemmas which, if not effectively addressed, may harm subjects. The high prevalence of SCA2 families in Cuba has offered great opportunities to carry intervention strategies in subjects in a preclinical state. SCA2 preclinical carriers revealed a high acceptation rate (97.5%) to be included in neurorehabilitation programs and/or clinical trials. Thus, Cuban SCA2 preclinical carriers have undergone early therapeutical approaches consisting in a rehabilitation program and an open-label clinical trial with vitamins, which improved both the subtle cerebellar manifestations and muscle cramps. Both treatments were safe in all subjects, minimizing the ethical dilemma associated with the drug side effects. Regarding the ethical concerns related to the placement of a preclinical carrier on a placebo group, all interviewed subjects that were referred agreed with these designs due to the possibility of receiving concomitant therapeutical options during the study and receiving the true drug after completion of the study, if it was effective and safe. In addition, the ethical dilemma of disease stigmatization were not observed in the treated SCA2 preclinical carriers, which could be explained by the long psychotherapeutical follow-up treatment that they received. In summary, the ethical concerns raised from the early interventions in prodromal SCA2 have led to new challenges for physicians, genetic counselors and researchers, which must be addressed via further investigations [37–39].

The cognitive impairment reported in 25% of patients is a common feature of Spinocerebellar Ataxia type 2 (SCA2), but has not been systematically studied, with no surrogate biomarkers having been described. In this context, Roberto Rodríguez-Labrada, also coming from the Ataxia Center in Cuba, exposed the results of a study guide to characterize new biomarkers of cognitive decline in SCA2 through clinical and electrophysiological assessments. The lecture, entitled "New biomarkers for Spinocerebellar Ataxia type 2: insight into physiopathology of cognitive decline", included the INECO frontal screening test and an antisaccadic eye movement paradigm in 40 SCA2 patients, 37 preclinical mutation carriers and 40 healthy controls. The results evidenced a significant decrease of mean INECO scores in SCA2 patients and preclinical carriers, when compared to controls. This score was inversely correlated to expanded CAG repeats and the SARA score in the SCA2 patients, and was directly correlated to the time to ataxia onset in the preclinical carriers. Regarding the antisaccadic assessment, both disease related groups exhibited increased antisaccadic error rates and latencies, but the percentage of antisaccadic errors correction was only reduced in the patients. SCA2 patients carrying larger CAG repeats showed poorer antisaccadic performances, while preclinical carriers with shorter times to ataxia onset exhibited larger antisaccadic latencies [40–42]. A conclusion of this study reveals the usefulness of INECO tests and antisaccadic movements as sensitive biomarkers of executive dysfunctions in SCA2 since the early stages of the disease, as well as offering new evidence on the role of the cerebellum in cognitive functions from a human model disease.

"Metabolic mismatches and spinocerebellar Ataxia type 2 clinical phenotype": Almaguer-Gotay Dennis from the Center for Research and Rehabilitation of Hereditary Ataxias (CIRAH) showed the results of his group, related to the characterization of the SCA2 metabolism in presymptomatic patients. They concluded that SCA2 have some metabolic mismatches beginning from the presymtomatic stages, which have a significant correlation with disease severity and progression markers [43,44]. Almaguer Mederos LE, from the same center (CIRAH), claimed that *MTHFR* C677T polymorphism is associated with disease progression in SCA 2. These results point to a possible implication of the folate metabolism in the pathophysiology of SCA2, having a role in disease progression but not in disease onset [43].

Prof. Ivón Pedroso Ibáñez delivered her lecture entitled "Erythropoietin induce neuroprotection in patients with Parkinson's disease". Dr. Pedroso discussed the results of a multicenter study at CIREN (International Center for Neurological Restauration), CIM (Center for Molecular Immunology) and CEMPALA (Center for Attention and Development of Animal for laboratory, Cuba), which showed that treatment strategies in Parkinson's disease (PD) have improved patients' quality of life without stopping their progression, and that different alternatives to modify the natural course of the disease have demonstrated neuroprotective properties of erythropoietin; particularly, Cuban recombinant form (EPOrh) and recombinant human erythropoietin with low sialic acid (NeuroEPO) have showed good results. This talk showed the results of two clinical trials for neuroprotection purposes performed by this group using patients with PD in the IV stages of the Hoenh and Yarh scale, who received an intranasal formulation of NeuroEPO. All patients were evaluated with a battery of neuropsychological scales Data showed that both molecules are tolerated by patients with Parkinson's disease, with only mild adverse effects and a positive response to the cognitive functions. Authors considered that more studies must be carry out to underline the real relevance of this new biotechnological product. Additionally, these results contribute to the necessary screening of these types of compounds, promising protective properties to neurodegenerative diseases [45,46].

In addition, the results of an intra-nasal administration of non-hematopoietic erythropoietin promoting a clinical benefit without toxicity in spinocerebellar ataxia type 2 patients were discussed from a double-blind experiment; a placebo-controlled phase 2 clinical trial presented by Prof. Luis Velázquez and colleagues from the Center for the Research and Rehabilitation of Hereditary Ataxias, Holguín, Cuba. This study demonstrated that NeuroEpo is safe, feasible, and it suggested that it might represent a new therapeutic strategy for SCA and other neurodegenerative diseases [46].

Currently the biotechnological industry offers novel potential molecules with neuroprotective properties. An area of the meeting was reserved for the presentations of Prof. Diogo O Souza, from UFRGS, Brasil, who showed the results of his group on the neuroprotective effect of guanosine in the experimental models of brain diseases. Glutamate is the main excitatory neurotransmitter in mammalian CNS, essential for most brain activities. However, the hyperactive activation of the glutamatergic system may be potentially neurotoxic, involving the pathogenesis of various acute and chronic brain injuries. Increased glutamate causes the sustained entry of calcium and its excessive accumulation inside the cell, firing various intracellular processes that eventually lead to cell death. This increase of calcium generates the formation of free radicals that promote lipid peroxidation at the level of the membranes and the synthesis of nitric oxide, which acts as feedback and powers the excitotoxic effect by increasing the release of glutamate.

ALS is an age-related neurodegenerative disorder that is believed to have complex genetic and environmental influences in pathogenesis, but the etiologies are unidentified for most patients. Until the major causes are better defined, drug development is directed at downstream pathophysiological mechanisms, which are themselves incompletely understood. For nearly 30 years, glutamate-induced excitotoxicity has lain at the core of theories behind the spiraling events, including mitochondrial dysfunction, oxidative stress, and protein aggregation, that lead to neurodegenerative cell death in ALS [47]. The main process responsible for maintaining the extracellular glutamate levels below the toxic concentration is the glutamate uptake exerted by glutamate transporters located in neural cell membranes, mainly in astrocytes. This group showed strong evidence that the guanine-based purinergic system is effectively neuroprotective against glutamate toxicity, in acute and chronic animal models from both in vitro and in vivo studies. These results indicate that the neuroprotective guanine-based purine is the nucleoside guanosine (Guo). In vivo studies showed that Guo (i.c.v., i.p. or orally administered) protects against seizures (induced by quinolinic acid), brain ischemia and hepatic encephalopathy. The group searched for mechanisms implicated in this neuroprotection and demonstrated that this compound stimulates the astrocytic glutamate uptake in astrocyte cultures, additionally exerting neuroprotective effects that avoid the decrease in glutamate uptake [23,24,48,49].

Other molecules with neuroprotective effects were exposed by Wong-Guerra Maylin from the Center for the Development and Research of Medications, Cuba, with her paper entitled "Neuroprotective effects of JM-20 on aluminium-chloride-induced learning impairments, mitochondrial dysfunction and neuronal death in adult rats". JM-20 is a hybrid benzodiazepine dihydropyridine molecule, with a neuroprotective effect demonstrated in brain disorders involving excitotoxicity, oxidative damage, inflammatory response and mitochondrial dysfunction. This paper showed that the treatment with JM-20 prevented the increase of the expression of pro-apoptotic signaling proteins, protecting neuronal loss and presumably cognitive impairment, and in this line of findings the authors suggested that JM-20 may prevent memory impairment via mitochondrial protection and the inhibition of the intrinsic apoptosis pathway, also suggesting a therapeutic benefit to neurodegenerative dementia like Alzheimer's disease. The results on the regional effects of transient cerebral ischemia on astrocytes reactivity and the PI3K/Akt survival pathway, and the role of JM-20, were shown by Ramírez-Sánchez Jeney [50,51].

A Cuban experiment on a novel tool of intervention, "Transcraneal Magnetic Stimulation", was presented by Prof. Lázaro Gómez's lecture, "Effects of Non-Invasive Brain Stimulation in children with Autism Spectrum Disorder: a short term outcome study".

From his approach, the core symptoms of ASD may improve with pharmacological and non-pharmacological interventions; but deficits in social interaction and language remain throughout the lifespan. Following this criteria, the study showed how non-invasive brain stimulation (NIBS) could be a valuable adjuvant therapy for ASD, from the evaluation of tolerability, safety and the clinical effect of NIBS in children with ASD. The Autism Diagnostic Interview Revisited (ADI-R), Autism Treatment Evaluation Checklist (ATEC) and the Autism Behaviour Checklist (ABC) were used to assess the intervention effects, comparing the scores before and one week, one month, three months and six months after completing all the sessions. The resting state EEG was based in the analysis of functional connectivity, which showed clear changes after treatment. A conclusion of this lecture was that both methods, tDCS and rTMS, were tolerable and safe for the patients included in the study, and that a remarkable clinical improvement in their autistic symptoms was found after treatment [52].

3. Conclusions

The prevalence of inflammatory processes became a major component in neurological disease, at time when a main focus in neuroscience is to look for both a major understanding of neuroimmune pathology in the context of these diseases, as well as more effective and earlier ways of intervention. Following this viewpoint, this meeting consistently highlighted the discussion of molecular mechanisms and therapeutic approaches related to a more effective neuromodulation in neurological diseases, with particular relevance to neurodevelopment and neurodegenerative diseases. Results on The TMS and NeuroEpo offered a good perspective on neuroprotectors and modulators of neuroplasticity, since the C-PC and PCB were shown to be useful and promising therapeutic options for MS, based in the remyelinating effect observed in EAE models. The microbiome was treated as a third player in MS pathogenesis. Single-target approaches are insufficient for these multifactorial diseases, and molecules are screened for different relevant targets and effects. As we observed before, natural products continue to be an important source of drugs with beneficial effects for NDs; the roles of oxidative stress and mitochondrial performance are strongly linked to AD pathogenesis; in silico research is the leading approach in drug discovery and it is being widely used, mainly for AD. The different methodologies and lines of research discussed in the symposium suggest new possible therapeutic options and provide further insights on NDs mechanisms, from basic to translational research, drug discovery (mainly from natural sources), and the use of high-technology methods. The hallmarks of the symposium were all focused on NDs and neurodevelopment disorders. The congress provided a framework for translational research to advance toward new promising neural disease-modifying therapies.

Author Contributions: M.d.l.A.R.-A. was President of the Organizing Committee of International Conference "CUBANNI 2017" and elaborated the conference report. L.L.P. was President of the Scientific Committee and participated writing and reviewing the conference report. O.R.S.-B. participated reviewing the conference report.

Acknowledgments: The authors want to acknowledge speakers as the main contributors of this paper and the editorial committee for this special issue.

References

1. Ader, R.; Kelley, K.W. A global view of twenty years of brain, behavior, and immunity. *Brain Behav. Immun.* **2007**, *21*, 20–22. [CrossRef] [PubMed]
2. Wekerle, H. T-cell autoimmunity in the central nervous system. *Intervirology* **1993**, *35*, 95–100. [CrossRef] [PubMed]

3. Schedlowski, M.; Pacheco-Lopez, G. The learned immune response: Pavlov and beyond. *Brain Behav. Immun.* **2010**, *24*, 176–185. [CrossRef] [PubMed]
4. Albring, A.; Wendt, L.; Benson, S.; Nissen, S.; Yavuz, Z.; Engler, H.; Witzke, O.; Schedlowski, M. Preserving learned immunosuppressive placebo response: Perspectives for clinical application. *Clin. Pharmacol. Ther.* **2014**, *96*, 247–255. [CrossRef] [PubMed]
5. Hohlfeld, R.; Dornmair, K.; Meinl, E.; Wekerle, H. The search for the target antigens of multiple sclerosis, part 1: Autoreactive $CD4^+$ T lymphocytes as pathogenic effectors and therapeutic targets. *Lancet Neurol.* **2016**, *15*, 198–209. [CrossRef]
6. Hohlfeld, R.; Dornmair, K.; Meinl, E.; Wekerle, H. The search for the target antigens of multiple sclerosis, part 2: $CD8^+$ T cells, B cells, and antibodies in the focus of reverse-translational research. *Lancet Neurol.* **2016**, *15*, 317–331. [CrossRef]
7. Hohlfeld, R.; Wekerle, H. Multiple sclerosis and microbiota. From genome to metagenome? *Nervenarzt* **2015**, *86*, 925–933. [CrossRef] [PubMed]
8. Wekerle, H. Brain autoimmunity and intestinal microbiota: 100 trillion game changers. *Trends Immunol.* **2017**, *38*, 483–497. [CrossRef] [PubMed]
9. Wekerle, H. The gut-brain connection: Triggering of brain autoimmune disease by commensal gut bacteria. *Rheumatology* **2016**, *55*, ii68–ii75. [CrossRef] [PubMed]
10. Belkaid, Y.; Artis, D. Immunity at the barriers. *Eur. J. Immunol.* **2013**, *43*, 3096–3097. [CrossRef] [PubMed]
11. Belkaid, Y.; Hand, T.W. Role of the microbiota in immunity and inflammation. *Cell* **2014**, *157*, 121–141. [CrossRef] [PubMed]
12. Catanzaro, R.; Anzalone, M.; Calabrese, F.; Milazzo, M.; Capuana, M.; Italia, A.; Occhipinti, S.; Marotta, F. The gut microbiota and its correlations with the central nervous system disorders. *Panminerva Med.* **2015**, *57*, 127–143. [PubMed]
13. Cekanaviciute, E.; Yoo, B.B.; Runia, T.F.; Debelius, J.W.; Singh, S.; Nelson, C.A.; Kanner, R.; Bencosme, Y.; Lee, Y.K.; Hauser, S.L.; et al. Gut bacteria from multiple sclerosis patients modulate human T cells and exacerbate symptoms in mouse models. *Proc. Natl. Acad. Sci. USA* **2017**, *114*, 10713–10718. [CrossRef] [PubMed]
14. Berer, K.; Gerdes, L.A.; Cekanaviciute, E.; Jia, X.; Xiao, L.; Xia, Z.; Liu, C.; Klotz, L.; Stauffer, U.; Baranzini, S.E.; et al. Gut microbiota from multiple sclerosis patients enables spontaneous autoimmune encephalomyelitis in mice. *Proc. Natl. Acad. Sci. USA* **2017**, *114*, 10719–10724. [CrossRef] [PubMed]
15. Gonzalez-Perez, G.; Hicks, A.L.; Tekieli, T.M.; Radens, C.M.; Williams, B.L.; Lamouse-Smith, E.S. Maternal antibiotic treatment impacts development of the neonatal intestinal microbiome and antiviral immunity. *J. Immunol.* **2016**, *196*, 3768–3779. [CrossRef] [PubMed]
16. Malys, M.K.; Campbell, L.; Malys, N. Symbiotic and antibiotic interactions between gut commensal microbiota and host immune system. *Medicina* **2015**, *51*, 69–75. [CrossRef] [PubMed]
17. Deczkowska, A.; Baruch, K.; Schwartz, M. Type I/II interferon balance in the regulation of brain physiology and pathology. *Trends Immunol.* **2016**, *37*, 181–192. [CrossRef] [PubMed]
18. Deczkowska, A.; Matcovitch-Natan, O.; Tsitsou-Kampeli, A.; Ben-Hamo, S.; Dvir-Szternfeld, R.; Spinrad, A.; Singer, O.; David, E.; Winter, D.R.; Smith, L.K.; et al. Mef2c restrains microglial inflammatory response and is lost in brain ageing in an IFN-I-dependent manner. *Nat. Commun.* **2017**, *8*, 717. [CrossRef] [PubMed]
19. Schwartz, M.; Deczkowska, A. Neurological disease as a failure of brain-immune crosstalk: The multiple faces of neuroinflammation. *Trends Immunol.* **2016**, *37*, 668–679. [CrossRef] [PubMed]
20. Baruch, K.; Ron-Harel, N.; Gal, H.; Deczkowska, A.; Shifrut, E.; Ndifon, W.; Mirlas-Neisberg, N.; Cardon, M.; Vaknin, I.; Cahalon, L.; et al. CNS-specific immunity at the choroid plexus shifts toward destructive TH2 inflammation in brain aging. *Proc. Natl. Acad. Sci. USA* **2013**, *110*, 2264–2269. [CrossRef] [PubMed]
21. Baruch, K.; Deczkowska, A.; Rosenzweig, N.; Tsitsou-Kampeli, A.; Sharif, A.M.; Matcovitch-Natan, O.; Kertser, A.; David, E.; Amit, I.; Schwartz, M. PD-1 immune checkpoint blockade reduces pathology and improves memory in mouse models of alzheimer's disease. *Nat. Med.* **2016**, *22*, 135–137. [CrossRef] [PubMed]
22. Michetti, F.; Corvino, V.; Geloso, M.C.; Lattanzi, W.; Bernardini, C.; Serpero, L.; Gazzolo, D. The S100B protein in biological fluids: More than a lifelong biomarker of brain distress. *J. Neurochem.* **2012**, *120*, 644–659. [CrossRef] [PubMed]

23. Bellaver, B.; Dos Santos, J.P.; Leffa, D.T.; Bobermin, L.D.; Roppa, P.H.A.; da Silva Torres, I.L.; Goncalves, C.A.; Souza, D.O.; Quincozes-Santos, A. Systemic inflammation as a driver of brain injury: The astrocyte as an emerging player. *Mol. Neurobiol.* **2017**, *55*, 2685–2695. [CrossRef] [PubMed]
24. Bellaver, B.; Souza, D.G.; Bobermin, L.D.; Goncalves, C.A.; Souza, D.O.; Quincozes-Santos, A. Guanosine inhibits LPS-induced pro-inflammatory response and oxidative stress in hippocampal astrocytes through the heme oxygenase-1 pathway. *Purinergic Signal.* **2015**, *11*, 571–580. [CrossRef] [PubMed]
25. De Souza, D.F.; Wartchow, K.; Hansen, F.; Lunardi, P.; Guerra, M.C.; Nardin, P.; Goncalves, C.A. Interleukin-6-induced S100B secretion is inhibited by haloperidol and risperidone. *Prog. Neuro-Psychopharmacol. Biol. Psychiatry* **2013**, *43*, 14–22. [CrossRef] [PubMed]
26. Guerra, M.C.; Tortorelli, L.S.; Galland, F.; Da Re, C.; Negri, E.; Engelke, D.S.; Rodrigues, L.; Leite, M.C.; Goncalves, C.A. Lipopolysaccharide modulates astrocytic S100B secretion: A study in cerebrospinal fluid and astrocyte cultures from rats. *J. Neuroinflamm.* **2011**, *8*, 128. [CrossRef] [PubMed]
27. Neves, J.D.; Aristimunha, D.; Vizuete, A.F.; Nicola, F.; Vanzella, C.; Petenuzzo, L.; Mestriner, R.G.; Sanches, E.F.; Goncalves, C.A.; Netto, C.A. Glial-associated changes in the cerebral cortex after collagenase-induced intracerebral hemorrhage in the rat striatum. *Brain Res. Bull.* **2017**, *134*, 55–62. [CrossRef] [PubMed]
28. Lorigados Pedre, L.; Morales Chacon, L.M.; Orozco Suarez, S.; Pavon Fuentes, N.; Estupinan Diaz, B.; Serrano Sanchez, T.; Garcia Maeso, I.; Rocha Arrieta, L. Inflammatory mediators in epilepsy. *Curr. Pharm. Des.* **2013**, *19*, 6766–6772. [CrossRef] [PubMed]
29. Lorigados Pedre, L.; Morales Chacon, L.M.; Pavon Fuentes, N.; Robinson Agramonte, M.L.A.; Serrano Sanchez, T.; Cruz-Xenes, R.M.; Diaz Hung, M.L.; Estupinan Diaz, B.; Baez Martin, M.M.; Orozco-Suarez, S. Follow-up of peripheral IL-1beta and IL-6 and relation with apoptotic death in drug-resistant temporal lobe epilepsy patients submitted to surgery. *Behav. Sci.* **2018**, *8*, 21. [CrossRef] [PubMed]
30. Lahiri, D.K.; Sokol, D.K.; Erickson, C.; Ray, B.; Ho, C.Y.; Maloney, B. Autism as early neurodevelopmental disorder: Evidence for an sappalpha-mediated anabolic pathway. *Front. Cell. Neurosci.* **2013**, *7*, 94. [CrossRef] [PubMed]
31. Sharma, S.; Woolfson, L.M.; Hunter, S.C. Maladaptive cognitive appraisals in children with high-functioning autism: Associations with fear, anxiety and theory of mind. *Autism Int. J. Res. Pract.* **2014**, *18*, 244–254. [CrossRef] [PubMed]
32. Inga Jacome, M.C.; Morales Chacon, L.M.; Vera Cuesta, H.; Maragoto Rizo, C.; Whilby Santiesteban, M.; Ramos Hernandez, L.; Noris Garcia, E.; Gonzalez Fraguela, M.E.; Fernandez Verdecia, C.I.; Vegas Hurtado, Y.; et al. Peripheral inflammatory markers contributing to comorbidities in autism. *Behav. Sci.* **2016**, *6*, 29. [CrossRef] [PubMed]
33. Nordahl, C.W.; Lange, N.; Li, D.D.; Barnett, L.A.; Lee, A.; Buonocore, M.H.; Simon, T.J.; Rogers, S.; Ozonoff, S.; Amaral, D.G. Brain enlargement is associated with regression in preschool-age boys with autism spectrum disorders. *Proc. Natl. Acad. Sci. USA* **2011**, *108*, 20195–20200. [CrossRef] [PubMed]
34. De Vries, P.J. Targeted treatments for cognitive and neurodevelopmental disorders in tuberous sclerosis complex. *Neurother. J. Am. Soc. Exp. NeuroTher.* **2010**, *7*, 275–282. [CrossRef] [PubMed]
35. Auburger, G.; Sen, N.E.; Meierhofer, D.; Basak, A.N.; Gitler, A.D. Efficient prevention of neurodegenerative diseases by depletion of starvation response factor ataxin-2. *Trends Neurosci.* **2017**, *40*, 507–516. [CrossRef] [PubMed]
36. Mei, Q.; Dvornyk, V. Evolution of pas domains and pas-containing genes in eukaryotes. *Chromosoma* **2014**, *123*, 385–405. [CrossRef] [PubMed]
37. Figueroa, K.P.; Coon, H.; Santos, N.; Velazquez, L.; Mederos, L.A.; Pulst, S.M. Genetic analysis of age at onset variation in spinocerebellar ataxia type 2. *Neurol. Genet.* **2017**, *3*, e155. [CrossRef] [PubMed]
38. Velazquez-Perez, L.; Rodriguez-Labrada, R.; Torres-Vega, R.; Montero, J.M.; Vazquez-Mojena, Y.; Auburger, G.; Ziemann, U. Central motor conduction time as prodromal biomarker in spinocerebellar ataxia type 2. *Mov. Disord. Off. J. Mov. Disord. Soc.* **2016**, *31*, 603–604. [CrossRef] [PubMed]
39. Velazquez-Perez, L.; Tunnerhoff, J.; Rodriguez-Labrada, R.; Torres-Vega, R.; Belardinelli, P.; Medrano-Montero, J.; Pena-Acosta, A.; Canales-Ochoa, N.; Vazquez-Mojena, Y.; Gonzalez-Zaldivar, Y.; et al. Corticomuscular coherence: A novel tool to assess the pyramidal tract dysfunction in spinocerebellar ataxia type 2. *Cerebellum* **2017**, *16*, 602–606. [CrossRef] [PubMed]

40. Rodriguez-Labrada, R.; Vazquez-Mojena, Y.; Canales-Ochoa, N.; Medrano-Montero, J.; Velazquez-Perez, L. Heritability of saccadic eye movements in spinocerebellar ataxia type 2: Insights into an endophenotype marker. *Cerebellum Ataxias* **2017**, *4*, 19. [CrossRef] [PubMed]
41. Rodriguez-Labrada, R.; Velazquez-Perez, L.; Aguilera-Rodriguez, R.; Seifried-Oberschmidt, C.; Pena-Acosta, A.; Canales-Ochoa, N.; Medrano-Montero, J.; Estupinan-Rodriguez, A.; Vazquez-Mojena, Y.; Gonzalez-Zaldivar, Y.; et al. Executive deficit in spinocerebellar ataxia type 2 is related to expanded cag repeats: Evidence from antisaccadic eye movements. *Brain Cogn.* **2014**, *91*, 28–34. [CrossRef] [PubMed]
42. Rodriguez-Labrada, R.; Velazquez-Perez, L.; Auburger, G.; Ziemann, U.; Canales-Ochoa, N.; Medrano-Montero, J.; Vazquez-Mojena, Y.; Gonzalez-Zaldivar, Y. Spinocerebellar ataxia type 2: Measures of saccade changes improve power for clinical trials. *Mov. Disord. Off. J. Mov. Disord. Soc.* **2016**, *31*, 570–578. [CrossRef] [PubMed]
43. Almaguer-Gotay, D.; Almaguer-Mederos, L.E.; Aguilera-Rodriguez, R.; Rodriguez-Labrada, R.; Cuello-Almarales, D.; Estupinan-Dominguez, A.; Velazquez-Perez, L.C.; Gonzalez-Zaldivar, Y.; Vazquez-Mojena, Y. Spinocerebellar ataxia type 2 is associated with the extracellular loss of superoxide dismutase but not catalase activity. *Front. Neurol.* **2017**, *8*, 276. [CrossRef] [PubMed]
44. Almaguer-Mederos, L.E.; Almaguer-Gotay, D.; Aguilera-Rodriguez, R.; Gonzalez-Zaldivar, Y.; Cuello-Almarales, D.; Laffita-Mesa, J.; Vazquez-Mojena, Y.; Zayas-Feria, P.; Rodriguez-Labrada, R.; Velazquez-Perez, L.; et al. Association of glutathione S-transferase omega polymorphism and spinocerebellar ataxia type 2. *J. Neurol. Sci.* **2017**, *372*, 324–328. [CrossRef] [PubMed]
45. Pedroso, I.; Bringas, M.L.; Aguiar, A.; Morales, L.; Alvarez, M.; Valdes, P.A.; Alvarez, L. Use of cuban recombinant human erythropoietin in parkinson's disease treatment. *MEDICC Rev.* **2012**, *14*, 11–17. [PubMed]
46. Santos-Morales, O.; Diaz-Machado, A.; Jimenez-Rodriguez, D.; Pomares-Iturralde, Y.; Festary-Casanovas, T.; Gonzalez-Delgado, C.A.; Perez-Rodriguez, S.; Alfonso-Munoz, E.; Viada-Gonzalez, C.; Piedra-Sierra, P.; et al. Nasal administration of the neuroprotective candidate neuroepo to healthy volunteers: A randomized, parallel, open-label safety study. *BMC Neurol.* **2017**, *17*, 129. [CrossRef] [PubMed]
47. Blasco, H.; Mavel, S.; Corcia, P.; Gordon, P.H. The glutamate hypothesis in als: Pathophysiology and drug development. *Curr. Med. Chem.* **2014**, *21*, 3551–3575. [CrossRef] [PubMed]
48. Hansel, G.; Ramos, D.B.; Delgado, C.A.; Souza, D.G.; Almeida, R.F.; Portela, L.V.; Quincozes-Santos, A.; Souza, D.O. The potential therapeutic effect of guanosine after cortical focal ischemia in rats. *PLoS ONE* **2014**, *9*, e90693. [CrossRef] [PubMed]
49. Quincozes-Santos, A.; Bobermin, L.D.; Tramontina, A.C.; Wartchow, K.M.; Tagliari, B.; Souza, D.O.; Wyse, A.T.; Goncalves, C.A. Oxidative stress mediated by NMDA, AMPA/KA channels in acute hippocampal slices: Neuroprotective effect of resveratrol. *Toxicol. In Vitro* **2014**, *28*, 544–551. [CrossRef] [PubMed]
50. Nunez-Figueredo, Y.; Pardo Andreu, G.L.; Oliveira Loureiro, S.; Ganzella, M.; Ramirez-Sanchez, J.; Ochoa-Rodriguez, E.; Verdecia-Reyes, Y.; Delgado-Hernandez, R.; Souza, D.O. The effects of JM-20 on the glutamatergic system in synaptic vesicles, synaptosomes and neural cells cultured from rat brain. *Neurochem. Int.* **2015**, *81*, 41–47. [CrossRef] [PubMed]
51. Ramirez-Sanchez, J.; Simoes Pires, E.N.; Nunez-Figueredo, Y.; Pardo-Andreu, G.L.; Fonseca-Fonseca, L.A.; Ruiz-Reyes, A.; Ochoa-Rodriguez, E.; Verdecia-Reyes, Y.; Delgado-Hernandez, R.; Souza, D.O.; et al. Neuroprotection by JM-20 against oxygen-glucose deprivation in rat hippocampal slices: Involvement of the AKT/GSK-3beta pathway. *Neurochem. Int.* **2015**, *90*, 215–223. [CrossRef] [PubMed]
52. Gomez, L.; Vidal, B.; Maragoto, C.; Morales, L.M.; Berrillo, S.; Vera Cuesta, H.; Baez, M.; Denis, M.; Marin, T.; Cabrera, Y.; et al. Non-invasive brain stimulation for children with autism spectrum disorders: A short-term outcome study. *Behav. Sci.* **2017**, *7*, 63. [CrossRef] [PubMed]

3

Oligodendrocyte Injury and Pathogenesis of HIV-1-Associated Neurocognitive Disorders

Han Liu, Enquan Xu, Jianuo Liu and Huangui Xiong *

Department of Pharmacology and Experimental Neuroscience, University of Nebraska Medical Center, Omaha, NE 68198-5880, USA; han.liu@unmc.edu (H.L.); enquan.xu@unmc.edu (E.X.); jnliu@unmc.edu (J.L.)

* Correspondence: hxiong@unmc.edu

Academic Editor: Donna Gruol

Abstract: Oligodendrocytes wrap neuronal axons to form myelin, an insulating sheath which is essential for nervous impulse conduction along axons. Axonal myelination is highly regulated by neuronal and astrocytic signals and the maintenance of myelin sheaths is a very complex process. Oligodendrocyte damage can cause axonal demyelination and neuronal injury, leading to neurological disorders. Demyelination in the cerebrum may produce cognitive impairment in a variety of neurological disorders, including human immunodeficiency virus type one (HIV-1)-associated neurocognitive disorders (HAND). Although the combined antiretroviral therapy has markedly reduced the incidence of HIV-1-associated dementia, a severe form of HAND, milder forms of HAND remain prevalent even when the peripheral viral load is well controlled. HAND manifests as a subcortical dementia with damage in the brain white matter (e.g., corpus callosum), which consists of myelinated axonal fibers. How HIV-1 brain infection causes myelin injury and resultant white matter damage is an interesting area of current HIV research. In this review, we tentatively address recent progress on oligodendrocyte dysregulation and HAND pathogenesis.

Keywords: HIV-1; dementia; oligodendrocyte; myelin sheath

1. Introduction

With the introduction of combined antiretroviral therapy (cART), there was a significant decline in human immunodeficiency virus type one (HIV-1)-associated neurocognitive disorders (HAND). As HIV-1-infected patients live a longer lifespan with a cART regimen, it is becoming increasingly evident that the prevalence of milder forms of HAND seems to be on the rise [1–3]. Many studies have revealed a preferential damage to subcortical white matter (e.g., corpus callosum) in the HIV-1-infected brain, and such damage is prevalent even in the era of cART and more severe in patients with HAND [4,5]. HIV-1-related white matter damage includes demyelination and axonal dysfunction and injury. The demyelination occurs when myelin sheaths of neuronal axons are impaired in the central nervous system (CNS) or peripheral nervous system (PNS). Myelination, formation of myelin sheaths by oligodendrocytes wrapping neuronal axons in the CNS or Schwann cells in the PNS, is highly regulated by neuronal and astrocytic signals and maintenance of myelin sheaths is a complex process. The oligodendrocyte injury is a hallmark in demyelination and white matter damage. Such damage can be induced by an alteration of genetics, viral infections, inflammation, autoimmunity, and other unknown factors. HIV-1-associated oligodendrocyte/myelin damage has been observed both in cell culture [6] and patients [7].

The earlier studies demonstrate that human polyomavirus JC (JCV) primarily causes demyelination in HIV-1-infected brain. Compared to HIV-1 infection of astrocytes and microglia in the brain, JCV predominately infects oligodendrocytes and, thus, causes oligodendrocyte damage and further demyelination. Additionally, JCV is also the main causative factor for progressive multifocal leukoencephalopathy (PML), a frequent opportunistic infection in the CNS and a common complication seen in AIDS patients [7,8]. Recent studies have shown that HIV-1 viral proteins per se can act on oligodendrocytes and produce detrimental effects, which are independent of JCV [6,9,10]. HIV-1 viral proteins, including the envelope glycoprotein 120 (gp120), trans-activator of transcription (Tat), and negative regulatory factor (Nef), have been implicated in HIV-1-associated oligodendrocyte injury [9,11–14]. Among these viral proteins, Tat has consistently been detected in both infected and uninfected oligodendrocytes in the brains of AIDS patients [7], and exhibited a synergistic detrimental effect with JCV or with addictive drugs, such as morphine. In this review, we tentatively address recent progress in HIV-1-associated oligodendrocyte pathophysiology, aiming at understanding the pathogenesis of milder forms of HAND.

2. Myelin/Oligodendrocyte Injury in HIV-1 Patients

The oligodendrocyte and myelin injury have been observed clinically from neurological imaging studies, serum biochemistry, and brain biopsies [15–18]. The diffusion tensor magnetic resonance imaging (DTI) promotes the investigations of white matter damage in early HAND and allows revealing the microstructures of myelin and oligodendrocytes. The changes of water molecules' diffusive parameters in brain white matter of HIV-1 patients, which indicate demyelination, have been detected in several DTI studies [15,19,20]. These findings were supported by a recent study on HIV-1-infected humanized mice that a decreased expression of myelin structural proteins was observed in whisker barrels, the corpus callosum, and the hippocampus, suggesting the loss of myelin elements [21]. In the sera and CSF of patients with HAND, antibody titers of myelin oligodendrocyte glycoprotein (MOG), an important myelin structural protein indicating CNS-specific autoimmune reaction for primary demyelination, are significantly higher compared with asymptomatic HAND patients and HIV-1-negative patients with other neurological diseases. In particular, the CSF anti-MOG antibodies exhibit a high sensitivity and specificity (85.7% and 76.2%) for discriminating patients with active HAND from those with asymptomatic HAND. The performance on HIV dementia scale tests is significantly worse and the viral loads in the CSF are higher in MOG immunopositive HAND patients than those in asymptomatic HAND patients [22], suggesting the dysfunction of oligodendrocytes is closely related with HIV-1 infection and HAND.

Compared to astrocytes that appear to promote recovery in response of injury, oligodendrocytes have a more passive role and tend to be damaged as a general response to insults [23]. In biopsy studies, the absolute number of nerve fibers and axons significantly decreased in HIV-1-infected brain, in particular in the frontal and occipital parts of the corpus callosum. The myelin sheath thickness diminished in corpus callosum as well [18]. Weighted gene co-expression network analysis showed that the oligodendrocyte-related genes are particularly elevated in the HIV encephalitis (HIVE) group, suggesting specific dysfunction of this cell type in those with HIVE [24].

In HIV-1 positive patients with PML, the myelin loss is apparent both macroscopically and microscopically [25]. Neuroimaging studies showed the myelin lesions were more frequently seen in the sub-cortical white matter areas [26]. PML is believed to be developed exclusively in immunosuppressive patients with significantly higher incidence in patients with AIDS, particularly in AIDS patients without cART and with a low $CD4^+$ lymphocyte count, than in patients with any other immunosuppressive conditions. Although cART has decreased the incidence of PML and improved patient survival [27], PML continues to occur in HIV-1-positive patients with good access to cART, and even with normal $CD4^+$ lymphocyte counts [28,29]. These findings suggest PML-related oligodendrocyte/myelin damage is often, but not necessarily, associated with severe immunosuppression or an immune reconstitution inflammatory syndrome (IRIS) in the cART era [30].

3. Fate of Oligodendrocytes in HIV-1-Infected Brain

Early publications reported that HIV-1 cannot be detected in oligodendrocytes [31,32] and this may due to the limitation of methodologies to identify oligodendrocytes. Dissenting results were found in purified human oligodendrocytes from temporal lobe resections, HIV-1 (IIIB and BaL) infectivity was confirmed by detection of p24gag antigen and PCR amplification [33]. It is well-known that HIV-1 attaches and infects human host cells through CD4 receptors, along with CXCR4 and CCR5 as co-receptors. The oligodendrocytes are CD4- and CCR5-negative, but do express CXCR4 [31,34,35], which designedly promote the oligodendrocyte progenitor cell (OPC) migration and remyelination [36], and may provide the anchor for HIV-1-induced oligodendrocyte injury. However, most investigators agree that HIV-1 primarily infects microglial cells in the brain, but not oligodendrocytes. HIV-1-associated oligodendrocyte injury is believed to be mediated through viral proteins shed off from virions or released from infected other cells [9,11,12].

In HIV-1 patients with PML complication, Tat and JCV both are present in oligodendrocytes. Tat has been shown to synergize with JCV, and facilitate of JCV gene transcription and replication, leading to robust JCV infection [37,38]. Tat stimulates JCV gene transcription by cooperating with SMAD proteins, the intracellular effectors of TGF-beta, at the JCV DNA control region [37]. The effectiveness of Tat on facilitating JCV transcription and replication varies from different HIV-1 clades [38]. Since Tat is expressed in the brain at relative high levels while the viral load is controlled in blood, this may, at least in part, explain why some HIV-1 patients still develop PML despite having a good access to cART [39]. In addition to the synergistic effect of Tat and JCV in oligodendrocytes, cytotoxic $CD8^+$ T cells aggregate at demyelinated lesion sites in the brain to engage JCV-infected oligodendrocytes, which tend to control JCV dissemination, but at the cost of oligodendrocyte death and further demyelination in PML [40].

In addition to Tat, gp120 seems to be also involved in HIV-1-associated oligodendrocytes/myelin injury. It has been shown that gp120 inhibits myelination in rat cerebral cortex culture [12] and induces functional dysregulation and apoptosis in cultured oligodendrocytes [11,41], which is discussed in a subsequent section. In addition to the primary oligodendrocyte injury, which leads to secondary axonal injury (outside-in) to further exacerbate neurocognitive impairments, oligodendrocyte injury can be caused by primary axonopathy as well (inside-out) [42]. The recent study has shown that gp120-induced β-APP accumulation and axon injury in the corpus callosum was attenuated by a CXCR4 antagonist, exampling HIV-1 injury of oligodendrocyte/myelin via CXCR4 [35]. Although it is not clear whether gp120 causes such a detrimental effect through an "outside-in" or "inside-out" mechanism, or both, CXCR4 expressed in oligodendrocytes can be a potential target [42].

4. Association between Blood-Brain Barrier (BBB) Disruption and Myelin Injury

Increasing evidence indicates that myelin injury may be associated with a dysregulated blood-brain barrier (BBB) since myelin pallor is often observed in perivascular sectors during white matter edema [43,44]. The BBB is a critically-protective barrier for the brain and serves as a highly selective layer that separates the CNS from the rest of the body. In HIV-1-infected brains, the BBB disruption is believed to be mediated by both viral and cellular factors, released from HIV-1-infected and immune-activated mononuclear phagocytes and endothelial cells [45,46]. The reported direct mechanisms underlying HIV-1-associated BBB disruption are often related to alterations of vascular tight junctions, direct toxicity of brain endothelial cells, production of matrix metalloproteinases, and N-Methyl-D-Aspartate (NMDA) receptor activation [47,48]. The disruption of BBB is essential for HIV-1 entrance to the brain, resulting in brain white matter damage and consequent neurologic deficits in patients with neuroHIV. This notion is supported by an observation that HIV-1 patients with impaired BBB showed poorer neurologic status than those with intact BBB [49]. However, myelin damage may also be related to BBB disruption without HIV-1 brain invasion. In a case report, diffuse myelin pallor in white matter and massive perivascular dilatation were observed in an AIDS patient without evidence of brain HIV-1 infection, significant inflammation, or microglial activation [50]. Postmortem studies on the brains of AIDS patients revealed discrete myelin pallor areas always associated with capillaries or venules [44]. These findings suggest that BBB breakdown may contribute to the observed oligodendrocyte/myelin/white matter injury.

Under physiological conditions, the BBB endothelial cells and components of the extracellular matrix support OPC survival, and promote neural progenitor cells (NPC) differentiate to neurons, astrocytes, and oligodendrocytes [51–53]. The critical function of BBB and the consequences of BBB disruption imply its involvement in HIV-1-associated oligodendrocyte/myelin injury. It is not surprising that the disrupted BBB promotes the entrance of viruses, infected T cells, and toxic substances from the blood to the brain, resulting in OPC/oligodendrocyte/myelin injury. Inhibition of OPC proliferation can be caused by plasma, serum, thrombin, and plasmin in primary culture. Thrombin also suppresses the differentiation of OPCs into mature oligodendrocytes [54]. In addition, elevated levels of TNF-α, an inflammatory cytokine promoting oligodendrocyte death [55], were detected in blood mononuclear phagocytes in HIV-infected patients [56]. HIV-1 infection also induces interleukin (IL)-1β production from mononuclear phagocytes [57]. IL-1β promotes oligodendrocyte death through glutamate excitotoxicity [58]. These findings suggest that BBB disruption contributes to HIV-1-associated myelin/oligodendrocyte damage.

5. Cellular Mechanisms for Oligodendrocyte Injury in HIV-1-Infected Brain

Apoptotic signal activation of oligodendrocytes has been observed in HAND patients [59]. Such an apoptotic activation of oligodendrocytes could be caused directly by HIV-1 viral proteins or induced indirectly by immune and inflammatory factors.

It is well-known that tumor suppressor p53 induces apoptosis by activating transcription of various pro-apoptotic genes [60]. Activation of p53 was detected in the oligodendrocyte lineage cells in the brains of HAND patients, but not in control brains [59]. Due to the difficulties in distinguishing the differentiating stages of oligodendrocyte lineage on autopsy samples, the detected p53 reactivity reflects apoptosis of mature oligodendrocytes and OPCs. These suggest that, in addition to oligodendrocyte injury, proliferation of OPCs is also impaired in HAND.

Gp120 was shown to cause slow but progressive oligodendrocyte cytosolic Ca^{2+} rise in a mixed culture of cerebellar cortex cells [41] and the rise of introcellular Ca^{2+} concentration may trigger oligodendrocytic apoptosis. Exposure of oligodendrocytes to Tat also produced a rapid increase in intracellular Ca^{2+} levels through NMDA and α-amino-3-hydroxy-5-methyl-4-isoxazolepropionic acid (AMPA) receptors, causing oligodendrocyte injury. It is worth mentioning that the roles of NMDA and AMPA receptors appear to be different and dependent on the stage of OPC differentiation. Tat-induced OPC death can be blocked by either NMDA or AMPA receptor antagonists. However, Tat's detrimental effects on mature oligodendrocytes can only be reversed by NMDA receptor antagonists, but not AMPA receptor blockade [6]. Tat was also found to cause oligodendrocyte apoptosis *in vitro* and myelin injury *ex vivo* by enhancing voltage-dependent K^+ channel (Kv) 1.3 activity [61]. The loss of K^+ ions may cause cell regulatory volume decrease (shrinkage), leading to cell apoptosis [62]. The involvement of Tat in oligodendrocyte apoptosis has been demonstrated in an HIV-1 Tat transgenic mouse model. The oligodendrocytes within the striatum exhibit a high sensitivity to morphine in HIV-1 Tat transgenic mice and they are the only apoptotic cell type in response to combined morphine exposure and Tat induction in Tat transgenic mice [9]. Tat also interacts with morphine to decrease the proliferation of OPCs [63]. Opioid abuse produces synergistic toxic activity in HIV-1-infected brains by direct actions on immature astrocytes and oligodendrocytes, which express μ-opioid or κ-opioid receptors [64].

In other viral-induced demyelination, there is clear evidence that mouse hepatitis virus (MHV) can directly infect and activate microglia during acute inflammation, which eventually causes phagocytosis of the myelin sheath, leading to demyelination during the chronic inflammation stage [65]. A similar theory has been proposed for multiple sclerosis, which is the most prevalent demyelinating disease, that immune-activated microglia strip the myelin. Recent evidence has shown that microglia become phagocytic in response to HIV-1 Tat [66,67]. It might be possible that the infected and activated microglia phagocyte oligodendrocytes and myelin sheath lead to the myelin damage and consequent HAND pathogenesis, although there is no direct evidence indicating microglia phagocytosis of oligodendrocyte in neuroHIV [68].

6. Myelin Maintenance and Remyelination in HIV-1-Infected Brain

Repair of the damaged myelin sheath, which is termed remyelination, is physiologically required to maintain myelin homeostasis. The myelin injury in neuroHIV may also be induced by abnormalities of remyelination, in addition to the loss of existing myelin sheath. Remyelination requires proliferation and survival of OPCs, migration of OPCs to the damaged site, and development of OPCs from immature to mature myelinating oligodendrocytes. HIV-1 disrupts OPC development, migration, and remyelination processes.

6.1. Alteration of OPC Proliferation and Differentiation in HIV-1-Infected Brains

In HIV-1-infected brains, mild degrees of myelin damage were associated with an increase in oligodendrocyte numbers, an initial reactive hyperplasia which was believed to represent an attempt to repair myelin damage. Such a change was reversed in the presence of severe myelin damage [69]. In agreement with the aforementioned results, mRNA levels of transcription factor Olig2, a marker expressed with higher levels in OPCs and lower levels in mature oligodendrocytes [70], are elevated in the front cortex of patients with HIVE [24], indicating an increase of OPC proliferation needed for repairing the damaged myelin sheath. Mature oligodendrocyte defects are also observed in animal models of secondary degeneration, which represents additional loss of neurons, myelin, and glial cells through toxic events. Early onset of secondary degeneration triggers OPC proliferation, but the cell numbers decrease in a long-term degenerative condition [71]. However, Tat exposure reduces the population of undifferentiated $Sox2^+$ NPC (ancestor of OPC) and $Olig2^+$ OPCs, but progenitor survival is unaffected [63], suggesting the proliferation was interrupted. Tat may inhibit NPC proliferation by downregulating cyclin D1, which is an important cell cycle component interacts with cyclin-dependent kinase 4 and 6 [72]. Over all, HIV-1 infection or viral protein exposure appears to incline NPC fate toward production of glia/astroglia at the expense of neurons and/or oligodendrocytes [63,73,74]. Thus, OPC differentiation and maturation are likely the key processes affected during remyelination in neuroHIV.

6.2. Imbalance of OPC Differentiation and Remyelination in HIV-1-Infected Brain

It has been shown that differentiation of OPCs into post-mitotic oligodendrocytes is a major checkpoint in the myelination process and such an oligodendrocyte differentiation is controlled by a number of factors, many of which act to inhibit myelination, including leucine-rich repeat and immunoglobulin domain-containing-1 (LINGO-1) [75,76], Notch-1 [77,78], and Wnt [79,80], whereas p38 MAPK [81,82] and AKT [83] have been shown to be required for oligodendrocyte differentiation and myelination. While molecular mechanisms in the regulation of developmental myelination are discussed in excellent review papers published elsewhere [84,85], the direct interaction between HIV-1 and these molecules remains largely unknown. It is, however, believed that HIV-1 may disturb the complex regulating network leading to the remyelination imbalance based on the following findings: (1) HIV-1 alters the cell cycle by Wnt signaling pathways and further impacts the cell proliferation and differentiation in different cell types, including peripheral blood mononuclear cells [86], HEK293 cells [87], and astrocytes [88]; (2) HIV-1 infection of astrocytes altered the astrocytic Wnt profile by elevating Wnt family members 2b and 10b [88]; (3) elevation of secreted Wnt from astrocytes may negatively regulate oligodendrocyte differentiation in neuroHIV; (4) Notch-1 signaling is permissive for OPC expansion, but inhibit differentiation and myelin formation [89]; and (5) in Kaposi's sarcoma cells, which is a neoplasm in HIV-1-infected individuals, overexpression of activated Notch-1 signaling is detected [90]. However, to our knowledge, there is no report yet on how OPC/oligodendrocyte Notch-1 signaling in responding to HIV-1. Moreover, CD44, a predominant hyaluronan receptor widely expressed in the nervous system, plays a negative role in OPC differentiation and myelination. Overexpression of CD44 in precursor cells inhibits differentiation toward oligodendrocytes and promotes differentiation into astrocytes, cause progressive demyelination in conditional transgenic mouse model [91,92]. In lymphocyte cell lines of Jurkat and U937 cells, HIV-1 infection-caused particle production is accompanied by CD44 upregulation [93]. In HIV-1-related diffuse large B-cell lymphoma patients, the CD44 levels significantly increased compared with HIV-1-unrelated diffuse large B-cell lymphoma patients (87% vs. 56%) [94]. These findings suggest CD44 may play a role in HIV-1-related remyelination failure.

Neurotrophins are important factors in the regulation of oligodendrocyte myelination and remyelination. The main cellular sources for neurotrophins in the brain are astrocytes, microglial cells, and neurons, in addition to lymphocytes' contribution through the blood circulation. Being aware of excellent reviews on the alteration of neurotrophins in HAND [95] and immunological communications between oligodendrocytes and microglia [96], we focus here on the HIV-1-induced alterations of neurotrophins that are potentially associated with oligodendrocyte abnormalities.

The platelet-derived growth factor (PDGF) is the most predominant mitogen for oligodendrocyte lineage cells. PDGF A and B chains both promote proliferation through activating PDGF receptor alpha (PDGFRα) expressed on OPCs, whereas the PDGF B chain appears to be more important for early NPC expansion [97,98]. It has been shown that PDGF regulates OPC development via glycogen synthase kinase-3β (GSK-3β) signaling pathway, which is a negative regulator of OPC differentiation and remyelination [99,100]. PDGF-BB prevents NPC from Tat-mediated proliferating impairment by inactivating GSK-3β / β-catenin pathways and, this effect is significantly inhibited by the p38 and JNK inhibitors [101]. The levels of fibroblast growth factor (FGF), which is an important pro-survival signal to stimulate OPC proliferation [102], increased in the sera of HIV-1-infected patients [103,104], but decreased in CSF [103]. FGF signaling complex is interrupted in HIV-1-infected brains, resulting in the abnormal activation of downstream signals, including GSK-3β [105,106], p38, ERK, and JNK cascades [107] in neurons through the surface receptors, such as NMDA receptor and CXCR4, which are also expressed on oligodendrocytes [36,108,109]. In addition, HIV-1 Tat and FGF-2 share a common core mechanism of unconventional secretion [110], although it is not clear whether they compete for the secretory routine. The brain-derived neurotrophic factor (BDNF), predominantly derived from astrocytes, has also been found to be essential for oligodendrocyte lineage development [68,111–113]. In rat primary neurons, gp120 promotes a time-dependent proBDNF accumulation at both intracellular and extracellular spaces by decreasing the expression level of intracellular furin, an enzyme required for cleavage and release of mature BDNF, leading to a reduction in mature BDNF. A similar imbalance in the ratio of proBDNF/mature BDNF was confirmed in postmortem brains of HAND patients [114]. These findings suggest that HIV-1 decreases the brain BDNF level by infecting astrocytes and gp120-associated neurotoxicity, resulting in downregulated remyelination. As BDNF is believed to protect neurons from HIV-1-induced apoptosis, thus, the reduction of BDNF may make the oligodendrocyte lose the support from neuronal axons that consequently cause myelin damage through the "inside-out" mechanism as proposed [42].

In addition to these signaling molecules, HIV-1 Tat interacting protein (TIP30), a co-factor that specifically enhances HIV-1 Tat-activated transcription [115], negatively regulates oligodendrocyte development. Overexpression of TIP30 dramatically inhibits the OPC differentiation, while knockdown of TIP30 enhances the differentiation of OPC remarkably [116]. The blockade of TIP30 may have dual benefits on inhibiting Tat-dependent gene transcription and promoting OPC differentiation, which is a potential therapeutic strategy for HIV-associated demyelination. Potassium channels are also involved in regulation of OPC development. Kv1.3 [117,118], Kv1.6 [117], Kv2.1 [119], and inward-rectified K^+ channel 4.1 [120,121] play crucial roles in regulation of OPC/oligodendrocyte proliferation and differentiation. Generally, channel expressions on oligodendrocyte lineage cells correlate with differentiating stages and are more complex in OPCs than in oligodendrocytes. Particularly, Kv1.3 channel plays an important role in G1/S transition in proliferating OPCs through regulating AKT signaling [118,122]. Moreover, L-type voltage-operated Ca^{2+} channel 1.2 knockdown induces a decrease in the proportion of oligodendrocytes expressing myelin proteins, and an increase in the population of immature oligodendrocyte [123].

Most recent studies proposed that myelin injury in HAND is partially due to the effects of antiretroviral drugs on oligodendrocyte survival and differentiation. The common prescribed antiretroviral drugs, ritonavir and lopinavir, impair both the differentiation of OPCs into myelin-producing oligodendrocytes and the maintenance of myelin proteins *in vivo*. Ritonavir induces accumulation of reactive oxygen species, which arrest the oligodendrocyte differentiation process [124,125]. Controversial results were reported in HIV-1-infected children in Africa that significant myelin loss in cART-naïve children was observed in comparison with cART-treated children. However, cART-treated children also exhibited a significant myelin loss in the corpus callosum [126]. Interestingly, myelin-related genes encoding myelin-associated oligodendrocyte basic protein, myelin transcription factor 1, and myelin basic protein are downregulated in both cART-treated and untreated HAND patients [127]. Apparently, the impact of antiretroviral drugs on oligodendrocyte pathophysiology requires further investigation.

7. Summary and Prospects

HIV-1 persists in the brain despite cART. The cART-treated subjects are not able to purge the virus from their brains and show concomitant and persistent white matter abnormalities. There are increasing interests in understanding how HIV-1 causes myelin sheath loss and white matter damage in HIV-1-infected brains. In this article, we try to address the clinical and postmortem manifestations of myelin damage in HAND patients and possible involvement of BBB integrity disruption, oligodendrocyte apoptosis mechanisms, and OPC regulation imbalance in HIV-1-induced oligodendrocyte/myelin abnormalities. The studies on direct toxicity of HIV-1 viral proteins on oligodendrocytes and OPCs are emerging. As the transcription of HIV-1 viral protein continues in the CNS, even when the viral load is at a low level [128], the persistence of the virus and viral proteins in the brain has changed the pattern of HAND pathogenesis, by which inflammation, encephalitis, and neurodegeneration have been significantly decreased by the advent of cART.

The methods of regulation of oligodendrocyte lineage cell development are well-established, including the extracellular pathways, cell to cell contact, and intracellular pathways. As $NG2^+$ cells are the largest population of progenitor cells in the human adult brain, a decrease of absolute cell number and proliferation of NPC and OPC may contribute less to myelin deficits in HAND. In contrast, HIV-1-related OPC differentiation and remyelination imbalance may better correlate with an impaired remyelination in HAND patients. The strategies for promoting axonal remyelination have been introduced especially in those demyelinating disease like multiple sclerosis. It is anticipated that those strategies for promoting axonal remyelination in other neurodegenerative disorders can be applied for HIV-1-associated oligodendrocyte/myelin injury, though studies are needed to elucidate the underlying mechanisms for HIV-1-associated brain white matter damage.

Further studies on understanding the mechanisms underlying HIV-1-associated oligodendrocyte/myelin injury may be hampered by the following potential difficulties: first, oligodendrocytes share many common extracellular signals and intracellular signaling pathways with neurons, the proposed "inside-out" and "outside-in" mechanisms for virus-induced demyelination are indistinguishable under these conditions [42]; and, second, the pro-proliferation signals for OPC are sometimes anti-maturative [129–131]. This will be a significant challenge to identify the certain time window to access proper remyelination in vivo. Overall, promoting remyelination could be an important therapeutic strategy for HAND and other neurodegenerative disorders in the future.

Acknowledgments: This work was supported by NIH grant R01 NS077873.

Author Contributions: H.L. and X.H. did literature research and wrote the paper, E.X. and J.L. participated in literature research and contributed to discussion in Sections 6 and 7.

References

1. Antinori, A.; Arendt, G.; Becker, J.T.; Brew, B.J.; Byrd, D.A.; Cherner, M.; Clifford, D.B.; Cinque, P.; Epstein, L.G.; Goodkin, K.; et al. Updated research nosology for HIV-associated neurocognitive disorders. *Neurology* **2007**, *69*, 1789–1799. [CrossRef] [PubMed]
2. Heaton, R.K.; Franklin, D.R.; Ellis, R.J.; McCutchan, J.A.; Letendre, S.L.; LeBlanc, S.; Corkran, S.H.; Duarte, N.A.; Clifford, D.B.; Woods, S.P. HIV-associated neurocognitive disorders before and during the era of combination antiretroviral therapy: Differences in rates, nature, and predictors. *J. Neurovirol.* **2011**, *17*, 3–16. [CrossRef] [PubMed]
3. Tozzi, V.; Balestra, P.; Bellagamba, R.; Corpolongo, A.; Salvatori, M.F.; Visco-Comandini, U.; Vlassi, C.; Giulianelli, M.; Galgani, S.; Antinori, A.; et al. Persistence of neuropsychologic deficits despite long-term highly active antiretroviral therapy in patients with HIV-related neurocognitive impairment: Prevalence and risk factors. *J. Acquir. Immune Defic. Syndr.* **2007**, *45*, 174–182. [CrossRef] [PubMed]
4. Chen, Y.; An, H.; Zhu, H.; Stone, T.; Smith, J.K.; Hall, C.; Bullitt, E.; Shen, D.; Lin, W. White matter abnormalities revealed by diffusion tensor imaging in non-demented and demented HIV+ patients. *Neuroimage* **2009**, *47*, 1154–1162. [CrossRef] [PubMed]
5. Gosztonyi, G.; Artigas, J.; Lamperth, L.; Webster, H.D. Human immunodeficiency virus (HIV) distribution in HIV encephalitis: Study of 19 cases with combined use of in situ hybridization and immunocytochemistry. *J. Neuropathol. Exp. Neurol.* **1994**, *53*, 521–534. [CrossRef] [PubMed]
6. Zou, S.; Fuss, B.; Fitting, S.; Hahn, Y.K.; Hauser, K.F.; Knapp, P.E. Oligodendrocytes are targets of HIV-1 tat: Nmda and ampa receptor-mediated effects on survival and development. *J. Neurosci.* **2015**, *35*, 11384–11398. [CrossRef] [PubMed]
7. Del Valle, L.; Croul, S.; Morgello, S.; Amini, S.; Rappaport, J.; Khalili, K. Detection of HIV-1 tat and JCV capsid protein, VP1, in AIDS brain with progressive multifocal leukoencephalopathy. *J. Neurovirol.* **2000**, *6*, 221–228. [CrossRef] [PubMed]
8. Bellizzi, A.; Nardis, C.; Anzivino, E.; Rodio, D.; Fioriti, D.; Mischitelli, M.; Chiarini, F.; Pietropaolo, V. Human polyomavirus JC reactivation and pathogenetic mechanisms of progressive multifocal leukoencephalopathy and cancer in the era of monoclonal antibody therapies. *J. Neurovirol.* **2012**, *18*, 1–11. [CrossRef] [PubMed]
9. Hauser, K.F.; Hahn, Y.K.; Adjan, V.V.; Zou, S.; Buch, S.K.; Nath, A.; Bruce-Keller, A.J.; Knapp, P.E. HIV-1 tat and morphine have interactive effects on oligodendrocyte survival and morphology. *Glia* **2009**, *57*, 194–206. [CrossRef] [PubMed]
10. Li, R.; Mi, H.; Zhao, J.; Yuan, D.; Ding, J.; Li, H. White matter damage and effects of nadir CD4+ count on patients with asymptomatic HIV associated dementia complex–A DTI study. *Radiol. Infect. Dis.* **2014**, *1*, 11–16. [CrossRef]
11. Bernardo, A.; Agresti, C.; Levi, G. HIV-gp120 affects the functional activity of oligodendrocytes and their susceptibility to complement. *J. Neurosci. Res.* **1997**, *50*, 946–957. [CrossRef]
12. Kimura-Kuroda, J.; Nagashima, K.; Yasui, K. Inhibition of myelin formation by HIV-1 gp120 in rat cerebral cortex culture. *Arch. Virol.* **1994**, *137*, 81–99. [CrossRef] [PubMed]
13. Nukuzuma, S.; Kameoka, M.; Sugiura, S.; Nakamichi, K.; Nukuzuma, C.; Miyoshi, I.; Takegami, T. Exogenous human immunodeficiency virus-1 protein, tat, enhances replication of JC virus efficiently in neuroblastoma cell lines. *J. Med. Virol.* **2012**, *84*, 555–561. [CrossRef] [PubMed]
14. Radja, F.; Kay, D.G.; Albrecht, S.; Jolicoeur, P. Oligodendrocyte-specific expression of human immunodeficiency virus type 1 NEF in transgenic mice leads to vacuolar myelopathy and alters oligodendrocyte phenotype in vitro. *J. Virol.* **2003**, *77*, 11745–11753. [CrossRef] [PubMed]
15. Correa, D.G.; Zimmermann, N.; Doring, T.M.; Wilner, N.V.; Leite, S.C.; Cabral, R.F.; Fonseca, R.P.; Bahia, P.R.; Gasparetto, E.L. Diffusion tensor mr imaging of white matter integrity in HIV-positive patients with planning deficit. *Neuroradiology* **2015**, *57*, 475–482. [CrossRef] [PubMed]
16. Gongvatana, A.; Schweinsburg, B.C.; Taylor, M.J.; Theilmann, R.J.; Letendre, S.L.; Alhassoon, O.M.; Jacobus, J.; Woods, S.P.; Jernigan, T.L.; Ellis, R.J.; et al. White matter tract injury and cognitive impairment in human immunodeficiency virus-infected individuals. *J. Neurovirol.* **2009**, *15*, 187–195. [CrossRef] [PubMed]
17. Uban, K.A.; Herting, M.M.; Williams, P.L.; Ajmera, T.; Gautam, P.; Huo, Y.; Malee, K.M.; Yogev, R.; Csernansky, J.G.; Wang, L.; et al. White matter microstructure among youth with perinatally acquired HIV is associated with disease severity. *AIDS* **2015**, *29*, 1035–1044. [CrossRef] [PubMed]

18. Wohlschlaeger, J.; Wenger, E.; Mehraein, P.; Weis, S. White matter changes in HIV-1 infected brains: A combined gross anatomical and ultrastructural morphometric investigation of the corpus callosum. *Clin. Neurol. Neurosurg.* **2009**, *111*, 422–429. [CrossRef] [PubMed]
19. Leite, S.C.; Correa, D.G.; Doring, T.M.; Kubo, T.T.; Netto, T.M.; Ferracini, R.; Ventura, N.; Bahia, P.R.; Gasparetto, E.L. Diffusion tensor mri evaluation of the corona radiata, cingulate gyri, and corpus callosum in HIV patients. *J. Magn. Reson. Imaging* **2013**, *38*, 1488–1493. [CrossRef] [PubMed]
20. Xuan, A.; Wang, G.B.; Shi, D.P.; Xu, J.L.; Li, Y.L. Initial study of magnetic resonance diffusion tensor imaging in brain white matter of early aids patients. *Chin. Med. J. (Engl.)* **2013**, *126*, 2720–2724. [PubMed]
21. Boska, M.D.; Dash, P.K.; Knibbe, J.; Epstein, A.A.; Akhter, S.P.; Fields, N.; High, R.; Makarov, E.; Bonasera, S.; Gelbard, H.A.; et al. Associations between brain microstructures, metabolites, and cognitive deficits during chronic HIV-1 infection of humanized mice. *Mol. Neurodegener.* **2014**, *9*, 58. [CrossRef] [PubMed]
22. Lackner, P.; Kuenz, B.; Reindl, M.; Morandell, M.; Berger, T.; Schmutzhard, E.; Eggers, C. Antibodies to myelin oligodendrocyte glycoprotein in HIV-1 associated neurocognitive disorder: A cross-sectional cohort study. *J. Neuroinflamm.* **2010**, *7*, 79. [CrossRef] [PubMed]
23. Fitting, S.; Booze, R.M.; Hasselrot, U.; Mactutus, C.F. Dose-dependent long-term effects of tat in the rat hippocampal formation: A design-based stereological study. *Hippocampus* **2010**, *20*, 469–480. [CrossRef] [PubMed]
24. Levine, A.J.; Miller, J.A.; Shapshak, P.; Gelman, B.; Singer, E.J.; Hinkin, C.H.; Commins, D.; Morgello, S.; Grant, I.; Horvath, S. Systems analysis of human brain gene expression: Mechanisms for HIV-associated neurocognitive impairment and common pathways with Alzheimer's disease. *BMC Med. Genom.* **2013**, *6*, 4. [CrossRef] [PubMed]
25. Berger, J.R.; Aksamit, A.J.; Clifford, D.B.; Davis, L.; Koralnik, I.J.; Sejvar, J.J.; Bartt, R.; Major, E.O.; Nath, A. Pml diagnostic criteria: Consensus statement from the aan neuroinfectious disease section. *Neurology* **2013**, *80*, 1430–1438. [CrossRef] [PubMed]
26. Del Valle, L.; Pina-Oviedo, S. HIV disorders of the brain: Pathology and pathogenesis. *Front. Biosci.* **2006**, *11*, 718–732. [CrossRef] [PubMed]
27. Sacktor, N. The epidemiology of human immunodeficiency virus-associated neurological disease in the era of highly active antiretroviral therapy. *J. Neurovirol.* **2002**, *8*, 115–121. [CrossRef] [PubMed]
28. Crossley, K.M.; Agnihotri, S.; Chaganti, J.; Rodriguez, M.L.; McNally, L.P.; Venna, N.; Turbett, S.E.; Gutman, M.; Morey, A.; Koralnik, I.J.; et al. Recurrence of progressive multifocal leukoencephalopathy despite immune recovery in two HIV seropositive individuals. *J. Neurovirol.* **2016**, *22*, 541–545. [CrossRef] [PubMed]
29. Mascarello, M.; Lanzafame, M.; Lattuada, E.; Concia, E.; Ferrari, S. Progressive multifocal leukoencephalopathy in an HIV patient receiving successful long-term haart. *J. Neurovirol.* **2011**, *17*, 196–199. [CrossRef] [PubMed]
30. Gates, T.M.; Cysique, L.A. The chronicity of HIV infection should drive the research strategy of neuroHIV treatment studies: A critical review. *CNS Drugs* **2016**, *30*, 53–69. [CrossRef] [PubMed]
31. Sharpless, N.; Gilbert, D.; Vandercam, B.; Zhou, J.M.; Verdin, E.; Ronnett, G.; Friedman, E.; Dubois-Dalcq, M. The restricted nature of HIV-1 tropism for cultured neural cells. *Virology* **1992**, *191*, 813–825. [CrossRef]
32. Takahashi, K.; Wesselingh, S.L.; Griffin, D.E.; McArthur, J.C.; Johnson, R.T.; Glass, J.D. Localization of HIV-1 in human brain using polymerase chain reaction/in situ hybridization and immunocytochemistry. *Ann. Neurol.* **1996**, *39*, 705–711. [CrossRef] [PubMed]
33. Albright, A.V.; Strizki, J.; Harouse, J.M.; Lavi, E.; O'Connor, M.; Gonzalez-Scarano, F. HIV-1 infection of cultured human adult oligodendrocytes. *Virology* **1996**, *217*, 211–219. [CrossRef] [PubMed]
34. Albright, A.; Lavi, E.; O'Connor, M.; González-Scarano, F. HIV-1 infection of a CD4-negative primary cell type: The oligodendrocyte. *Perspect. Drug Discov. Des.* **1996**, *5*, 43–50. [CrossRef]
35. Zhang, J.; Liu, J.; Katafiasz, B.; Fox, H.; Xiong, H. HIV-1 gp120-induced axonal injury detected by accumulation of β-amyloid precursor protein in adult rat corpus callosum. *J. Neuroimmune Pharmacol.* **2011**, *6*, 650–657. [CrossRef] [PubMed]
36. Patel, J.R.; McCandless, E.E.; Dorsey, D.; Klein, R.S. CXCR4 promotes differentiation of oligodendrocyte progenitors and remyelination. *Proc. Natl. Acad. Sci. USA* **2010**, *107*, 11062–11067. [CrossRef] [PubMed]

37. Stettner, M.R.; Nance, J.A.; Wright, C.A.; Kinoshita, Y.; Kim, W.K.; Morgello, S.; Rappaport, J.; Khalili, K.; Gordon, J.; Johnson, E.M. Smad proteins of oligodendroglial cells regulate transcription of JC virus early and late genes coordinately with the tat protein of human immunodeficiency virus type 1. *J. Gen. Virol.* **2009**, *90*, 2005–2014. [CrossRef] [PubMed]
38. Wright, C.A.; Nance, J.A.; Johnson, E.M. Effects of tat proteins and tat mutants of different human immunodeficiency virus type 1 clades on glial JC virus early and late gene transcription. *J. Gen. Virol.* **2013**, *94*, 514–523. [CrossRef] [PubMed]
39. Cinque, P.; Pierotti, C.; Vigano, M.G.; Bestetti, A.; Fausti, C.; Bertelli, D.; Lazzarin, A. The good and evil of haart in HIV-related progressive multifocal leukoencephalopathy. *J. Neurovirol.* **2001**, *7*, 358–363. [PubMed]
40. Martin-Blondel, G.; Bauer, J.; Cuvinciuc, V.; Uro-Coste, E.; Debard, A.; Massip, P.; Delisle, M.B.; Lassmann, H.; Marchou, B.; Mars, L.T.; et al. In situ evidence of jc virus control by CD8+ t cells in pml-iris during HIV infection. *Neurology* **2013**, *81*, 964–970. [CrossRef] [PubMed]
41. Codazzi, F.; Menegon, A.; Zacchetti, D.; Ciardo, A.; Grohovaz, F.; Meldolesi, J. HIV-1 gp120 glycoprotein induces $[Ca^{2+}]i$ responses not only in type-2 but also type-1 astrocytes and oligodendrocytes of the rat cerebellum. *Eur. J. Neurosci.* **1995**, *7*, 1333–1341. [CrossRef] [PubMed]
42. Tsunoda, I.; Fujinami, R.S. Inside-out versus outside-in models for virus induced demyelination: Axonal damage triggering demyelination. *Springer Semin. Immunopathol.* **2002**, *24*, 105–125. [CrossRef] [PubMed]
43. Langford, T.D.; Letendre, S.L.; Marcotte, T.D.; Ellis, R.J.; McCutchan, J.A.; Grant, I.; Mallory, M.E.; Hansen, L.A.; Archibald, S.; Jernigan, T.; et al. Severe, demyelinating leukoencephalopathy in AIDS patients on antiretroviral therapy. *AIDS* **2002**, *16*, 1019–1029. [CrossRef] [PubMed]
44. Smith, T.W.; DeGirolami, U.; Henin, D.; Bolgert, F.; Hauw, J.J. Human immunodeficiency virus (HIV) leukoencephalopathy and the microcirculation. *J. Neuropathol. Exp. Neurol.* **1990**, *49*, 357–370. [CrossRef] [PubMed]
45. Miller, F.; Afonso, P.V.; Gessain, A.; Ceccaldi, P.E. Blood-brain barrier and retroviral infections. *Virulence* **2012**, *3*, 222–229. [CrossRef] [PubMed]
46. Strazza, M.; Pirrone, V.; Wigdahl, B.; Nonnemacher, M.R. Breaking down the barrier: The effects of HIV-1 on the blood-brain barrier. *Brain Res.* **2011**, *1399*, 96–115. [CrossRef] [PubMed]
47. Louboutin, J.P.; Strayer, D.S. Blood-brain barrier abnormalities caused by HIV-1 gp120: Mechanistic and therapeutic implications. *ScientificWorldJournal* **2012**, *2012*. [CrossRef] [PubMed]
48. Titulaer, M.J.; Dalmau, J. Antibodies to nmda receptor, blood-brain barrier disruption and schizophrenia: A theory with unproven links. *Mol. Psychiatry* **2014**, *19*, 1054. [CrossRef] [PubMed]
49. Avison, M.; Nath, A.; Avison, R.; Schmitt, F.; Greenberg, R.; Berger, J. Viremia in the presence of blood-brain barrier compromise increases severity of HIV-associated neurocognitive impairment. In *Annals of Neurology*; Wiley-Liss Div John Wiley & Sons Inc.: New York, NY, USA, 2003; p. S49.
50. Gray, F.; Belec, L.; Chretien, F.; Dubreuil-Lemaire, M.L.; Ricolfi, F.; Wingertsmann, L.; Poron, F.; Gherardi, R. Acute, relapsing brain oedema with diffuse blood-brain barrier alteration and axonal damage in the acquired immunodeficiency syndrome. *Neuropathol. Appl. Neurobiol.* **1998**, *24*, 209–216. [CrossRef] [PubMed]
51. Chintawar, S.; Cayrol, R.; Antel, J.; Pandolfo, M.; Prat, A. Blood-brain barrier promotes differentiation of human fetal neural precursor cells. *Stem Cells* **2009**, *27*, 838–846. [CrossRef] [PubMed]
52. Plane, J.M.; Andjelkovic, A.V.; Keep, R.F.; Parent, J.M. Intact and injured endothelial cells differentially modulate postnatal murine forebrain neural stem cells. *Neurobiol. Dis.* **2010**, *37*, 218–227. [CrossRef] [PubMed]
53. Relucio, J.; Menezes, M.J.; Miyagoe-Suzuki, Y.; Takeda, S.; Colognato, H. Laminin regulates postnatal oligodendrocyte production by promoting oligodendrocyte progenitor survival in the subventricular zone. *Glia* **2012**, *60*, 1451–1467. [CrossRef] [PubMed]
54. Juliet, P.A.; Frost, E.E.; Balasubramaniam, J.; Del Bigio, M.R. Toxic effect of blood components on perinatal rat subventricular zone cells and oligodendrocyte precursor cell proliferation, differentiation and migration in culture. *J. Neurochem.* **2009**, *109*, 1285–1299. [CrossRef] [PubMed]
55. Antel, J.P.; Williams, K.; Blain, M.; McRea, E.; McLaurin, J. Oligodendrocyte lysis by CD4+ T cells independent of tumor necrosis factor. *Ann. Neurol.* **1994**, *35*, 341–348. [CrossRef] [PubMed]
56. Navikas, V.; Link, J.; Persson, C.; Olsson, T.; Hojeberg, B.; Ljungdahl, A.; Link, H.; Wahren, B. Increased mrna expression of IL-6, IL-10, TNF-α, and perforin in blood mononuclear cells in human HIV infection. *J. Acquir. Immune Defic. Syndr. Hum. Retrovirol.* **1995**, *9*, 484–489. [CrossRef] [PubMed]

57. Guo, H.; Gao, J.; Taxman, D.J.; Ting, J.P.; Su, L. HIV-1 infection induces interleukin-1beta production via TLR8 protein-dependent and NLRP3 inflammasome mechanisms in human monocytes. *J. Biol. Chem.* **2014**, *289*, 21716–21726. [CrossRef] [PubMed]
58. Takahashi, J.L.; Giuliani, F.; Power, C.; Imai, Y.; Yong, V.W. Interleukin-1β promotes oligodendrocyte death through glutamate excitotoxicity. *Ann. Neurol.* **2003**, *53*, 588–595. [CrossRef] [PubMed]
59. Jayadev, S.; Yun, B.; Nguyen, H.; Yokoo, H.; Morrison, R.S.; Garden, G.A. The glial response to CNS HIV infection includes p53 activation and increased expression of p53 target genes. *J. Neuroimmune Pharmacol.* **2007**, *2*, 359–370. [CrossRef] [PubMed]
60. Amaral, J.D.; Xavier, J.M.; Steer, C.J.; Rodrigues, C.M. The role of p53 in apoptosis. *Discov. Med.* **2010**, *9*, 145–152. [PubMed]
61. Liu, H.; Xiong, H.; University of Nebraska Medical Center, Omaha, NE, USA. Unpublished work, 2016.
62. Remillard, C.V.; Yuan, J.X. Activation of k^+ channels: An essential pathway in programmed cell death. *Am. J. Physiol. Lung Cell Mol. Physiol.* **2004**, *286*, L49–L67. [CrossRef] [PubMed]
63. Hahn, Y.K.; Podhaizer, E.M.; Hauser, K.F.; Knapp, P.E. HIV-1 alters neural and glial progenitor cell dynamics in the central nervous system: Coordinated response to opiates during maturation. *Glia* **2012**, *60*, 1871–1887. [CrossRef] [PubMed]
64. Buch, S.K.; Khurdayan, V.K.; Lutz, S.E.; Knapp, P.E.; El-Hage, N.; Hauser, K.F. Glial-restricted precursors: Patterns of expression of opioid receptors and relationship to human immunodeficiency virus-1 tat and morphine susceptibility in vitro. *Neuroscience* **2007**, *146*, 1546–1554. [CrossRef] [PubMed]
65. Chatterjee, D.; Biswas, K.; Nag, S.; Ramachandra, S.G.; Das Sarma, J. Microglia play a major role in direct viral-induced demyelination. *Clin. Dev. Immunol.* **2013**, *2013*. [CrossRef] [PubMed]
66. Marker, D.F.; Puccini, J.M.; Mockus, T.E.; Barbieri, J.; Lu, S.M.; Gelbard, H.A. LRRK2 kinase inhibition prevents pathological microglial phagocytosis in response to HIV-1 Tat protein. *J. Neuroinflamm.* **2012**, *9*, 261. [CrossRef] [PubMed]
67. Tremblay, M.E.; Marker, D.F.; Puccini, J.M.; Muly, E.C.; Lu, S.M.; Gelbard, H.A. Ultrastructure of microglia-synapse interactions in the HIV-1 Tat-injected murine central nervous system. *Commun. Integr. Biol.* **2013**, *6*, e27670. [CrossRef] [PubMed]
68. Fulmer, C.G.; VonDran, M.W.; Stillman, A.A.; Huang, Y.; Hempstead, B.L.; Dreyfus, C.F. Astrocyte-derived bdnf supports myelin protein synthesis after cuprizone-induced demyelination. *J. Neurosci.* **2014**, *34*, 8186–8196. [CrossRef] [PubMed]
69. Esiri, M.M.; Morris, C.S.; Millard, P.R. Fate of oligodendrocytes in HIV-1 infection. *AIDS* **1991**, *5*, 1081–1088. [CrossRef] [PubMed]
70. Bradl, M.; Lassmann, H. Oligodendrocytes: Biology and pathology. *Acta Neuropathol.* **2010**, *119*, 37–53. [CrossRef] [PubMed]
71. Payne, S.C.; Bartlett, C.A.; Savigni, D.L.; Harvey, A.R.; Dunlop, S.A.; Fitzgerald, M. Early proliferation does not prevent the loss of oligodendrocyte progenitor cells during the chronic phase of secondary degeneration in a cns white matter tract. *PLoS ONE* **2013**, *8*, e65710. [CrossRef] [PubMed]
72. Mishra, M.; Taneja, M.; Malik, S.; Khalique, H.; Seth, P. Human immunodeficiency virus type 1 Tat modulates proliferation and differentiation of human neural precursor cells: Implication in neuroaids. *J. Neurovirol.* **2010**, *16*, 355–367. [CrossRef] [PubMed]
73. Hahn, Y.K.; Vo, P.; Fitting, S.; Block, M.L.; Hauser, K.F.; Knapp, P.E. β-chemokine production by neural and glial progenitor cells is enhanced by HIV-1 Tat: Effects on microglial migration. *J. Neurochem.* **2010**, *114*, 97–109. [CrossRef] [PubMed]
74. Peng, H.; Sun, L.; Jia, B.; Lan, X.; Zhu, B.; Wu, Y.; Zheng, J. HIV-1-infected and immune-activated macrophages induce astrocytic differentiation of human cortical neural progenitor cells via the stat3 pathway. *PLoS ONE* **2011**, *6*, e19439. [CrossRef] [PubMed]
75. Mi, S.; Lee, X.; Shao, Z.; Thill, G.; Ji, B.; Relton, J.; Levesque, M.; Allaire, N.; Perrin, S.; Sands, B.; et al. Lingo-1 is a component of the nogo-66 receptor/p75 signaling complex. *Nat. Neurosci.* **2004**, *7*, 221–228. [CrossRef] [PubMed]
76. Mi, S.; Miller, R.H.; Lee, X.; Scott, M.L.; Shulag-Morskaya, S.; Shao, Z.; Chang, J.; Thill, G.; Levesque, M.; Zhang, M.; et al. Lingo-1 negatively regulates myelination by oligodendrocytes. *Nat. Neurosci.* **2005**, *8*, 745–751. [CrossRef] [PubMed]

77. Bongarzone, E.R.; Byravan, S.; Givogri, M.I.; Schonmann, V.; Campagnoni, A.T. Platelet-derived growth factor and basic fibroblast growth factor regulate cell proliferation and the expression of notch-1 receptor in a new oligodendrocyte cell line. *J. Neurosci. Res.* **2000**, *62*, 319–328. [CrossRef]
78. Kim, H.; Shin, J.; Kim, S.; Poling, J.; Park, H.C.; Appel, B. Notch-regulated oligodendrocyte specification from radial glia in the spinal cord of zebrafish embryos. *Dev. Dyn.* **2008**, *237*, 2081–2089. [CrossRef] [PubMed]
79. Shimizu, T.; Kagawa, T.; Wada, T.; Muroyama, Y.; Takada, S.; Ikenaka, K. Wnt signaling controls the timing of oligodendrocyte development in the spinal cord. *Dev. Biol.* **2005**, *282*, 397–410. [CrossRef] [PubMed]
80. Zhang, Z.-H.; Li, J.-J.; Wang, Q.-J.; Zhao, W.-Q.; Hong, J.; Lou, S.-j.; Xu, X.-H. WNK1 is involved in Nogo66 inhibition of OPC differentiation. *Mol. Cell. Neurosci.* **2015**, *65*, 135–142. [CrossRef] [PubMed]
81. Bhat, N.R.; Zhang, P.; Mohanty, S.B. P38 map kinase regulation of oligodendrocyte differentiation with creb as a potential target. *Neurochem. Res.* **2007**, *32*, 293–302. [CrossRef] [PubMed]
82. Chew, L.J.; Coley, W.; Cheng, Y.; Gallo, V. Mechanisms of regulation of oligodendrocyte development by p38 mitogen-activated protein kinase. *J. Neurosci.* **2010**, *30*, 11011–11027. [CrossRef] [PubMed]
83. Flores, A.I.; Narayanan, S.P.; Morse, E.N.; Shick, H.E.; Yin, X.; Kidd, G.; Avila, R.L.; Kirschner, D.A.; Macklin, W.B. Constitutively active akt induces enhanced myelination in the cns. *J. Neurosci.* **2008**, *28*, 7174–7183. [CrossRef] [PubMed]
84. Mitew, S.; Hay, C.M.; Peckham, H.; Xiao, J.; Koenning, M.; Emery, B. Mechanisms regulating the development of oligodendrocytes and central nervous system myelin. *Neuroscience* **2014**, *276*, 29–47. [CrossRef] [PubMed]
85. Tanaka, T.; Yoshida, S. Mechanisms of remyelination: Recent insight from experimental models. *Biomol. Concepts* **2014**, *5*, 289–298. [CrossRef] [PubMed]
86. Wu, J.Q.; Saksena, M.M.; Soriano, V.; Vispo, E.; Saksena, N.K. Differential regulation of cytotoxicity pathway discriminating between HIV, HCV mono-and co-infection identified by transcriptome profiling of PBMCs. *Virol. J.* **2015**, *12*, 1–16. [CrossRef] [PubMed]
87. Weiser, K.; Barton, M.; Gershoony, D.; DasGupta, R.; Cardozo, T.; Tang, S.-J. HIV's nef interacts with β-catenin of the wnt signaling pathway in hek293 cells. *PLoS ONE* **2013**, *8*, e77865. [CrossRef] [PubMed]
88. Richards, M.H.; Narasipura, S.D.; Kim, S.; Seaton, M.S.; Lutgen, V.; Al-Harthi, L. Dynamic interaction between astrocytes and infiltrating PBMCs in context of neuroAIDS. *Glia* **2015**, *63*, 441–451. [CrossRef] [PubMed]
89. Zhang, Y.; Argaw, A.T.; Gurfein, B.T.; Zameer, A.; Snyder, B.J.; Ge, C.; Lu, Q.R.; Rowitch, D.H.; Raine, C.S.; Brosnan, C.F.; et al. Notch1 signaling plays a role in regulating precursor differentiation during CNS remyelination. *Proc. Natl. Acad. Sci. USA* **2009**, *106*, 19162–19167. [CrossRef] [PubMed]
90. Curry, C.L.; Reed, L.L.; Golde, T.E.; Miele, L.; Nickoloff, B.J.; Foreman, K.E. Gamma secretase inhibitor blocks notch activation and induces apoptosis in kaposi's sarcoma tumor cells. *Oncogene* **2005**, *24*, 6333–6344. [CrossRef] [PubMed]
91. Liu, Y.; Han, S.S.; Wu, Y.; Tuohy, T.M.; Xue, H.; Cai, J.; Back, S.A.; Sherman, L.S.; Fischer, I.; Rao, M.S. CD44 expression identifies astrocyte-restricted precursor cells. *Dev. Biol.* **2004**, *276*, 31–46. [CrossRef] [PubMed]
92. Tuohy, T.M.; Wallingford, N.; Liu, Y.; Chan, F.H.; Rizvi, T.; Xing, R.; Bebo, B.; Rao, M.S.; Sherman, L.S. CD44 overexpression by oligodendrocytes: A novel mouse model of inflammation-independent demyelination and dysmyelination. *Glia* **2004**, *47*, 335–345. [CrossRef] [PubMed]
93. Suyama, M.; Daikoku, E.; Goto, T.; Sano, K.; Morikawa, Y. Reactivation from latency displays HIV particle budding at plasma membrane, accompanying CD44 upregulation and recruitment. *Retrovirology* **2009**, *6*, 63. [CrossRef] [PubMed]
94. Chao, C.; Silverberg, M.J.; Xu, L.; Chen, L.H.; Castor, B.; Martinez-Maza, O.; Abrams, D.I.; Zha, H.D.; Haque, R.; Said, J. A comparative study of molecular characteristics of diffuse large b-cell lymphoma from patients with and without human immunodeficiency virus infection. *Clin. Cancer Res.* **2015**, *21*, 1429–1437. [CrossRef] [PubMed]
95. Fields, J.; Dumaop, W.; Langford, T.D.; Rockenstein, E.; Masliah, E. Role of neurotrophic factor alterations in the neurodegenerative process in HIV associated neurocognitive disorders. *J. Neuroimmune Pharmacol.* **2014**, *9*, 102–116. [CrossRef] [PubMed]
96. Peferoen, L.; Kipp, M.; van der Valk, P.; van Noort, J.M.; Amor, S. Oligodendrocyte-microglia cross-talk in the central nervous system. *Immunology* **2014**, *141*, 302–313. [CrossRef] [PubMed]

97. Erlandsson, A.; Brannvall, K.; Gustafsdottir, S.; Westermark, B.; Forsberg-Nilsson, K. Autocrine/paracrine platelet-derived growth factor regulates proliferation of neural progenitor cells. *Cancer Res.* **2006**, *66*, 8042–8048. [CrossRef] [PubMed]
98. Jiang, Y.; Boije, M.; Westermark, B.; Uhrbom, L. PDGF-B can sustain self-renewal and tumorigenicity of experimental glioma-derived cancer-initiating cells by preventing oligodendrocyte differentiation. *Neoplasia* **2011**, *13*, 492–503. [CrossRef] [PubMed]
99. Azim, K.; Butt, A.M. GSK3β negatively regulates oligodendrocyte differentiation and myelination in vivo. *Glia* **2011**, *59*, 540–553. [CrossRef] [PubMed]
100. Luo, F.; Burke, K.; Kantor, C.; Miller, R.H.; Yang, Y. Cyclin-dependent kinase 5 mediates adult OPC maturation and myelin repair through modulation of Akt and GSK-3β signaling. *J. Neurosci.* **2014**, *34*, 10415–10429. [CrossRef] [PubMed]
101. Chao, J.; Yang, L.; Yao, H.; Buch, S. Platelet-derived growth factor-BB restores HIV Tat -mediated impairment of neurogenesis: Role of GSK-3β/β-catenin. *J. Neuroimmune Pharmacol.* **2014**, *9*, 259–268. [CrossRef] [PubMed]
102. Frederick, T.J.; Min, J.; Altieri, S.C.; Mitchell, N.E.; Wood, T.L. Synergistic induction of cyclin D1 in oligodendrocyte progenitor cells by IGF-I and FGF-2 requires differential stimulation of multiple signaling pathways. *Glia* **2007**, *55*, 1011–1022. [CrossRef] [PubMed]
103. Albrecht, D.; Garcia, L.; Cartier, L.; Kettlun, A.M.; Vergara, C.; Collados, L.; Valenzuela, M.A. Trophic factors in cerebrospinal fluid and spinal cord of patients with tropical spastic paraparesis, HIV, and creutzfeldt-jakob disease. *AIDS Res. Hum. Retrovir.* **2006**, *22*, 248–254. [CrossRef] [PubMed]
104. Ascherl, G.; Sgadari, C.; Bugarini, R.; Bogner, J.; Schatz, O.; Ensoli, B.; Sturzl, M. Serum concentrations of fibroblast growth factor 2 are increased in HIV type 1-infected patients and inversely related to survival probability. *AIDS Res. Hum. Retrovir.* **2001**, *17*, 1035–1039. [CrossRef] [PubMed]
105. Maggirwar, S.B.; Tong, N.; Ramirez, S.; Gelbard, H.A.; Dewhurst, S. HIV-1 tat-mediated activation of glycogen synthase kinase-3β contributes to Tat-mediated neurotoxicity. *J. Neurochem.* **1999**, *73*, 578–586. [CrossRef] [PubMed]
106. Sui, Z.; Sniderhan, L.F.; Fan, S.; Kazmierczak, K.; Reisinger, E.; Kovacs, A.D.; Potash, M.J.; Dewhurst, S.; Gelbard, H.A.; Maggirwar, S.B. Human immunodeficiency virus-encoded tat activates glycogen synthase kinase-3β to antagonize nuclear factor-kappab survival pathway in neurons. *Eur. J. Neurosci.* **2006**, *23*, 2623–2634. [CrossRef] [PubMed]
107. Lannuzel, A.; Barnier, J.V.; Hery, C.; Huynh, V.T.; Guibert, B.; Gray, F.; Vincent, J.D.; Tardieu, M. Human immunodeficiency virus type 1 and its coat protein gp120 induce apoptosis and activate JNK and ERK mitogen-activated protein kinases in human neurons. *Ann. Neurol.* **1997**, *42*, 847–856. [CrossRef] [PubMed]
108. Cavaliere, F.; Benito-Muñoz, M.; Panicker, M.; Matute, C. Nmda modulates oligodendrocyte differentiation of subventricular zone cells through pkc activation. *Front. Cell. Neurosci.* **2013**, *7*, 261. [CrossRef] [PubMed]
109. Lundgaard, I.; Luzhynskaya, A.; Stockley, J.H.; Wang, Z.; Evans, K.A.; Swire, M.; Volbracht, K.; Gautier, H.O.; Franklin, R.J.; Attwell, D.; et al. Neuregulin and BDNF induce a switch to nmda receptor-dependent myelination by oligodendrocytes. *PLoS Biol.* **2013**, *11*, e1001743. [CrossRef] [PubMed]
110. Zeitler, M.; Steringer, J.P.; Muller, H.M.; Mayer, M.P.; Nickel, W. HIV-tat forms phosphoinositide dependent membrane pores implicated in unconventional protein secretion. *J. Biol. Chem.* **2015**, *290*, 21976–21984. [CrossRef] [PubMed]
111. Ramos-Cejudo, J.; Gutierrez-Fernandez, M.; Otero-Ortega, L.; Rodriguez-Frutos, B.; Fuentes, B.; Vallejo-Cremades, M.T.; Hernanz, T.N.; Cerdan, S.; Diez-Tejedor, E. Brain-derived neurotrophic factor administration mediated oligodendrocyte differentiation and myelin formation in subcortical ischemic stroke. *Stroke* **2015**, *46*, 221–228. [CrossRef] [PubMed]
112. Tsiperson, V.; Huang, Y.; Bagayogo, I.; Song, Y.; VonDran, M.W.; DiCicco-Bloom, E.; Dreyfus, C.F. Brain-derived neurotrophic factor deficiency restricts proliferation of oligodendrocyte progenitors following cuprizone-induced demyelination. *ASN Neuro* **2015**, *7*. [CrossRef] [PubMed]
113. Vondran, M.W.; Clinton-Luke, P.; Honeywell, J.Z.; Dreyfus, C.F. BDNF+/− mice exhibit deficits in oligodendrocyte lineage cells of the basal forebrain. *Glia* **2010**, *58*, 848–856. [CrossRef] [PubMed]
114. Bachis, A.; Avdoshina, V.; Zecca, L.; Parsadanian, M.; Mocchetti, I. Human immunodeficiency virus type 1 alters brain-derived neurotrophic factor processing in neurons. *J. Neurosci.* **2012**, *32*, 9477–9484. [CrossRef] [PubMed]

115. Xiao, H.; Tao, Y.; Greenblatt, J.; Roeder, R.G. A cofactor, tip30, specifically enhances HIV-1 tat-activated transcription. *Proc. Natl. Acad. Sci. USA* **1998**, *95*, 2146–2151. [CrossRef] [PubMed]
116. Yang, W.; Xiao, L.; Li, C.; Liu, X.; Liu, M.; Shao, Q.; Wang, D.; Huang, A.; He, C. Tip30 inhibits oligodendrocyte precursor cell differentiation via cytoplasmic sequestration of olig1. *Glia* **2015**, *63*, 684–698. [CrossRef] [PubMed]
117. Attali, B.; Wang, N.; Kolot, A.; Sobko, A.; Cherepanov, V.; Soliven, B. Characterization of delayed rectifier kv channels in oligodendrocytes and progenitor cells. *J. Neurosci.* **1997**, *17*, 8234–8245. [PubMed]
118. Chittajallu, R.; Chen, Y.; Wang, H.; Yuan, X.; Ghiani, C.A.; Heckman, T.; McBain, C.J.; Gallo, V. Regulation of kv1 subunit expression in oligodendrocyte progenitor cells and their role in g1/s phase progression of the cell cycle. *Proc. Natl. Acad. Sci. USA* **2002**, *99*, 2350–2355. [CrossRef] [PubMed]
119. Peretz, A.; Gil-Henn, H.; Sobko, A.; Shinder, V.; Attali, B.; Elson, A. Hypomyelination and increased activity of voltage-gated k^+ channels in mice lacking protein tyrosine phosphatase epsilon. *EMBO J.* **2000**, *19*, 4036–4045. [CrossRef] [PubMed]
120. Kalsi, A.S.; Greenwood, K.; Wilkin, G.; Butt, A.M. Kir4.1 expression by astrocytes and oligodendrocytes in CNS white matter: A developmental study in the rat optic nerve. *J. Anat.* **2004**, *204*, 475–485. [CrossRef] [PubMed]
121. Neusch, C.; Rozengurt, N.; Jacobs, R.E.; Lester, H.A.; Kofuji, P. Kir4.1 potassium channel subunit is crucial for oligodendrocyte development and in vivo myelination. *J. Neurosci.* **2001**, *21*, 5429–5438. [PubMed]
122. Tegla, C.A.; Cudrici, C.; Rozycka, M.; Soloviova, K.; Ito, T.; Singh, A.K.; Khan, A.; Azimzadeh, P.; Andrian-Albescu, M.; Niculescu, F.; et al. C5b-9-activated, k(v)1.3 channels mediate oligodendrocyte cell cycle activation and dedifferentiation. *Exp. Mol. Pathol.* **2011**, *91*, 335–345. [CrossRef] [PubMed]
123. Cheli, V.T.; Santiago Gonzalez, D.A.; Spreuer, V.; Paez, P.M. Voltage-gated Ca^{2+} entry promotes oligodendrocyte progenitor cell maturation and myelination in vitro. *Exp. Neurol.* **2015**, *265*, 69–83. [CrossRef] [PubMed]
124. French, H.M.; Reid, M.; Mamontov, P.; Simmons, R.A.; Grinspan, J.B. Oxidative stress disrupts oligodendrocyte maturation. *J. Neurosci. Res.* **2009**, *87*, 3076–3087. [CrossRef] [PubMed]
125. Jensen, B.K.; Monnerie, H.; Mannell, M.V.; Gannon, P.J.; Espinoza, C.A.; Erickson, M.A.; Bruce-Keller, A.J.; Gelman, B.B.; Briand, L.A.; Pierce, R.C.; et al. Altered oligodendrocyte maturation and myelin maintenance: The role of antiretrovirals in HIV-associated neurocognitive disorders. *J. Neuropathol. Exp. Neurol.* **2015**, *74*, 1093–1118. [CrossRef] [PubMed]
126. Hoare, J.; Fouche, J.P.; Phillips, N.; Joska, J.A.; Paul, R.; Donald, K.A.; Thomas, K.G.; Stein, D.J. White matter micro-structural changes in art-naive and art-treated children and adolescents infected with HIV in south Africa. *AIDS* **2015**, *29*, 1793–1801. [CrossRef] [PubMed]
127. Borjabad, A.; Morgello, S.; Chao, W.; Kim, S.Y.; Brooks, A.I.; Murray, J.; Potash, M.J.; Volsky, D.J. Significant effects of antiretroviral therapy on global gene expression in brain tissues of patients with HIV-1-associated neurocognitive disorders. *PLoS Pathog.* **2011**, *7*, e1002213. [CrossRef] [PubMed]
128. Heaton, R.K.; Clifford, D.B.; Franklin, D.R., Jr.; Woods, S.P.; Ake, C.; Vaida, F.; Ellis, R.J.; Letendre, S.L.; Marcotte, T.D.; Atkinson, J.H.; et al. HIV-associated neurocognitive disorders persist in the era of potent antiretroviral therapy: Charter study. *Neurology* **2010**, *75*, 2087–2096. [CrossRef] [PubMed]
129. Baas, D.; Bourbeau, D.; Sarlieve, L.L.; Ittel, M.E.; Dussault, J.H.; Puymirat, J. Oligodendrocyte maturation and progenitor cell proliferation are independently regulated by thyroid hormone. *Glia* **1997**, *19*, 324–332. [CrossRef]
130. Grinspan, J.B.; Stern, J.L.; Franceschini, B.; Pleasure, D. Trophic effects of basic fibroblast growth factor (bFGF) on differentiated oligodendroglia: A mechanism for regeneration of the oligodendroglial lineage. *J. Neurosci. Res.* **1993**, *36*, 672–680. [CrossRef] [PubMed]
131. Miller, R.H. Regulation of oligodendrocyte development in the vertebrate CNS. *Prog. Neurobiol.* **2002**, *67*, 451–467. [CrossRef]

4

Impact of Increased Astrocyte Expression of IL-6, CCL2 or CXCL10 in Transgenic Mice on Hippocampal Synaptic Function

Donna Gruol

Molecular and Cellular Neuroscience Department, The Scripps Research Institute, La Jolla, CA 92037, USA; gruol@scripps.edu

Academic Editor: Balapal S. Basavarajappa

Abstract: An important aspect of CNS disease and injury is the elevated expression of neuroimmune factors. These factors are thought to contribute to processes ranging from recovery and repair to pathology. The complexity of the CNS and the multitude of neuroimmune factors that are expressed in the CNS during disease and injury is a challenge to an understanding of the consequences of the elevated expression relative to CNS function. One approach to address this issue is the use of transgenic mice that express elevated levels of a specific neuroimmune factor in the CNS by a cell type that normally produces it. This approach can provide basic information about the actions of specific neuroimmune factors and can contribute to an understanding of more complex conditions when multiple neuroimmune factors are expressed. This review summarizes studies using transgenic mice that express elevated levels of IL-6, CCL2 or CXCL10 through increased astrocyte expression. The studies focus on the effects of these neuroimmune factors on synaptic function at the Schaffer collateral to CA1 pyramidal neuron synapse of the hippocampus, a brain region that plays a key role in cognitive function.

Keywords: pyramidal neurons; Schaffer collaterals; LTP; neuroimmune; alcohol; field potential recordings; cytokine; chemokine

---

1. Introduction

Several lines of evidence have confirmed the existence of a neuroimmune system in the CNS, and a role for neuroimmune communication in CNS homeostasis, function, and pathology. Glial cells, and in particular astrocytes and microglia, are the main cellular components of the CNS neuroimmune system. Glial cells initiate neuroimmune communication primarily through the production of small protein signaling factors with distinct structure and function. These neuroimmune factors include members of the cytokine superfamily such as proinflammatory cytokines and chemokines. Typically, proinflammatory cytokines and chemokines are present at low levels in the normal CNS, while elevate levels are associated with CNS disease and injury. For example, elevated levels of proinflammatory cytokines and/or chemokines in the CNS are typical hallmarks of CNS inflammatory and neurodegenerative diseases such as HIV infection [1], Alzheimer's disease [2], epilepsy [3], multiple sclerosis [4], alcoholism and fetal alcohol spectrum disorders [5–7], and psychiatric disorders (e.g., autism spectrum disorders, schizophrenia, depression) [8–10]. The elevated levels are thought contribute to pathological processes occurring in these conditions, although protective actions could also play a role. Elevated levels of these neuroimmune factors also occur in normal aging, and may play a role in cognitive decline that can occur with normal aging [11,12].

CNS glial cells are capable of producing a variety of proinflammatory cytokines and chemokines, but the specific biological actions and roles of these neuroimmune factors have yet to be fully elucidated, and are likely to depend on the cell source and physiological or pathological context. During conditions associated with CNS disease and injury, multiple neuroimmune factors are commonly, and often chronically produced. The complexity of this situation makes it difficult to identify the actions of specific neuroimmune factors and the cell source, especially if pharmacological, biological, or other types of tools are lacking. A number of approaches have been used to circumvent this problem. This article focuses on one approach, the use of transgenic mice that endogenously produce elevated levels of a specific neuroimmune factor in the CNS by a cell type that normally produces it, and within the anatomical integrity and physiological pathways of the CNS. The transgenic mice of interest in this review express elevated levels of the proinflammatory cytokine Interleukin-6 (IL-6), the chemokine CCL2 (CC chemokine ligand 2, previously known as monocyte chemoattractant protein-1 or MCP-1), or the chemokine CXCL10 (previously known as interferon-gamma inducible protein 10 or IP10) through increased astrocyte expression. The review summarizes studies on the consequences of the increased astrocyte expression on a basic mechanism of CNS function, synaptic function, and in particular, hippocampal synaptic function. The hippocampus plays a critical role in learning and memory, and alterations in hippocampal synaptic function can significantly affect cognition [13]. Studies in experimental models have shown that altered hippocampal synaptic function is associated with CNS conditions known to involve elevated expression of neuroimmune factors (e.g., [14–26]). The transgenic mice have also been a useful model for a number of other types of studies related to CNS conditions during disease and injury, a topic that is not addressed in this review (e.g., [27–34]).

2. Astrocytes Are a Primary Source of Neuroimmune Factors in the CNS

Astrocytes are the most abundant cell type in the CNS and a key component of the neuroimmune system of the CNS [35]. Astrocytes play a variety of roles in the CNS, as regulators/mediators of normal physiology and responders to adverse conditions, such as those occurring during injury and infection, when astrocytes contribute to repair and recovery processes [36,37]. A large number of cytokines and chemokines are produced by astrocytes, including IL-6, CCL2, and CXCL10, but relatively little is known about the specific roles and biological actions of these factors under physiological or pathophysiological conditions when astrocytes are the initial cell source of these factors. Astrocytes are in close association with neurons and synapses, making them ideally positioned to influence neuronal circuit activity, which is essential for normal CNS function and is often compromised in CNS disorders [38,39]. In this review, studies on the consequence of elevated astrocyte expression IL-6, CCL2, or CXCL10 on synaptic function at the Schaffer collateral to CA1 pyramidal neuron synapse of the hippocampus are summarized. The Schaffer collateral to CA1 pyramidal neuron synapse is one of the most highly studied synapse in the CNS [40]. Output from the CA1 region provides important input to other brain regions and plays a key role in learning, memory, and other cognitive functions.

3. Signal Transduction Pathways

IL-6, CCL2 and CXCL10 initiate biological actions through the activation of specific membrane receptors, IL-6R, CCR2, and CXCR3, respectively. However, downstream signal transduction pathways differ. CCR2 and CXCR3 are G-protein coupled receptors (GPCRs), whereas IL-6R is linked to a tyrosine kinase signal transduction pathway (Figure 1). Moreover, IL-6R associated signal transduction can occur through two pathways, a classic pathway and trans-signaling [41] (Figure 1).

The classic IL-6 pathway involves membrane bound IL-6R, which interacts with another membrane bound protein, gp130, the signaling subunit of IL-6R and other cytokine receptors. Trans-signaling involves IL-6R that has been released from cells into the extracellular fluid and is referred to as soluble IL-6R. Soluble IL-6R can bind to IL-6 in the extracellular fluid and the ligand/receptor complex can then bind to membrane bound gp130. Because gp130 is ubiquitously expressed in CNS cells, trans-signaling can occur in cells that do not express membrane bound IL-6R, and consequently trans-signaling greatly expands the target area of IL-6 actions. Trans-signaling appears to be the primary pathway involved in the pathological actions of IL-6 in the CNS [42].

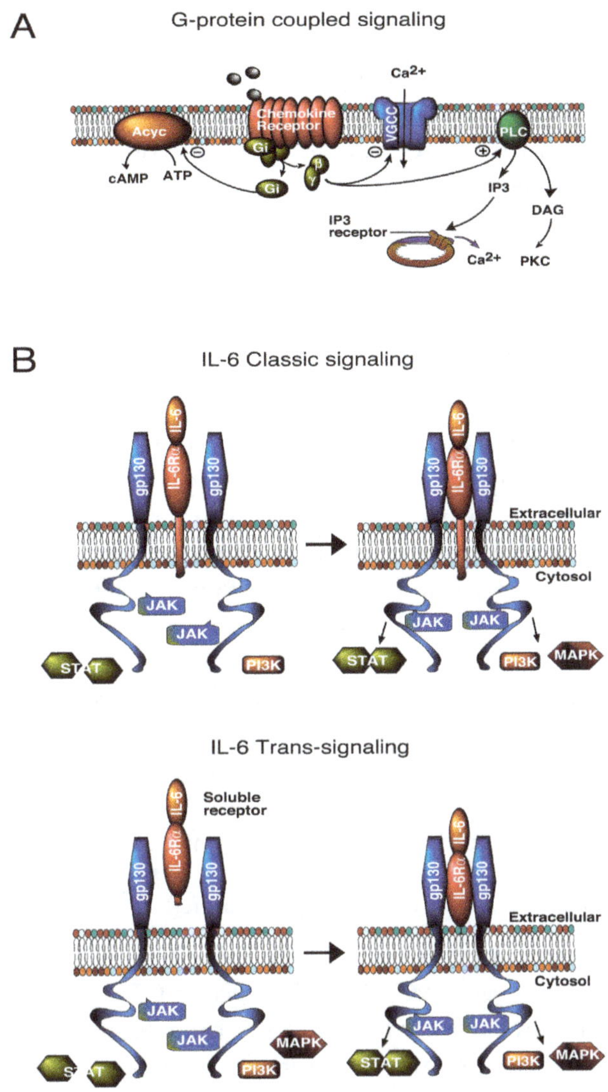

Figure 1. Diagrams showing signal transduction pathways used by chemokines and the proinflammatory cytokine IL-6. A plus sign within a circle indicates activation of the target molecule and a minus sign within a circle indicates inhibition of the target molecule. (**A**) Agonist binding to the G-protein coupled receptors (GPCR) initiates dissociation of the G-protein heterotrimer coupled to the receptor into Gα and Gβγ subunits. The Gα and Gβγ subunits then activate or inhibit downstream effectors. These effectors include ion channels, such as voltage-gated calcium channels (VGCC), and signal transduction molecules including phospholipase C (PLC) and adenylate cyclase (Acyc). Activation of PLC leads to the production of other signaling molecules including diacylglycerol (DAG) and inositol trisphosphate (IP3), and downstream activation of protein kinase C (PKC) and inositol trisphosphate receptors (IP3R), which regulate the release of calcium from intracellular stores; (**B**) IL-6 can signal through either a membrane bound (classic signaling) or a soluble (trans-signaling) IL-6R. The IL-6/IL-6R complex interacts with gp130 to activate the JAK/STAT signaling pathway. In addition, the IL-6/IL-6R/gp130 complex can activate RAS/mitogen-activated protein kinase (p44/42 MAPK, also called ERK1/2; MAPK) and phosphatidylinositol-3 kinase (PI3K) signaling pathways. All three signaling pathways activate additional downstream signaling molecules and effectors.

The differences in signal transduction pathways utilized by IL-6 and chemokines could indicate different biological actions. However, signal transduction pathways downstream of the G-protein and tyrosine kinase step can merge at common pathway partners or targets and lead to similar biological actions. Thus, it is not surprising that all three neuroimmune factors have neuronal or synaptic actions, although the actions are not identical.

Both neurons and glial cells express receptors and signal transduction pathways utilized by IL-6R [41,43], CCR2 [44–46], and CXCR3 [47,48], and are potential downstream cellular targets of the astrocyte produced neuroimmune factors. Because of the close association of astrocytes with neurons and synapses [39], actions of cytokines or chemokines on either cell type could potentially alter neuronal and synaptic function. Downstream molecular targets of GPCR and IL-6R pathways can regulate gene expression, which may be instrumental in directing neuroadaptive changes associated with elevated expression of IL-6, CCL2, and CXCL10 in the CNS of the transgenic mice.

4. IL-6, CCL2, or CXCL10 Transgenic Mice

All three lines of transgenic mice with increased astrocyte expression of IL-6, CCL2, or CXCL10 were generated by a similar approach, insertion of the transgene (mouse or human) for the neuroimmune factor under transcriptional control of the glial fibrillary acidic protein (GFAP) gene promoter [29,34,49,50]. GFAP is an intermediate filament protein expressed almost exclusively by astrocytes in the adult CNS and commonly used as a marker for astrocytes [50,51]. More than one line was generated for each neuroimmune factor. Heterozygotes from the following lines were used for the studies discussed in this review: IL-6 transgenic line 167 (IL-6 tg), CXCL10 transgenic line CXCL10-10 (CXCL10 tg), CCL2 transgenic line on a SJL background (CCL2-tg SJL mice), and CCL2 transgenic line on a C57Bl/6J background (CCL2-tg), which were developed from the CCL2-tg SJL mice. Non-transgenic littermates of the respective transgenic line were used as controls. In general, elevated expression of other neuroimmune factors was not evident, or at low level in these transgenic lines [29,34,52], enabling investigation of the consequences of elevated expression of the transgene alone or in combination with other experimental manipulations.

4.1. Expression of IL-6, CCL2, or CXCL10 in the Transgenic Mice

Because transgene expression in the transgenic mice is under control of the GFAP promoter, elevated expression of IL-6, CCL2, or CXCL10 is linked to GFAP expression. GFAP expression in astrocytes is initiated during the developmental period, which occurs primarily during the first 3 weeks of postnatal life in mice. GFAP expression in the mouse hippocampus is evident at 1 day postnatal, increases with age until 6 days postnatal, and then levels off and remains stable through adulthood [53]. Thus, neuronal/synaptic exposure to these neuroimmune factors in the transgenic mice occurs during an important period of structural and synaptic development and could affect developmental patterns. Evidence is limited on this topic, but in general, neuropathology in the hippocampus of the IL-6, CCL2, and CXCL10 heterozygous mice is absent or minimal up to 3–6 months of age, although homozygous mice can show pathology at early ages [29,32,54,55]. Thus, if the elevated expression of IL-6, CCL2, or CXCL10 altered CNS development in the transgenic mice, the effects on development were not pathological or were compensated for by other changes. In this review, discussion of the transgenic mice refers to the heterozygotes.

CNS expression of IL-6, CCL2, or CXCL10 has been quantified in the respective transgenic mice at the mRNA and/or protein levels. Studies of IL-6-tg mice showed that IL-6 mRNA was evident in the CNS at 7 days postnatal, increased with age and reached a peak at 3 months postnatal (adult stage), after which a decline was observed [52]. IL-6 transgene expression was demonstrated in hippocampal astrocytes by expression of the lacZ reporter gene and immunohistochemical detection of β-gal [55]. Constitutive secretion of IL-6 from astrocytes was demonstrated in studies of astrocyte cultures prepared from CNS of the IL-6 tg mice [49]. IL-6 levels were ~150 pg/mL in the supernatant from astrocyte cultures prepared from CNS of IL-6 tg mice, compared with <5 pg/mL for supernatant from astrocyte cultures prepared from CNS of non-tg mice. Interestingly, ELISA analysis of IL-6 levels in the hippocampus have revealed low levels and no differences between the IL-6 tg and non-tg hippocampus, although higher levels and genotypic differences were noted in the cerebellum [52,56]. The cerebellum is the CNS region with the highest level of IL-6 mRNA expression in the transgenic mice, particularly in the Bergman glial [49]. These results may indicate that IL-6 produced by hippocampal astrocytes *in vivo* is rapidly released and degraded. Others have noted difficulty in measuring IL-6 levels in CNS tissue using commercial ELISA kits, which may mean that there are technical issues to be resolved [57]. In spite of the lack of differences in measureable levels of IL-6 protein, increase expression of IL-6 regulated genes (e.g., GFAP, eb22, Socs3) and elevated levels of STAT3 and the activated form of STAT3 (phosphoSTAT3), the downstream partner of IL-6 signal transduction through which IL-6 acts to increase GFAP [58–60], were observed in the CNS of IL-6 tg mice. These results are consistent with actions of elevated levels of IL-6 in the IL-6 tg CNS.

Protein measurements in the CNS of the two CCL2 transgenic lines showed that the older CCL2-tg SJL mice express higher levels of CCL2 in the hippocampus than in the CCL2-tg mice. CCL2 levels measured by ELISA were ~1.3 ng/mL at 3–4 months of age and ~3.0 ng/mL at 7–9 months of age in hippocampal homogenate from the CCL2-tg SJL mice [61]. In the CCL2-tg mice, CCL2 levels measured by ELISA were ~1.2 ng/mL at 3–5 months of age and ~1.5 ng/mL at 7–9 [58]. CCL2 levels were ~0.2 ng/mL in hippocampal homogenates from the non-tg mice from both the CCL2-tg and CCL2-tg SJL lines. Studies of supernatants from astrocyte cultures prepared from CNS of CCL2-tg SJL mice showed that astrocytes constitutively secrete large amounts of CCL2 (e.g., ~3.5 ng/mL) [34].

Expression of CXCL-10 in the CNS of CXCL10-tg mice has been characterized at the mRNA level by *in situ* hybridization [29]. The highest levels of CXCL10 mRNA were observed in the hippocampus, olfactory bulb, periventricular zone, cortical areas, cerebellum, and choroid plexus of the CXCL10-tg CNS (mice 5–6 months of age). Western blot studies confirmed high levels of CXCL10 protein in the hippocampus, and immunohistochemical staining confirmed expression of CXCL10 protein in astrocytes [29]. No CXCL10 mRNA or protein expression was observed in non-tg mice. Levels of CXCL10 protein in the CNS of CXCL10-tg mice have not been measured by ELISA.

Elevated levels of neuroimmune factors are typically associated with pathological conditions, whereas low levels appear to exist under physiological conditions. However, the range of protein levels expressed during physiological and pathophysiological conditions has yet to be fully elucidated for most neuroimmune factors. Although elevated levels IL-6, CCL2 and CXCL-10 mRNA and/or protein have been documented in the CNS of the respective transgenic mice, it is unknown if protein levels for the three transgenic lines are functionally comparable. However, mRNA or protein levels were shown to be within the range associated with experimentally induced pathophysiological conditions in the CNS of IL-6 tg [62], CXCL10-tg [29] and CCL2-tg SJL mice [34].

4.2. *Neuropathology*

In general, before 3–6 months of age, the heterozygous IL-6, CCL2, and CXCL10 transgenic mice show relatively little neuropathology. In the IL-6 tg mice, the cerebellum shows the highest levels of IL-6 mRNA expression in the CNS of the IL-6 tg mice and greatest neuropathological changes, the most prominent being neovascularization [49,63]. Age-dependent neuropathological changes in the cortex and hippocampus of the IL-6 tg mice were evident in immunohistochemical studies of synaptic and cellular proteins. The neuropathological changes included reduced immunostaining for the presynaptic protein synapsin I indicative of synaptic damage (cortex, 12 months of age), reduced immunostaining for microtubule associated protein-2 (MAP-2) indicative of dendritic damage (cortex at 3 and 12 months of age), reduced immunostaining for parvalbumin, a calcium binding protein expressed by inhibitory interneurons (hippocampus at 3 and 12 months of age), and eventual loss of the interneurons, and reduced immunostaining for calbindin, a calcium binding protein expressed by inhibitory interneurons (cortex, 12 months of age) [49,54].

Histological studies of the CNS of CCL2-tg and CXCL10-tg mice are limited. However, CCL2-tg SJL mice have been reported to be free of neurological impairment before 6 month of age [34]. Routine histological analysis of the CNS of the CXCL10 mice showed no apparent neuropathological changes relative to the CNS of the non-tg mice [29].

5. Synaptic Function in the Hippocampus from IL-6, CCL2, and CXCL10 Transgenic Mice

For all three transgenic lines, physiological studies to assess synaptic function have been carried out at the Schaffer collateral to CA1 pyramidal neuron synapse of the hippocampus using a similar protocol that involved extracellular field potential recordings from acutely isolated slices of hippocampus (Figure 2). This approach has been extensively used for physiological studies of hippocampal synaptic function. One potential limitation to this approach is that the normal level of neuroimmune factors could be altered by the slice preparation and recording procedures. However, such effects would presumably also occur in the non-tg slices and thus be controlled for.

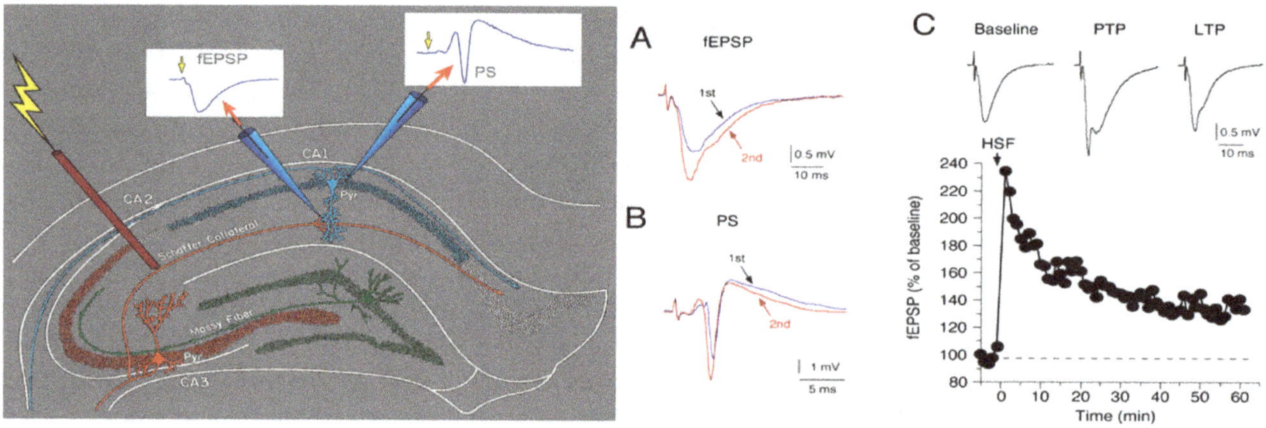

Figure 2. Measurement of synaptic function using extracellular recordings in hippocampal slices. (**Left Panel**) Simplified diagram showing the placement of stimulating and recording electrodes and recorded responses in a field potential recording of synaptic transmission at the Schaffer collateral to CA1 pyramidal neuron synapse in a hippocampal slice. Synaptic transmission is initiated experimentally by electrical stimulation of Schaffer collaterals, axons of the CA3 pyramidal neurons of the hippocampus. Stimulation of the Schaffer collateral elicits a fEPSP in the dendritic region and, depending on the strength of the stimulation, a PS in the somatic region; (**Right panel**) Repetitive stimulation can result in a change in the magnitude of synaptic responses. (**A**) Repetitive stimulation with a 40 ms interval between the first and second stimulation resulted in an enhancement of the fEPSP (2nd) evoked by the second stimulation relative to the fEPSP (1st) evoked by the first stimulation; (**B**) Repetitive stimulation with a 10 ms interval between the first and second stimulation resulted in an enhancement the PS (2nd) evoked by the second stimulation relative to the PS (1st) evoked by the first stimulation in this slice; (**C**) High frequency stimulation (HSF) induces a long-term enhancement of the fEPSP. The graph shows the magnitude of the fEPSP enhancement relative to baseline levels before high frequency stimulation was applied (at the arrow). The initial, large enhancement of the fEPSP is referred to as post-tetanic potentiation (PTP). The delayed, stable increase in the magnitude of the fEPSP is referred to as long-term potentiation (LTP). Representative recordings are shown above the graph.

Synaptic transmission to CA1 pyramidal neurons was elicited by electrical stimulation of the Schaffer collaterals. Both baseline synaptic transmission elicited by single stimulations and synaptic plasticity elicited by repetitive stimulation were studied. The response to synaptic transmission was measured in the dendritic region of the CA1 neurons as a field excitatory postsynaptic potential (fEPSP), which reflects the membrane depolarization produced by synaptic transmission in a population of CA1 neurons (Figure 2). In some studies, recordings were also made in the somatic region of the CA1 pyramidal neurons, where population spikes (PS) were recorded (Figure 2). The PS reflects action potentials occurring in the soma/dendritic region that were generated by synaptic depolarizations in a population of CA1 pyramidal neurons. Data from hippocampal slices from the transgenic mice were compared to data from hippocampal slices from the respective non-tg littermate controls. Results are summarized in Table 1. In addition to the studies of IL-6 tg mice discussed in this review, two other studies of synaptic function in the hippocampus have appeared, both in the dentate region [64,65]. In addition, one study on synaptic function in the cerebellum has appeared [66].

Table 1. Genotypic differences in synaptic function in the hippocampus.

Measurement	**IL-6 tg *vs.* Non-tg**		**CCL2-tg *vs.* Non-tg**	**CCL2-tg SJL *vs.* Non-tg**	**CXCL10-tg *vs.* Non-tg**
Age (months)	1–2	3–6	2–3	7–12	5–6
Synaptic transmission					
-fEPSP	↑	↑	no Δ	↓	no Δ
-PS	↑	↑	↑	↓	no Δ
P-P synaptic plasticity					
-fEPSP (PPF)	no Δ	no Δ	no Δ	↑	no Δ
-PS (PPR)	no Δ	no Δ	no Δ	↑	no Δ
Long-term synaptic plasticity					
-PTP	↓	no Δ	no Δ	↑	no Δ
-LTP	no Δ	no Δ	no Δ	no Δ	no Δ
Reference	[60]		[67]	[61]	[68]

↓ = decrease, ↑ = increase, no Δ = no difference.

5.1. Synaptic Transmission

The hippocampus from the IL-6 tg mice was studied at two ages, young mice 1–2 months of age and adult mice 3–6 months of age. Results were similar for the two age groups and showed that the fEPSP was enhanced in the hippocampus from the IL-6 tg mice compared to the hippocampus from non-tg mice of the same age group [60]. As a consequence of the enhanced fEPSP, the PS was also enhanced in the IL-6 tg hippocampus [60].

There was no difference in the fEPSP magnitude between the hippocampus from the CCL2-tg and non-tg mice at 2–3 months of age, whereas the PS was significantly larger in the hippocampus from the CCL2-tg mice [67]. Thus, the hippocampus from both the IL-6 tg and CCL2-tg mice showed an increase in the PS, indicative of increased excitability. However the increased PS in the hippocampus from the IL-6 tg mice could be explained by a larger fEPSP, but the increased PS in the hippocampus from the CCL2-tg mice could not. This difference indicates that although the functional consequence at the level of the PS was similar for the IL-6 tg and CCL2-tg hippocampus, different underlying mechanisms were involved. The increased excitability in the IL-6 tg mice could underlie the enhanced sensitivity to glutamate receptor agonists-induced seizure activity [69] and enhanced alcohol withdrawal hyperexcitability [70] observed in the IL-6 tg mice compared to the non-tg mice. The CCL2-tg mice did not show the enhanced alcohol withdrawal hyperexcitability observed in the IL-6 tg mice [70]. Effects glutamate receptor agonist on seizure activity has not been tested in the CCL2-tg mice.

In contrast to the CCL2-tg mice where only the PS was altered and an enhancement was observed, in the hippocampus from the CCL2-tg SJL mice at 7–12 months of age, both the fEPSP and PS showed a reduction in magnitude compared to non-tg hippocampus [61]. This difference between CCL2-tg and CCL2-tg SJL hippocampus may be due to the older age or the higher level of CCL2 expression in the CCL2-tg SJL hippocampus. In contrast to the IL-6 tg, CCL2-tg and CCL2-tg SJL hippocampus, there was no significant difference in the magnitude of the fEPSP or PS between the CXCL10 tg and non-tg hippocampus from 5–6 months old mice [68].

5.2. *Synaptic Plasticity in IL-6 tg, CCL2-tg and CXCL-10 tg Mice*

Synaptic plasticity is a change in the magnitude of synaptic responses that results when a synapse is repetitively stimulated. Synaptic plasticity is considered to be an important cellular mechanism of memory and learning [71]. Short-term and/or long-term synaptic plasticity at the Schaffer collateral to CA1 pyramidal neuron synapse has been studied in one or more of the transgenic lines. Results are summarized in Table 1.

5.2.1. Short-Term Synaptic Plasticity

In this form of synaptic plasticity, repetitive activation of a synapse at short intervals (<1 s) elicits a transient increase or decrease in the magnitude of the synaptic response. Short-term synaptic plasticity is experimentally determined by applying repetitive stimulation to the Schaffer collaterals using a paired-pulse (P-P) paradigm. The magnitude of the plasticity is indicated by the paired-pulse ratio (PPR, magnitude of the response to the 2nd stimulation divided by magnitude of the response to the 1st stimulation). At the Schaffer collateral to CA1 pyramidal neuron synapse the paired-pulse protocol results in an enhancement the fEPSP (*i.e.*, a PPR greater than 1, Figure 2A). This enhancement is referred to as paired-pulse facilitation (PPF). PPF reflects greater transmitter release with the 2nd stimulation due to actions of residue Ca^{2+} on the probably of transmitter release in the presynaptic terminals of the Schaffer collaterals [72–74].

There was no difference in PPF of the fEPSP between the hippocampus from IL-6 tg and non-tg mice at either age studied (1–2 and 3–6 months of age) [60]. The hippocampus from CCL2-tg and non-tg mice studied at 2–3 months of age also showed no difference in PPF of the fEPSP [67]. In the 7–12 months CCL2-tg SJL mice, PPF of the fEPSP was increased at the 40 ms paired-pulse interval but not at longer intervals compared to the hippocampus from non-tg mice, indicating activity-induced presynaptic changes that impact excitatory synaptic transmission in a limited manner [61]. There was no significant difference in the PPF between the CXCL10 tg and non-tg hippocampus from 5–6 months old mice [68].

A second form of short-term plasticity induced by synaptic activation occurs in the somatic region of the CA1 neurons and affects the PS that is generated by the fEPSP. Plasticity of the PS can result in a PPR greater than one (less inhibition; Figure 2B) or less than one (more inhibition) depending on the relative contribution of somatic/dendritic excitability and recurrent inhibition to the somatic region. There was no difference in PPR of the PS between the hippocampus from IL-6 tg and non-tg mice at either age studied (1–2 and 3–5 months of age) [60], or between the hippocampus from CCL2-tg and non-tg mice at 2–3 months of age [67]. PPR of the PS in the hippocampus from 7–12 months old CCL2-tg SJL mice was increased compared to the hippocampus from non-tg mice, indicating decreased inhibitory influences in the soma/dendritic region [61]. There was no significant difference in PPR of the PS between the CXCL10 tg and non-tg hippocampus from 5–6 months old mice [68].

5.2.2. Long-Term Synaptic Plasticity

Long-lasting changes in synaptic transmission are also observed at the Schaffer collateral to CA1 pyramidal neuron synapse. These changes can involve an increase in the magnitude of the synaptic response, referred to as long-term potentiation (LTP), or a decrease in the magnitude of the synaptic response, referred to as long-term depression (LTD). LTP is experimentally induced by brief, high frequency stimulation of the Schaffer collaterals, whereas LTD is induced experimentally by prolonged stimulation of the Schaffer collaterals at low frequency. LTP has been studied in hippocampal slices from the IL-6 tg, CCL2-tg, CCL2-tg SJL and CXCL10-tg mice, but studies on LTD have not appeared.

High frequency stimulation (HFS) of the Schaffer collaterals induces an immediate and dramatic increase in the amplitude of the fEPSP, after which the enhancement declines somewhat to a steady, stable level reflecting LTP (Figure 2C). The initial enhancement is a shorter form of synaptic plasticity referred to as post-tetanic potentiation (PTP). PTP results from the impact of HFS on presynaptic mechanisms involved in transmitter release. LTP, the delayed, persistent, stable increase in the magnitude of the fEPSP is primarily a result of activity-induced changes in post-synaptic mechanisms. Results from studies of long-term synaptic plasticity are shown in Table 1.

In the IL-6 tg line, there was no genotypic difference in LTP between IL-6 and non-tg hippocampus from both young (1–2 months of age) and adult (3–6 months of age) mice. PTP was reduced in the hippocampus from young (1–2 months of age) IL-6 tg mice compared to the hippocampus from non-tg mice, indicating changes in presynaptic function, a genotypic effect that was not observed for IL-6 and non-tg hippocampus from adult mice (3–6 months of age) [60]. In both the CCL2-tg and CXCL10-tg lines, no genotypic effect on PTP or LTP was observed between the hippocampus from transgenic *vs.* non-tg mice [67,68]. PTP was enhanced in the hippocampus from the CCL2-tg SJL mice compared with the hippocampus from the non-tg mice, but there was no genotypic difference in LTP.

5.3. *Effect of Acute Application of Neuroimmune Factors on Synaptic Function*

In addition to studies of the hippocampus from transgenic mice, studies on the effects of acute, exogenous applied IL-6 or CXCL10 on synaptic transmission and plasticity at the Schaffer collateral to CA1 pyramidal synapse have been carried out in hippocampal slices from rat or mice. The effect of acute exposure is of interest because it presumably reflects to some degree the actions of the endogenous cytokine or chemokine during the initial stages of elevated expression in the transgenic mice. Results are summarized in Table 2. There was no significant effect of exogenously applied IL-6 on the fEPSP or PS of rat hippocampal slices. There was also no significant effect of exogenously applied CXCL10 on the fEPSP in hippocampal slices from the CXCL10 tg and non-tg mice [68]. The effect of acute, exogenous applied CCL2 on synaptic transmission was studied in the rat hippocampal slices using whole cell voltage clamp techniques. CCL2 enhanced the excitatory postsynaptic currents elicited by stimulation of the Schaffer collaterals, an effect shown to result from actions of CCL2 on presynaptic mechanisms [75,76].

Although acute, exogenous application of IL-6 or CXCL10 had no effect on baseline synaptic transmission, IL-6 significantly reduced PTP and LTP in rat hippocampal slices [77,78]. Exogenous application of CXCL-10 also significantly reduced both PTP and LTP hippocampal slices from the non-tg mice, but only LTP in hippocampal slices from CXCL10-tg mice [68]. The lack of effect of CXCL-10 on PTP in the CXCL10-tg hippocampus, suggest neuroadaptive changes in the CXCL10-tg mice that prevent the actions of acute CXCL-10.

Table 2. Effects of exogenous application of neuroimmune factor on synaptic function in hippocampus.

Measurement	Neuroimmune Factor				
	IL-6		CCL2	CXCL10 non-tg	CXCL10 tg
species	rat	rat	rat	mouse	mouse
Age (months) or weight (gm)	2–3 months	200–250 gm	0.5–1 month	5–6 months	5–6 months
Concentration	1, 5, 50 ng/mL	50–2000 U/mL	2.3 nM	10 ng/mL	10 ng/mL
Synaptic transmission					
-fEPSP or EPSC	nd	no Δ	↑	no Δ	nd
-Population spike	no Δ	nd	nd	nd	nd
Short-term synaptic plasticity					
-fEPSP (PPF)	no Δ	nd	nd	↑	no Δ
-Population spike (PPR)	nd	nd	nd	nd	nd
Long-term synaptic plasticity					
-PTP	↓	↓	nd	↓	no Δ
-LTP	↓	↓	nd	↓	↓
Reference	[79]	[78]	[75]	[68]	

↓ = decrease, ↑ = increase, no Δ = no difference, nd = not determined. EPSC = excitatory postsynaptic current.

Taken together, these results show that mechanisms that induce LTP and PTP are sensitive to acute exposure to IL-6 or CXCL10. Thus, the lack of genotypic differences in LTP and PTP between the IL-6 tg and non-tg hippocampus and the CXCL10-tg and non-tg hippocampus may reflect neuroadaptive changes in mechanisms that induce LTP and PTP. These neuroadaptive changes produced an apparent normalization of function. Effects of acute, exogenous application of CCL2 on PTP and LTP have not been reported.

6. Protein Levels in Hippocampus

IL-6, CCL2, and CXCL10 signal transduction pathways can lead to downstream effects on gene expression and, consequently, changes in the levels of important cellular and synaptic proteins. Changes in protein levels could also occur through other regulatory mechanisms. Such neuroadaptive changes could impact synaptic function. Western blot studies were carried out to identify potential changes in protein levels in the hippocampus from IL-6 tg and CCL2-tg mice. CXCL10-tg mice have not examined. Relatively few changes in protein levels were observed in the hippocampus from the IL-6 tg and CCL2-tg mice compared to hippocampus from their respective non-tg mice, as shown in Table 3. These results are consistent with the relative lack of neuropathological changes observed in the hippocampus from the IL-6 tg and CCL2-tg mice at the ages studied. However, some differences were observed that could affect synaptic function.

Table 3. Genotypic differences on protein levels in hippocampus.

Measurement	IL-6 tg *vs.* Non-tg		CCL2-tg *vs.* Non-tg		CCL2-tg SJL *vs.* Non-tg	
Age (months)	1–2	3–5	1–3	3–5	3–4	7–9
Housekeeping proteins						
-β-actin	no Δ	no Δ	no Δ	no Δ	no Δ	no Δ
Astrocyte proteins						
-GFAP	↑	↑	no Δ	no Δ	no Δ	↑
-Glutamine synthetase	no Δ	no Δ	no Δ	no Δ	nd	nd
Microglial protein						
-CD11b	nd	no Δ	no Δ	nd	↑	no Δ
Neuronal proteins						
-Enolase	no Δ	no Δ	no Δ	no Δ	no Δ	no Δ
-GAD65/67	no Δ	↓	no Δ	no Δ	no Δ	no Δ
Synaptic proteins						
-Synapsin 1	no Δ	no Δ	no Δ	↑	no Δ	no Δ
-VGLUT1	nd	no Δ	no Δ	nd	nd	nd
-GluA1	no Δ	no Δ	no Δ	no Δ	no Δ	no Δ
-GluN1	no Δ	no Δ	↑	↑	no Δ	no Δ
Signal transduction						
-STAT3	↑	↑	no Δ	nd	nd	nd
-p42/44 MAPK	no Δ	no Δ	no Δ	no Δ	nd	nd
Reference	[58,60]		[58,67]		[61]	

↓ = decrease, ↑ = increase, no Δ = no difference, nd = not determined.

Compared to the hippocampus from non-tg mice, the hippocampus from IL-6 tg mice showed elevated levels of GFAP and STAT3, the signal transduction molecule that is involved in IL-6 regulation of GFAP gene expression [59,60]. The level of phosphorylated (*i.e.*, activated) STAT3 was also elevated in the hippocampus from IL-6 tg mice [59,60]. Another astrocytic protein, glutamate synthetase, which is involved in glutamate cycling, an important aspect of excitatory synaptic transmission [80], was not altered in the hippocampus from the IL-6 tg mice [60], suggesting that the increased levels of GFAP do not reflect a general action of IL-6 on astrocytic protein levels. The increased levels of activated STAT3 in the hippocampus of IL-6 tg mice could affect synaptic function. STAT3 has been shown to be highly expressed in CNS neurons, where it is present in the postsynaptic density, and to regulate synaptic plasticity (LTD) in the hippocampus [1]. In addition to increased levels of GFAP and STAT3, reduced levels of GAD65/67, the synthetic enzyme for the inhibitory transmitter GABA, were observed in the IL-6 tg hippocampus [60], consistent with the immunohistochemical studies indicating a negative effect of the elevated levels of IL-6 on the structure of inhibitory interneurons [49,54].

Compared to the hippocampus from non-tg mice, the hippocampus from CCL2-tg mice showed elevated levels of synapsin 1, a presynaptic protein involved in transmitter release, and GluN1, the essential subunit of NMDA receptors [58,67]. NMDA receptors play a critical role in neuronal development, synaptic plasticity, and neuronal toxicity, and are an important target site for therapeutic intervention in a number of neurological disorders [81,82]. The neuroadaptive changes in synapsin 1 and GluN1 levels were not evident in the CCL2-tg SJL hippocampus, where the only changes were an increase in CD11b and GFAP [61]. Taken together, these results show that neuroadaptive changes occur at the level of synaptic proteins in the IL-6 tg and CCL2-tg hippocampus. The differences in proteins targeted in the IL-6 tg and CCL2-tg hippocampus could contribute to differences in the synaptic properties altered in the two transgenic lines.

7. Behavioral Studies

Alterations in synaptic function can result in changes in behavior. Two behavioral tests that evaluate the functioning of the hippocampus are the avoidance learning test and the contextual fear conditioning test. These behavioral tests were used examine hippocampal function in the IL-6 tg or CCL2-tg lines. Behavior has not been tested in the CXCL10-tg line. The IL-6 tg mice did not show a behavioral deficit compared to non-tg mice in the avoidance learning when tested at 3 months of age. However, by 6 months of age the IL-6 tg mice exhibited a significant deficit in their ability to learn the avoidance response, which declined further by 12 months of age [54]. The CCL2-tg mice were examined in behavioral tests for contextual fear conditioning at 2–3 months of age. There were no significant differences between the CCL2-tg and non-tg mice in these tests [67]. These results suggest the lack of significant hippocampal dysfunction at 3 months of age in both the IL-6 tg and CCL2 tg mice, at least under baseline conditions in these tests.

8. Covert Neuroadaptive Changes

Taken together, studies of synaptic function and protein expression in the hippocampus from IL-6 tg and CCL2-tg mice revealed relatively few neuroadaptive changes produced by the respective neuroimmune factor under baseline conditions, although the observed changes could significantly alter CNS function depending on physiological or pathological context. However, studies on the effects of acute alcohol on synaptic function in the hippocampus from IL-6 tg and CCL2-tg mice and their respective non-tg controls revealed covert neuroadaptive changes that resulted in an altered the response to alcohol (Table 4). For example, although there was no difference in the magnitude of PTP and LTP in hippocampal slices from IL-6 tg or CCL2-tg mice compared to their respective non-tg controls under baseline conditions, exposure to acute alcohol (60 mM) depressed PTP and LTP in hippocampal slices from non-tg mice from both the IL-6 and CCL-2 lines, while PTP and LTP in hippocampal slices from the IL-6 tg and CCL2-tg hippocampus were resistant to this effect of acute alcohol [67,70]. Thus, the hippocampus from the IL-6 tg and CCL2-tg mice showed a similar resistance to the depressing effects of alcohol on LTP and PTP. Differences in the response to alcohol were also observed between IL-6 tg and CCL2-tg mice in the effects of alcohol on the fEPSP and PS. For example, 60 mM acute alcohol reduced the fEPSP and PS in hippocampal slices from non-tg mice from the IL-6 and CCL2 lines and in hippocampal slices from CCL2-tg mice, whereas in hippocampal slices from IL-6 tg mice the same dose of alcohol increased the fEPSP and PS [67,70]. 60 mM alcohol is a pharmacologically relevant dose that would produce severe intoxication in humans.

Table 4. Effects of alcohol on synaptic function in hippocampus.

Measurement	60 mM Alcohol *vs.* Baseline			
	Non-tg	IL-6 tg	Non-tg	CCL2-tg
Synaptic transmission				
-fEPSP	↓	↑	↓	↓
-PS	↓	↑	↓	↓
P-P synaptic plasticity				
-fEPSP (PPF)	no Δ	no Δ	no Δ	no Δ
-PS (PPR)	↑	no Δ	↑	no Δ
Long-term synaptic plasticity				
-PTP	↓	no Δ	↓	no Δ
-LTP	↓	no Δ	↓	no Δ
Reference	[70]		[67]	

↓ = decrease, ↑ = increase, no Δ = no difference.

A difference in response to alcohol was also observed in behavioral studies of alcohol actions. In one study of alcohol withdrawal hyperexcitability, IL-6 tg and CCL2-tg mice and their non-tg littermates were exposed to an acute, high dose of alcohol (4 gm/kg, i.p.), which initially causes sedation, but during the phase of declining blood alcohol levels, CNS hyperexcitability is produced. The hyperexcitability was measured by handling induced convulsions (HIC) [83,84]. The IL-6 tg mice showed significantly higher HIC scores than their non-tg controls, indicating greater hyperexcitability, whereas CCL2-tg and their non-tg mice showed similar HIC scores [70]. In behavioral tests for contextual fear conditioning, there were no significant differences between the CCL2-tg and non-tg mice under baseline conditions. Acute alcohol (1 gm/kg, i.p.) significantly impaired the non-tg mice but not the CCL2-tg mice in this behavioral test [67]. In contrast, in the rotorod test, which is considered primarily a cerebellar mediated behavior, CCL2-tg and non-tg mice show no difference in recovery from the effects of acute alcohol (2 gm/kg, i.p.) [67]. A similar result was obtained for the effects of acute alcohol (2 gm/kg, i.p.) on IL-6 tg and non-tg mice in the rotarod test (recovery time = 176.2 $\pm$ 9.3 min for non-tg and 171.2 $\pm$ 9.0 min for IL-6 tg).

Covert changes were also revealed in other studies of the IL-6 tg mice. Systemic exposure (i.p. injection) to a low dose of kainate or NMDA induced prominent seizures and lethality in IL-6-tg mice but not in the non-tg mice, which required a higher dose to produce such effects [69]. Also, basal plasma corticosterone levels were normal in IL-6-tg mice but, after restraint stress, abnormally increased levels were observed in the IL-6 tg mice compared to non-tg mice [85]. Thus, in addition to the detected neuroadaptive changes in baseline functions and behavior, covert neuroadaptive changes are produced by the chronic exposure to IL-6 and CCL2 and can be revealed within certain contexts. Such neuroadaptive changes could play an important role in pathophysiological conditions.

9. Conclusions

Although a large literature has demonstrated elevated CNS expression of cytokines and chemokines in CNS disease and injury, a relatively small number of studies have examined the consequences of the elevated expression at the synaptic level. The transgenic approach provides tools for such studies. Transgenic models that target astrocyte production of neuroimmune factors have enabled studies that provide a basic understanding of the synaptic consequence of persistent elevated expression of a specific neuroimmune factor by this CNS cell type. This information can facilitate identification of potential contributions of the neuroimmune factor to a more complex condition when multiple neuroimmune factors are expressed. This information may also be useful for identification of the actions/role of specific neuroimmune factors in CNS physiology. The astrocyte targeted transgenic models complement traditional approaches involving knock out (KO) models. In the KO model, all cell types are affected and, therefore, the KO models provide more global information about the involvement of a specific neuroimmune factor in CNS development, function or dysfunction. One caveat to these models is that expression in the transgenic model or lack of expression in the KO model occurs over the lifespan of the animal, which could influence CNS development. It is unclear if or how potential development effects would impact studies in adult animals. However, emerging research on the actions of neuroimmune factors on CNS development is starting to provide answers to this question.

Overall, the studies of synaptic function in the hippocampus from the three transgenic lines revealed relatively few alterations. This result is consistent with the relative lack of neuropathology in the hippocampus of the transgenic mice at the ages studied, and raises the possibility that additional factors may be necessary when pathology is observed. Both similarities and differences were observed in the effects of the three neuroimmune factors on synaptic function, suggesting that similarities and differences exist in underlying mechanisms, and are likely to be reflected in the consequences of elevated expression under different pathological contexts.

Although only a limited number of neuroadaptive changes in synaptic function were identified under basal conditions, several experimental manipulations revealed that covert neuroadaptive changes were produced by elevated expression of the neuroimmune factors. These covert neuroadaptive changes may have been responsible for the apparent normalization of function under baseline conditions such that genotypic differences were not observed. The identification of covert actions illustrates the importance of physiological or pathological context in the consequence of cytokine or chemokine actions in the CNS. Both the identified and covert neuroadaptive changes resulting from increased astrocyte production of the neuroimmune factors could contribute to cognitive impairment in a pathological context.

The mechanisms and molecular targets underlying the neuroadaptive changes produced by IL-6, CCL2, and CXCL10 have yet to be elucidated. Studies to address these issues are an important future direction, and are essential for a more complete understanding of the actions and roles of IL-6, CCL2 and CXCL10 in CNS physiology and pathology. The level of expression, duration of exposure, presence of other neuroimmune factors, and biological context are all likely to be important variables, and their biological impact will also need to be resolved in future studies. Taken together, such information could reveal new targets for therapeutic intervention for a range of pathophysiological conditions that are associated with increased expression of IL-6, CCL2 and/or CXCL10 in the CNS.

Acknowledgments: Supported by NIAAA Grant AA019261.

References

1. Nicolas, C.S.; Peineau, S.; Amici, M.; Csaba, Z.; Fafouri, A.; Javalet, C.; Collett, V.J.; Hildebrandt, L.; Seaton, G.; Choi, S.L.; *et al.* The JAK/STAT pathway is involved in synaptic plasticity. *Neuron* **2012**, *73*, 374–390. [CrossRef] [PubMed]
2. Zheng, C.; Zhou, X.W.; Wang, J.Z. The dual roles of cytokines in Alzheimer's disease: Update on interleukins, TNF-α, TGF-β and IFN-γ. *Transl. Neurodegener.* **2016**. [CrossRef] [PubMed]
3. De Vries, E.E.; van den Munckhof, B.; Braun, K.P.; van Royen-Kerkhof, A.; de Jager, W.; Jansen, F.E. Inflammatory mediators in human epilepsy: A systematic review and meta-analysis. *Neurosci. Biobehav. Rev.* **2016**, *63*, 177–190. [CrossRef] [PubMed]
4. Rothhammer, V.; Quintana, F.J. Control of autoimmune CNS inflammation by astrocytes. *Semin. Immunopathol.* **2015**, *37*, 625–638. [CrossRef] [PubMed]
5. Crews, F.T.; Vetreno, R.P. Neuroimmune basis of alcoholic brain damage. *Int. Rev. Neurobiol.* **2014**, *118*, 315–357. [PubMed]
6. Drew, P.D.; Kane, C.J. Fetal alcohol spectrum disorders and neuroimmune changes. *Int. Rev. Neurobiol.* **2014**, *118*, 41–80. [PubMed]
7. Chastain, L.G.; Sarkar, D.K. Role of microglia in regulation of ethanol neurotoxic action. *Int. Rev. Neurobiol.* **2014**, *118*, 81–103. [PubMed]

8. Tomasik, J.; Rahmoune, H.; Guest, P.C.; Bahn, S. Neuroimmune biomarkers in schizophrenia. *Schizophr. Res.* **2014**. in press.
9. Shie, F.S.; Chen, Y.H.; Chen, C.H.; Ho, I.K. Neuroimmune pharmacology of neurodegenerative and mental diseases. *J. Neuroimmune Pharmacol.* **2011**, *6*, 28–40. [CrossRef] [PubMed]
10. Gottfried, C.; Bambini-Junior, V.; Francis, F.; Riesgo, R.; Savino, W. The impact of neuroimmune alterations in autism spectrum disorder. *Front. Psychiatry* **2015**. [CrossRef] [PubMed]
11. Hein, A.M.; O'Banion, M.K. Neuroinflammation and cognitive dysfunction in chronic disease and aging. *J. Neuroimmune Pharmacol.* **2012**, *7*, 3–6. [CrossRef] [PubMed]
12. Patterson, S.L. Immune dysregulation and cognitive vulnerability in the aging brain: Interactions of microglia, IL-1β, BDNF and synaptic plasticity. *Neuropharmacology* **2015**, *96*, 11–18. [CrossRef] [PubMed]
13. Eichenbaum, H. Hippocampus: Cognitive processes and neural representations that underlie declarative memory. *Neuron* **2004**, *44*, 109–120. [CrossRef] [PubMed]
14. Di Filippo, M.; Chiasserini, D.; Gardoni, F.; Viviani, B.; Tozzi, A.; Giampa, C.; Costa, C.; Tantucci, M.; Zianni, E.; Boraso, M.; *et al.* Effects of central and peripheral inflammation on hippocampal synaptic plasticity. *Neurobiol. Dis.* **2013**, *52*, 229–236. [CrossRef] [PubMed]
15. Zink, W.E.; Anderson, E.; Boyle, J.; Hock, L.; Rodriguez-Sierra, J.; Xiong, H.; Gendelman, H.E.; Persidsky, Y. Impaired spatial cognition and synaptic potentiation in a murine model of human immunodeficiency virus type 1 encephalitis. *J. Neurosci.* **2002**, *22*, 2096–2105. [PubMed]
16. Savanthrapadian, S.; Wolff, A.R.; Logan, B.J.; Eckert, M.J.; Bilkey, D.K.; Abraham, W.C. Enhanced hippocampal neuronal excitability and LTP persistence associated with reduced behavioral flexibility in the maternal immune activation model of schizophrenia. *Hippocampus* **2013**, *23*, 1395–1409. [CrossRef] [PubMed]
17. Mosayebi, G.; Soleyman, M.R.; Khalili, M.; Mosleh, M.; Palizvan, M.R. Changes in synaptic transmission and long-term potentiation induction as a possible mechanism for learning disability in an animal model of multiple sclerosis. *Int. Neurourol. J.* **2016**, *20*, 26–32. [CrossRef] [PubMed]
18. Fernandez-Fernandez, D.; Dorner-Ciossek, C.; Kroker, K.S.; Rosenbrock, H. Age-related synaptic dysfunction in tg2576 mice starts as a failure in early long-term potentiation which develops into a full abolishment of late long-term potentiation. *J. Neurosci. Res.* **2016**, *94*, 266–281. [CrossRef] [PubMed]
19. Imamura, Y.; Wang, H.; Matsumoto, N.; Muroya, T.; Shimazaki, J.; Ogura, H.; Shimazu, T. Interleukin-1β causes long-term potentiation deficiency in a mouse model of septic encephalopathy. *Neuroscience* **2011**, *187*, 63–69. [CrossRef] [PubMed]
20. Batti, L.; O'Connor, J.J. Tumor necrosis factor-α impairs the recovery of synaptic transmission from hypoxia in rat hippocampal slices. *J. Neuroimmunol.* **2010**, *218*, 21–27. [CrossRef] [PubMed]
21. Rossi, S.; Motta, C.; Studer, V.; Barbieri, F.; Buttari, F.; Bergami, A.; Sancesario, G.; Bernardini, S.; de Angelis, G.; Martino, G.; *et al.* Tumor necrosis factor is elevated in progressive multiple sclerosis and causes excitotoxic neurodegeneration. *Mult. Scler.* **2014**, *20*, 304–312. [CrossRef] [PubMed]
22. Bateup, H.S.; Johnson, C.A.; Denefrio, C.L.; Saulnier, J.L.; Kornacker, K.; Sabatini, B.L. Excitatory/inhibitory synaptic imbalance leads to hippocampal hyperexcitability in mouse models of tuberous sclerosis. *Neuron* **2013**, *78*, 510–522. [CrossRef] [PubMed]
23. Costa, C.; Sgobio, C.; Siliquini, S.; Tozzi, A.; Tantucci, M.; Ghiglieri, V.; di Filippo, M.; Pendolino, V.; de Iure, A.; Marti, M.; *et al.* Mechanisms underlying the impairment of hippocampal long-term potentiation and memory in experimental Parkinson's disease. *Br. J. Neurol.* **2012**, *135*, 1884–1899. [CrossRef] [PubMed]
24. Scott-McKean, J.J.; Costa, A.C. Exaggerated NMDA mediated LTD in a mouse model of down syndrome and pharmacological rescuing by memantine. *Learn. Mem.* **2011**, *18*, 774–778. [CrossRef] [PubMed]
25. Roberto, M.; Nelson, T.E.; Ur, C.L.; Gruol, D.L. Long-term potentiation in the rat hippocampus is reversibly depressed by chronic intermittent ethanol exposure. *J. Neurophysiol.* **2002**, *87*, 2385–2397. [PubMed]
26. Biber, K.; Pinto-Duarte, A.; Wittendorp, M.C.; Dolga, A.M.; Fernandes, C.C.; von Frijtag Drabbe Kunzel, J.; Keijser, J.N.; de Vries, R.; Ijzerman, A.P.; Ribeiro, J.A.; *et al.* Interleukin-6 upregulates neuronal adenosine A1 receptors: Implications for neuromodulation and neuroprotection. *Neuropsychopharmacology* **2008**, *33*, 2237–2250. [CrossRef] [PubMed]
27. Penkowa, M.; Giralt, M.; Lago, N.; Camats, J.; Carrasco, J.; Hernandez, J.; Molinero, A.; Campbell, I.L.; Hidalgo, J. Astrocyte-targeted expression of IL-6 protects the CNS against a focal brain injury. *Exp. Neurol.* **2003**, *181*, 130–148. [CrossRef]

28. Millington, C.; Sonego, S.; Karunaweera, N.; Rangel, A.; Aldrich-Wright, J.R.; Campbell, I.L.; Gyengesi, E.; Munch, G. Chronic neuroinflammation in Alzheimer's disease: New perspectives on animal models and promising candidate drugs. *BioMed Res. Int.* **2014**. [CrossRef] [PubMed]
29. Boztug, K.; Carson, M.J.; Pham-Mitchell, N.; Asensio, V.C.; DeMartino, J.; Campbell, I.L. Leukocyte infiltration, but not neurodegeneration, in the CNS of transgenic mice with astrocyte production of the CXC chemokine ligand 10. *J. Immunol.* **2002**, *169*, 1505–1515. [CrossRef] [PubMed]
30. Kiyota, T.; Yamamoto, M.; Xiong, H.; Lambert, M.P.; Klein, W.L.; Gendelman, H.E.; Ransohoff, R.M.; Ikezu, T. CCL2 accelerates microglia-mediated Aβ oligomer formation and progression of neurocognitive dysfunction. *PLoS ONE* **2009**, *4*, e6197. [CrossRef] [PubMed]
31. Elhofy, A.; Wang, J.; Tani, M.; Fife, B.T.; Kennedy, K.J.; Bennett, J.; Huang, D.; Ransohoff, R.M.; Karpus, W.J. Transgenic expression of CCL2 in the central nervous system prevents experimental autoimmune encephalomyelitis. *J. Leukoc. Biol.* **2005**, *77*, 229–237. [CrossRef] [PubMed]
32. Huang, D.; Wujek, J.; Kidd, G.; He, T.T.; Cardona, A.; Sasse, M.E.; Stein, E.J.; Kish, J.; Tani, M.; Charo, I.F.; *et al.* Chronic expression of monocyte chemoattractant protein-1 in the central nervous system causes delayed encephalopathy and impaired microglial function in mice. *FASEB J.* **2005**, *19*, 761–772. [CrossRef] [PubMed]
33. Almolda, B.; Villacampa, N.; Manders, P.; Hidalgo, J.; Campbell, I.L.; Gonzalez, B.; Castellano, B. Effects of astrocyte-targeted production of interleukin-6 in the mouse on the host response to nerve injury. *Glia* **2014**, *62*, 1142–1161. [CrossRef] [PubMed]
34. Huang, D.; Tani, M.; Wang, J.; Han, Y.; He, T.T.; Weaver, J.; Charo, I.F.; Tuohy, V.K.; Rollins, B.J.; Ransohoff, R.M. Pertussis toxin-induced reversible encephalopathy dependent on monocyte chemoattractant protein-1 overexpression in mice. *J. Neurosci.* **2002**, *22*, 10633–10642. [PubMed]
35. Jensen, C.J.; Massie, A.; de Keyser, J. Immune players in the CNS: The astrocyte. *J. Neuroimmune Pharmacol.* **2013**, *8*, 824–839. [CrossRef] [PubMed]
36. Ransom, B.R.; Ransom, C.B. Astrocytes: Multitalented stars of the central nervous system. *Methods Mol. Biol.* **2012**, *814*, 3–7. [PubMed]
37. Finsterwald, C.; Magistretti, P.J.; Lengacher, S. Astrocytes: New targets for the treatment of neurodegenerative diseases. *Curr. Pharma. Des.* **2015**, *21*, 3570–3581. [CrossRef]
38. Halassa, M.M.; Fellin, T.; Haydon, P.G. The tripartite synapse: Roles for gliotransmission in health and disease. *Trends Mol. Med.* **2007**, *13*, 54–63. [CrossRef] [PubMed]
39. Ota, Y.; Zanetti, A.T.; Hallock, R.M. The role of astrocytes in the regulation of synaptic plasticity and memory formation. *Neural Plast.* **2013**. [CrossRef] [PubMed]
40. Gruart, A.; Delgado-Garcia, J.M. Activity-dependent changes of the hippocampal CA3-CA1 synapse during the acquisition of associative learning in conscious mice. *Genes Brain Behav.* **2007**, *6*, 24–31. [CrossRef] [PubMed]
41. Gruol, D.L. IL-6 regulation of synaptic function in the CNS. *Neuropharmacology* **2015**. [CrossRef] [PubMed]
42. Campbell, I.L.; Erta, M.; Lim, S.L.; Frausto, R.; May, U.; Rose-John, S.; Scheller, J.; Hidalgo, J. Trans-signaling is a dominant mechanism for the pathogenic actions of interleukin-6 in the brain. *J. Neurosci.* **2014**, *34*, 2503–2513. [CrossRef] [PubMed]
43. Vollenweider, F.; Herrmann, M.; Otten, U.; Nitsch, C. Interleukin-6 receptor expression and localization after transient global ischemia in gerbil hippocampus. *Neurosci. Lett.* **2003**, *341*, 49–52. [CrossRef]
44. Chang, G.Q.; Karatayev, O.; Leibowitz, S.F. Prenatal exposure to ethanol stimulates hypothalamic CCR2 chemokine receptor system: Possible relation to increased density of orexigenic peptide neurons and ethanol drinking in adolescent offspring. *Neuroscience* **2015**, *310*, 163–175. [CrossRef] [PubMed]
45. Van der Meer, P.; Ulrich, A.M.; Gonzalez-Scarano, F.; Lavi, E. Immunohistochemical analysis of CCR2, CCR3, CCR5, and CXCR4 in the human brain: Potential mechanisms for HIV dementia. *Exp. Mol. Pathol.* **2000**, *69*, 192–201. [CrossRef] [PubMed]
46. Banisadr, G.; Gosselin, R.D.; Mechighel, P.; Rostene, W.; Kitabgi, P.; Parsadaniantz, S.M. Constitutive neuronal expression of CCR2 chemokine receptor and its colocalization with neurotransmitters in normal rat brain: Functional effect of MCP-1/CCL2 on calcium mobilization in primary cultured neurons. *J. Comp. Neurol.* **2005**, *492*, 178–192. [CrossRef] [PubMed]
47. Ragozzino, D. CXC chemokine receptors in the central nervous system: Role in cerebellar neuromodulation and development. *J. Neurovirol.* **2002**, *8*, 559–572. [CrossRef] [PubMed]

48. Xia, M.Q.; Bacskai, B.J.; Knowles, R.B.; Qin, S.X.; Hyman, B.T. Expression of the chemokine receptor CXCR3 on neurons and the elevated expression of its ligand IP-10 in reactive astrocytes: *In vitro* ERK1/2 activation and role in Alzheimer's disease. *J. Neuroimmunol.* **2000**, *108*, 227–235. [CrossRef]
49. Campbell, I.L.; Abraham, C.R.; Masliah, E.; Kemper, P.; Inglis, J.D.; Oldstone, M.B.; Mucke, L. Neurologic disease induced in transgenic mice by cerebral overexpression of interleukin 6. *Proc. Natl. Acad. Sci. USA* **1993**, *90*, 10061–10065. [CrossRef] [PubMed]
50. Brenner, M.; Messing, A. GFAP transgenic mice. *Methods* **1996**, *10*, 351–364. [CrossRef] [PubMed]
51. Su, M.; Hu, H.; Lee, Y.; D'Azzo, A.; Messing, A.; Brenner, M. Expression specificity of GFAP transgenes. *Neurochem. Res.* **2004**, *29*, 2075–2093. [CrossRef] [PubMed]
52. Chiang, C.S.; Stalder, A.; Samimi, A.; Campbell, I.L. Reactive gliosis as a consequence of interleukin-6 expression in the brain: Studies in transgenic mice. *Dev. Neurosci.* **1994**, *16*, 212–221. [CrossRef] [PubMed]
53. Kim, J.S.; Kim, J.; Kim, Y.; Yang, M.; Jang, H.; Kang, S.; Kim, J.C.; Kim, S.H.; Shin, T.; Moon, C. Differential patterns of nestin and glial fibrillary acidic protein expression in mouse hippocampus during postnatal development. *J. Vet. Sci.* **2011**, *12*, 1–6. [CrossRef] [PubMed]
54. Heyser, C.J.; Masliah, E.; Samimi, A.; Campbell, I.L.; Gold, L.H. Progressive decline in avoidance learning paralleled by inflammatory neurodegeneration in transgenic mice expressing interleukin 6 in the brain. *Proc. Natl. Acad. Sci. USA* **1997**, *94*, 1500–1505. [CrossRef] [PubMed]
55. Vallieres, L.; Campbell, I.L.; Gage, F.H.; Sawchenko, P.E. Reduced hippocampal neurogenesis in adult transgenic mice with chronic astrocytic production of interleukin-6. *J. Neurosci.* **2002**, *22*, 486–492. [PubMed]
56. Gruol, D.L.; Vo, K.; Bray, J.G.; Roberts, A.J. CCL2-ethanol interactions and hippocampal synaptic protein expression in a transgenic mouse model. *Front. Integr. Neurosci.* **2014**. [CrossRef] [PubMed]
57. Quintana, A.; Erta, M.; Ferrer, B.; Comes, G.; Giralt, M.; Hidalgo, J. Astrocyte-specific deficiency of interleukin-6 and its receptor reveal specific roles in survival, body weight and behavior. *Brain Behav. Immun.* **2013**, *27*, 162–173. [CrossRef] [PubMed]
58. Gruol, D.L.; Vo, K.; Bray, J.G. Increased astrocyte expression of IL-6 or CCL2 in transgenic mice alters levels of hippocampal and cerebellar proteins. *Front. Cell Neurosci.* **2014**. [CrossRef] [PubMed]
59. Sanz, E.; Hofer, M.J.; Unzeta, M.; Campbell, I.L. Minimal role for stat1 in interleukin-6 signaling and actions in the murine brain. *Glia* **2008**, *56*, 190–199. [CrossRef] [PubMed]
60. Nelson, T.E.; Engberink, A.O.; Hernandez, R.; Puro, A.; Huitron-Resendiz, S.; Hao, C.; de Graan, P.N.; Gruol, D.L. Altered synaptic transmission in the hippocampus of transgenic mice with enhanced central nervous systems expression of interleukin-6. *Brain Behav. Immun.* **2012**, *26*, 959–971. [CrossRef] [PubMed]
61. Nelson, T.E.; Hao, C.; Manos, J.; Ransohoff, R.M.; Gruol, D.L. Altered hippocampal synaptic transmission in transgenic mice with astrocyte-targeted enhanced CCL2 expression. *Brain Behav. Immun.* **2011**, *25* (Suppl. S1), S106–S119. [CrossRef] [PubMed]
62. Campbell, I.L. Structural and functional impact of the transgenic expression of cytokines in the CNS. *Annu. N. Y. Acad. Sci.* **1998**, *840*, 83–96. [CrossRef]
63. Brett, F.M.; Mizisin, A.P.; Powell, H.C.; Campbell, I.L. Evolution of neuropathologic abnormalities associated with blood-brain barrier breakdown in transgenic mice expressing interleukin-6 in astrocytes. *J. Neuropathol. Exp. Neurol.* **1995**, *54*, 766–775. [CrossRef] [PubMed]
64. Steffensen, S.C.; Campbell, I.L.; Henriksen, S.J. Site-specific hippocampal pathophysiology due to cerebral overexpression of interleukin-6 in transgenic mice. *Brain Res.* **1994**, *652*, 149–153. [CrossRef]
65. Bellinger, F.P.; Madamba, S.G.; Campbell, I.L.; Siggins, G.R. Reduced long-term potentiation in the dentate gyrus of transgenic mice with cerebral overexpression of interleukin-6. *Neurosci. Lett.* **1995**, *198*, 95–98. [CrossRef]
66. Nelson, T.E.; Campbell, I.L.; Gruol, D.L. Altered physiology of purkinje neurons in cerebellar slices from transgenic mice with chronic central nervous system expression of interleukin-6. *Neuroscience* **1999**, *89*, 127–136. [CrossRef]
67. Bray, J.G.; Reyes, K.C.; Roberts, A.J.; Ransohoff, R.M.; Gruol, D.L. Synaptic plasticity in the hippocampus shows resistance to acute ethanol exposure in transgenic mice with astrocyte-targeted enhanced CCL2 expression. *Neuropharmacology* **2013**, *67*, 115–125. [CrossRef] [PubMed]
68. Vlkolinsky, R.; Siggins, G.R.; Campbell, I.L.; Krucker, T. Acute exposure to cxc chemokine ligand 10, but not its chronic astroglial production, alters synaptic plasticity in mouse hippocampal slices. *J. Neuroimmunol.* **2004**, *150*, 37–47. [CrossRef] [PubMed]

69. Samland, H.; Huitron-Resendiz, S.; Masliah, E.; Criado, J.; Henriksen, S.J.; Campbell, I.L. Profound increase in sensitivity to glutamatergic- but not cholinergic agonist-induced seizures in transgenic mice with astrocyte production of IL-6. *J. Neurosci. Res.* **2003**, *73*, 176–187. [CrossRef] [PubMed]
70. Hernandez, R.V.; Puro, A.C.; Manos, J.C.; Huitron-Resendiz, S.; Reyes, K.C.; Liu, K.; Vo, K.; Roberts, A.J.; Gruol, D.L. Transgenic mice with increased astrocyte expression of IL-6 show altered effects of acute ethanol on synaptic function. *Neuropharmacology* **2015**, *103*, 27–43. [CrossRef] [PubMed]
71. Lynch, M.A. Long-term potentiation and memory. *Physiol. Rev.* **2004**, *84*, 87–136. [CrossRef] [PubMed]
72. Wu, L.G.; Saggau, P. Presynaptic calcium is increased during normal synaptic transmission and paired-pulse facilitation, but not in long-term potentiation in area ca1 of hippocampus. *J. Neurosci.* **1994**, *14*, 645–654. [PubMed]
73. Zucker, R.S.; Regehr, W.G. Short-term synaptic plasticity. *Annu. Rev Physiol.* **2002**, *64*, 355–405. [CrossRef] [PubMed]
74. Jackman, S.L.; Turecek, J.; Belinsky, J.E.; Regehr, W.G. The calcium sensor synaptotagmin 7 is required for synaptic facilitation. *Nature* **2016**, *529*, 88–91. [CrossRef] [PubMed]
75. Zhou, Y.; Tang, H.; Liu, J.; Dong, J.; Xiong, H. Chemokine CCL2 modulation of neuronal excitability and synaptic transmission in rat hippocampal slices. *J. Neurochem.* **2011**, *116*, 406–414. [CrossRef] [PubMed]
76. Zhou, Y.; Tang, H.; Xiong, H. Chemokine CCL2 enhances nmda receptor-mediated excitatory postsynaptic current in rat hippocampal slices-a potential mechanism for HIV-1-associated neuropathy? *J. Neuroimmune Pharmacol.* **2016**, *11*, 306–315. [CrossRef] [PubMed]
77. Tancredi, V.; D'Antuono, M.; Cafe, C.; Giovedi, S.; Bue, M.C.; D'Arcangelo, G.; Onofri, F.; Benfenati, F. The inhibitory effects of interleukin-6 on synaptic plasticity in the rat hippocampus are associated with an inhibition of mitogen-activated protein kinase erk. *J. Neurochem.* **2000**, *75*, 634–643. [CrossRef] [PubMed]
78. Li, A.J.; Katafuchi, T.; Oda, S.; Hori, T.; Oomura, Y. Interleukin-6 inhibits long-term potentiation in rat hippocampal slices. *Brain Res.* **1997**, *748*, 30–38. [CrossRef]
79. Tancredi, V.; D'Arcangelo, G.; Grassi, F.; Tarroni, P.; Palmieri, G.; Santoni, A.; Eusebi, F. Tumor necrosis factor alters synaptic transmission in rat hippocampal slices. *Neurosci. Lett.* **1992**, *146*, 176–178. [CrossRef]
80. Rose, C.F.; Verkhratsky, A.; Parpura, V. Astrocyte glutamine synthetase: Pivotal in health and disease. *Biochem. Soc. Trans.* **2013**, *41*, 1518–1524. [CrossRef] [PubMed]
81. Gonzalez, J.; Jurado-Coronel, J.C.; Avila, M.F.; Sabogal, A.; Capani, F.; Barreto, G.E. NMDARs in neurological diseases: A potential therapeutic target. *Int. J. Neurosci.* **2015**, *125*, 315–327. [CrossRef] [PubMed]
82. Zhou, Q.; Sheng, M. NMDA receptors in nervous system diseases. *Neuropharmacology* **2013**, *74*, 69–75. [CrossRef] [PubMed]
83. Goldstein, D.B.; Pal, N. Alcohol dependence produced in mice by inhalation of ethanol: Grading the withdrawal reaction. *Science* **1971**, *172*, 288–290. [CrossRef] [PubMed]
84. Metten, P.; Crabbe, J.C. Alcohol withdrawal severity in inbred mouse (mus musculus) strains. *Behav. Neurosci.* **2005**, *119*, 911–925. [CrossRef] [PubMed]
85. Raber, J.; O'Shea, R.D.; Bloom, F.E.; Campbell, I.L. Modulation of hypothalamic-pituitary-adrenal function by transgenic expression of interleukin-6 in the CNS of mice. *J. Neurosci.* **1997**, *17*, 9473–9480. [PubMed]

5

Non-Invasive Brain Stimulation for Children with Autism Spectrum Disorders

Lázaro Gómez [1,4,*], Belkis Vidal [2], Carlos Maragoto [1,3], Lilia Maria Morales [4], Sheyla Berrillo [4], Héctor Vera Cuesta [1,3], Margarita Baez [4], Marlén Denis [1,3], Tairí Marín [1,3], Yaumara Cabrera [1,3], Abel Sánchez [1], Celia Alarcón [4], Maribel Selguera [2], Yaima Llanez [3], Lucila Dieguez [4] and María Robinson [5]

1 Non Invasive Brain Stimulation Unit, International Center for Neurological Restoration, 25th Ave, Playa, Havana 15805, Cuba; maragoto@neuro.ciren.cu (C.M.); verac@neuro.ciren.cu (H.V.C.); mdenis@neuro.ciren.cu (M.D.); tairi@neuro.ciren.cu (T.M.); yaumara@neuro.ciren.cu (Y.C.); abel@neuro.ciren.cu (A.S.)

2 Child and Adolescent Mental Health Service, Borrás-Marfán Hospital, G and 27 Street., Vedado, Havana 10400, Cuba; bvidalm@infomed.sld.cu (B.V.); marser@infomed.sld.cu (M.S.)

3 Neuropediatric Clinic, International Center for Neurological Restoration, 25th Ave. Playa, Havana 15805, Cuba; yllanez@neuro.ciren.cu

4 Clinical Neurophysiology Lab., International Center for Neurological Restoration, 25th Ave. Playa, Havana 15805, Cuba; lily@neuro.ciren.cu (L.M.M.); sheyla@neuro.ciren.cu (S.B.); minou@neuro.ciren.cu (M.B.); calarcon@neuro.ciren.cu (C.A.); lucila@neuro.ciren.cu (L.D.)

5 Clinical Immunology Lab., International Center for Neurological Restoration, 25th Ave. Playa, Havana 15805, Cuba; robin@neuro.ciren.cu

* Correspondence: lazarog@neuro.ciren.cu

Abstract: Non-Invasive Brain Stimulation (NIBS) is a relatively new therapeutic approach that has shown beneficial effects in Autism Spectrum Disorder (ASD). One question to be answered is how enduring its neuromodulatory effect could be. Twenty-four patients with ASD (mean age: 12.2 years) received 20 sessions of NIBS over the left dorsolateral prefrontal cortex (L-DLPFC). They were randomized into two groups with two (G1) or three (G2) clinical evaluations before NIBS. Both groups had a complete follow-up at six months after the intervention, with the aim of determining the short-term outcome using the total score on the Autism Behavior Checklist, Autism Treatment Evaluation Checklist, and the Autism Diagnostic Interview. Transcranial Direct Current Stimulation (tDCS) was used in ASD patients aged <11 years, and repetitive Transcranial Magnetic Stimulation (rTMS) for 11–13-year-olds. Observation points were at one, three, and six months after completing all the sessions of NIBS. A significant reduction in the total score on the three clinical scales was observed and maintained during the first six months after treatment, with a slight and non-significant tendency to increase the scores in the last evaluation. Twenty sessions of NIBS over the L-DLPFC improves autistic symptoms in ASD children, with a lasting effect of six months.

Keywords: autism; transcranial direct current stimulation; repetitive transcranial magnetic stimulation

---

1. Introduction

Autism Spectrum Disorders (ASD) still pose challenges for neuroscience for many reasons; one of these is how to apply the advances in neuroscience to understanding and treating ASD by improving diagnosis, interventions, and treatments. To date, diagnosis is made on clinical bases in the absence of a true biomarker for diagnosis and a better therapeutic approach. Different pharmacological and non-pharmacological therapies have shown positive results but are far from leading to a significant improvement in the core symptoms of patients with ASD. A high incidence of brain anomalies had been described by different methods in autistic patients in comparison with neurotypical patients, including MRI techniques and anatomic studies [1–3]. One interesting feature described by Casanova et al. was the abnormal structure in cortical mini-columns, with poor neuropil development in ASD patients, which probably accounts for intracortical inhibitory dysfunction [1,4]. Alterations in the GABAergic signaling pathway may characterize autistic neurobiology, which seems to not simply be related to a decreased GABA concentration, but probably to perturbations in key components of the GABAergic pathway beyond GABA levels, such as receptors and inhibitory neuronal density [5].

There is also some research exploring functional intracortical inhibition in motor areas of ASD patients that reinforce these ideas; nevertheless, its functional expression in terms of modulation by means of paired pulse stimulation protocol with TMS is really less remarkable than was expected, and it has been demonstrated in only a fraction of the ASD population [6]. In other experiments, indirect evidence has been described related to an aberrant plasticity based on an imbalanced excitatory and inhibitory cortical tone as well as biased GABAergic dysfunction [7].

Casanova et al. were the first to propose the use of Non-Invasive Brain Stimulation (NIBS) for ASD patients, based on the possibility that low-frequency repetitive TMS could somehow improve GABAergic neurotransmission; in their case, low-frequency repetitive Transcranial Magnetic Stimulation (rTMS) was used as a way to improve intracortical inhibition in ASD patients. They applied one weekly session over 12 weeks in a group of 25 ASD patients and described an increase in gamma activity in the EEG evoked by a visual processing paradigm, with changes in Event Related Potential (ERP), improved error monitoring, and correction function in a visual recognition task after the intervention [8,9]. There are just a few other studies providing evidence of the potential efficacy of both rTMS and transcranial direct current stimulation (tDCS) in ASD (excluding case reports). Unfortunately, most of the trials are limited to a low number of sessions (not more than 15 in the best-case scenario), and it was not known how enduring the modulatory effect was [10–13].

Dorsolateral prefrontal cortex (DLPFC) is the preferred target for many other clinical conditions, thus also in ASD based on its connections with other cortical and subcortical structures. Nevertheless, other considerations are valid about the feasibility for the selection of other targets [1,14]. Studies in ASD patients using low-frequency rTMS over the left DLPFC (L-DLPFC) have shown a significant improvement in some components of event-related cortical potentials (N200 and P300) as well as a significant reduction in response errors during cognitive tasks, repetitive behavior, and irritability [9]. Other authors using cathodal tDCS over the L-DLPFC have also reported beneficial effects for ASD in young adults. Curiously, there is also a published work of a trial with anodal stimulation over DLPFC reporting improvement in autistic symptomatology [10,11].

If we accept the hypothesis that an intra-cortical inhibitory dysfunction exists in ASD patients that can contribute to several dysfunctions in the motor, sensorial, and cognitive domains, we can expect some improvement in autistic behavior after applying brain-stimulating protocols that may potentiate intracortical inhibition, probably increasing the amount of available endogenous GABA in neuronal networks related to the stimulation target. In previous experiments, low-frequency rTMS and cathodal stimulation over the left DLPFC in children with ASD were associated with an improvement in autistic behavior one week after completing 20 sessions of transcranial stimulation [15,16]. One important question is how lasting this effect would be; in the present study, we describe the short-term clinical response during the first six months after treatment. We hypothesized that 20 sessions of NIBS over the L-DLPFC are expected to have a lasting positive neuromodulatory effect in patients with ASD.

2. Materials and Methods

2.1. Study Design

A controlled, randomized, and partial crossover trial was carried out in 24 children with ASD. Fifteen patients received the intervention after two clinical evaluations within one month (group 1, G1); nine patients started receiving the intervention after two months with three evaluation points at one-month intervals (group 2, G2). We assume that according to the stimulation protocol to be used (one daily session, up to a total of 20), it would be difficult to determine a washout period and patients from G2 ran in parallel to patients from G1 while they were receiving the intervention.

2.2. Sample Selection and Group Distribution

Children with ASD were recruited from the ambulatory service of the International Center for Neurological Restoration and Marfán-Borrás Hospital, from November 2015 to October 2016. Their diagnosis was made based on DSM-V diagnostic criteria, with the consensus of a multidisciplinary team including two Child Psychiatrists and two Neuropediatric Specialists. Only patients with a slight or moderate grade of severity were included according to their clinical characteristics, with stability during the last two months, and no changes in their therapeutic scheme in either pharmacologic or non-pharmacologic interventions. Diagnosis was confirmed by the results of the Childhood Autism Rating Scale (CARS) [17] and the Autism Diagnostic Interview, Revisited Edition (ADI-R, diagnostic algorithm) [18].

Patients with severe autistic behavior were excluded, as well as patients with concurrent epilepsy. Patients with unclear diagnosis or with diagnostic disagreement between neurologist and psychiatrist opinion were also excluded. If any change was needed in their therapeutic scheme, the patient was also excluded from the trial. We applied a simple randomization technique to assign patients to G1 (early intervention group, after one month of follow-up) or G2 (intervention after two months of follow-up).

2.3. Clinical Evaluation

Three main clinical scales were used as outcome measurements for all patients, according to their parent opinions: ADI-R (algorithm for current condition), the Autism Behavioral Checklist (ABC) [19], and the Autism Treatment Evaluation Checklist (ATEC) [20]. All the scales were applied by a Child Psychiatrist who was not involved in the intervention, and patients were evaluated at one, three, and six months after completing the 20 sessions. The Global Clinical Impression Scale (GCIS) [21] was also applied as a complementary, more qualitative evaluation. The Wilcoxon matched pair test and Mann–Whitney U test were used either for intra- or between-group comparisons at the different evaluation moments ($\alpha = 0.05$).

2.4. Neurophysiological Evaluation

2.4.1. Functional Brain Connectivity

An electroencephalogram (EEG) based connectivity analysis was carried out in all the ASD patients, but only 15 good-quality EEG recording were obtained for connectivity analysis (nine from the tDCS group and six from the rTMS group). EEG traces taken one week before starting the intervention and one week after finishing it were analyzed. Significant windows were selected from the EEG trace in open eyes state (38 from each patient), because they were more often artifact-free than the closed-eyes state.

We used a 19-electrode montage including Fp1, Fp2, F7, F8, F3, F4, C3, C4, T5, T6, T3, T4, P3, P4, O1, O2, Fz, Cz, and Pz, from the 10/20 system. Electrode Impedance was kept below 5 kΩ. Functional connectivity was analyzed based on the synchronization likelihood between electrodes for the five frequency bands: δ (1–3.9 Hz), θ (4–7.9 Hz) α (8–12.9 Hz), β (13–29.9 Hz), and γ (30–35 Hz) [22]. Mathematical analysis was developed with connectivity algorithms implemented in MATLAB v.7.7

R2008b. Significant connectivity ($p < 0.05$) in each frequency band was represented on an X/Y coordinate according to the 10/20 system for each brain stimulation modality independently, and the results by group were represented over the scalp surface map.

2.4.2. Event-Related Potentials

Only in six children was it possible to carry out a passive oddball paradigm for P300 Event-Related Potentials (ERPs) before the intervention; four of them received tDCS and two rTMS. Patients were seated in a sound- and light-attenuated room while a paradigm was conducted consisting of 200 stimuli, 80% frequent (500 Hz) and 20% infrequent target (1000 Hz) tones, delivered through headphones while children were watching a silent movie. In the passive version of the oddball task the subject´s attention is usually directed away from the sequence of standard and deviant tones toward another, moderately demanding task, usually in a different modality [23]. We proposed a version of this paradigm considering the characteristics of the autistic children, with poor collaboration. All stimuli (50 ms; 5 ms rise and fall time) were presented binaurally with an inter-stimulus interval of 1300 ms.

To record the auditory P300 ERPs, 19 surface electrodes (Ag/ClAg) were attached to the scalp according to the international electrode placement 10–20 system (Fp1, Fp2, F3, F4, F7, F8, C3, C4, T3, T4, T5, T6, P3, P4, O1, O2, Fz, Cz, Pz), with additional electrodes for EOG (lateral to the outer canthus of the right eye and above the middle of the left eyebrow), and referenced to the linked earlobe. The electrode impedance was kept below 5 kΩ. EEG data were off-line averaged (100 ms prior and 700 ms after stimulus onset), and P300 latency and amplitude were quantified at Fz, Cz, and Pz. A continuous acquisition system was employed (Medicid 5, Neuronic SA, Cuba) and EEG data were EOG-corrected offline. The sampling rate of all channels was 200 Hz. To assure auditory system normality, Auditory Brainstem Response was previously recorded. The stimuli were 0.1 ms alternating clicks delivered through a headphone (DR-531B-7, Elegas Acous Co. Ltd., Tokyo, Japan). The records were obtained using the evoked potentials measuring system Neuropack M1 (Nihon Kohden, Tokyo, Japan).

P300 ERPs were obtained before and after NIBS, and P300 latency and amplitude values from the two evaluations were compared (from Fz electrode position; Wilcoxon matched pairs test, $\alpha < 0.05$). All measurements were of the difference wave (infrequent wave minus frequent wave) and in this case, due to the low number of patients' recordable P300, the analysis was performed considering all patients as a single group.

2.5. *Intervention*

Patients received one daily session of NIBS, from Monday to Friday, for a total of 20 sessions. tDCS was used in patients 10 years old or younger, and rTMS in patients 11 and older. The reason for using tDCS in younger children instead of rTMS was that in this case a major degree of collaboration is needed to assure effective focal stimulation over the selected target (left dorsolateral prefrontal cortex, L-DLPFC). During the stimulation sessions patients, were comfortably seated while watching TV cartoons of their preference or listening to music and playing with small, simple toys.

2.5.1. Transcranial Direct Current Stimulation (tDCS)

tDCS was only used in patients 10 years old or younger (Neuroconn tDCS stimulator, München, Germany). A cathode was positioned over F3 (10/20 international EEG electrode system), and an anode over the proximal right arm. The stimulation intensity was 1 mA, and was maintained for 20 min. Each electrode pad was humidified with a 0.9% NaCl solution.

2.5.2. Repetitive Transcranial Magnetic Stimulation (rTMS)

rTMS was used in patients older than 10 years and 11 months (MagStim Rapid^2, Whitland, UK). A butterfly coil with air cooling system (MagStim Double 70 mm Air Film Coil) was used. The center of the coil was located over F3, back handed 45° from the midline, and a total of 1500 pulses were delivered in each session, at 1 Hz of frequency and an intensity of 90% of the resting motor threshold (i.e., the minimum stimulation intensity required to elicit a discernible hand muscle response in at least three of five consecutive pulses) [24]. Sessions were subdivided into four trains of 375 pulses, with a 1-min interval between each allowing for free movement of the head and neck. Most of the patients rejected the use of earplugs, and in the best-case scenario they agreed to listen to music by wearing headphones from their own devices.

2.6. Ethical Considerations

All the procedures followed the rules of the Declaration of Helsinki of 1975 for human research, and the study was approved by the scientific and ethics committee from the International Center for Neurological Restoration (CIREN37/2015). Parents gave written informed consent for their children to be considered for inclusion in the study, and where possible children also gave their consent.

3. Results

3.1. Change in Clinical Scales One Month after the Intervention

As a global result (G1 + G2), a significant decrease in the total score was observed in ADI-R, ABC, and ATEC scales one month after the intervention (Wilcoxon matched pair test; ABC, Z = 3.823, $p = 0.000131$; ADI-R, 3.337, $p = 0.000846$; ATEC, Z = 3.723, $p = 0.000196$). Figure 1a represents the global scores for the three main clinical scales we applied for the evaluation of autism behavior. The values are in correspondence with qualitative changes described by their relative uniqueness in socialization and communication domains, and with the GCIS (pre-intervention: 3.47 ± 0.6; post-intervention: 2.95 ± 0.2. Wilcoxon pair series test: Z = 2.803, $p = 0.005062$). All of the patients' autistic behavior improved according to the scale results observed one month after the intervention. A comparison between the change in the total score of clinical scales did not show any significant differences correlated with the use of tDCS and rTMS (Mann–Whitney *U* Test, $p > 0.05$). Initial evaluation did not show any differences in the total score between groups when we looked for any evidence of age-dependent characteristics in both groups. The clinical response to NIBS was apparently independent of group age and type of intervention (See Figure 1b).

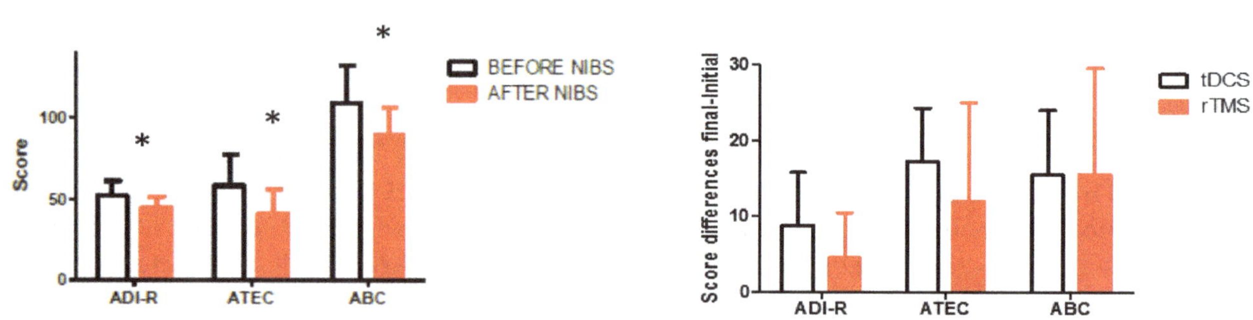

(a) (b)

Figure 1. (**a**) Comparison of pre- intervention and one-month post-intervention scores in clinical scales; (**b**) no significant differences in the clinical effect with the use of rTMS or tDCS according to the score differences (Initial–Final) (* $p < 0.05$).

Figure 2 shows that no significant differences were observed between G1 and G2 in the initial clinical scale scores before the intervention (Mann–Whitney *U* test, $p > 0.05$); but values observed in G1 after NIBS showed a very important change when compared with the initial values (Wilcoxon; ABC, Z = 3.823, $p = 0.000132$; ADI-R, Z = 3.550, $p = 0.000385$;ATEC, Z = 5.526, $p = 0.000241$); the same behavior was seen in G2 after the intervention (Wilcoxon; ABC, Z = 3.295, $p = 0.000982$; ADI-R, Z = 3.588, $p = 0.009633$; ATEC, Z = 3.179, $p = 0.001474$).

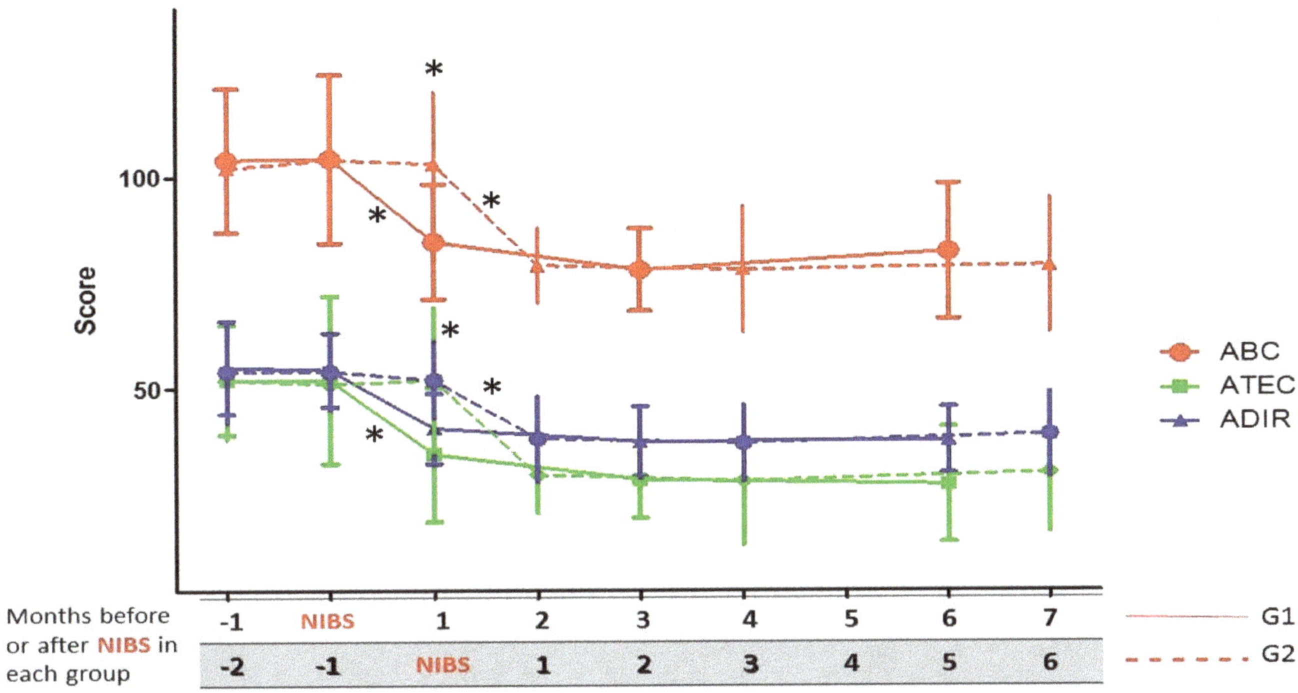

Figure 2. Short-term outcome based on clinical scale scores until six months of follow-up after NIBS in group 1 (G1) and group 2 (G2). * $p < 0.05$ (significant differences; comparisons between and within each group with scale scores before and after NIBS).

3.2. Change in Clinical Scales during the First Six Months after the Intervention

Post-intervention follow-up was extended over six months. For both groups G1 and G2, NIBS induced a significant change in clinical scale scores (See Figure 2), and both groups maintained approximately the same values until the sixth month after NIBS, when there was a slight tendency for the total score in ABC, ADI-R, and ATEC to increase, but their punctuation remained lower than the observed values before treatment (See Figure 2). According to their parents' opinion, stereotypes intensity and variety increased in frequency and number in many patients around the sixth month, but in clinical scales there were not any significant changes in specific domains.

Group 1 had lower values for all the scales one month after NIBS (solid lines); the same happened with G2 patients running in parallel, but only since the fourth month and ahead of follow-up (also one month after NIBS; dashed lines).

3.3. EEG-Based Brain Functional Connectivity Analysis

An increase in brain functional connectivity was observed after NIBS for patients who received either tDCS or rTMS, especially for higher frequencies: α, β, and γ bands showed the greatest increase, with a large increment in the number of 10/20 system points functionally related. The analysis of the effect in functional connectivity showed that the group that received rTMS accounted for the most significant changes when initial and final values were compared (see Figure 3).

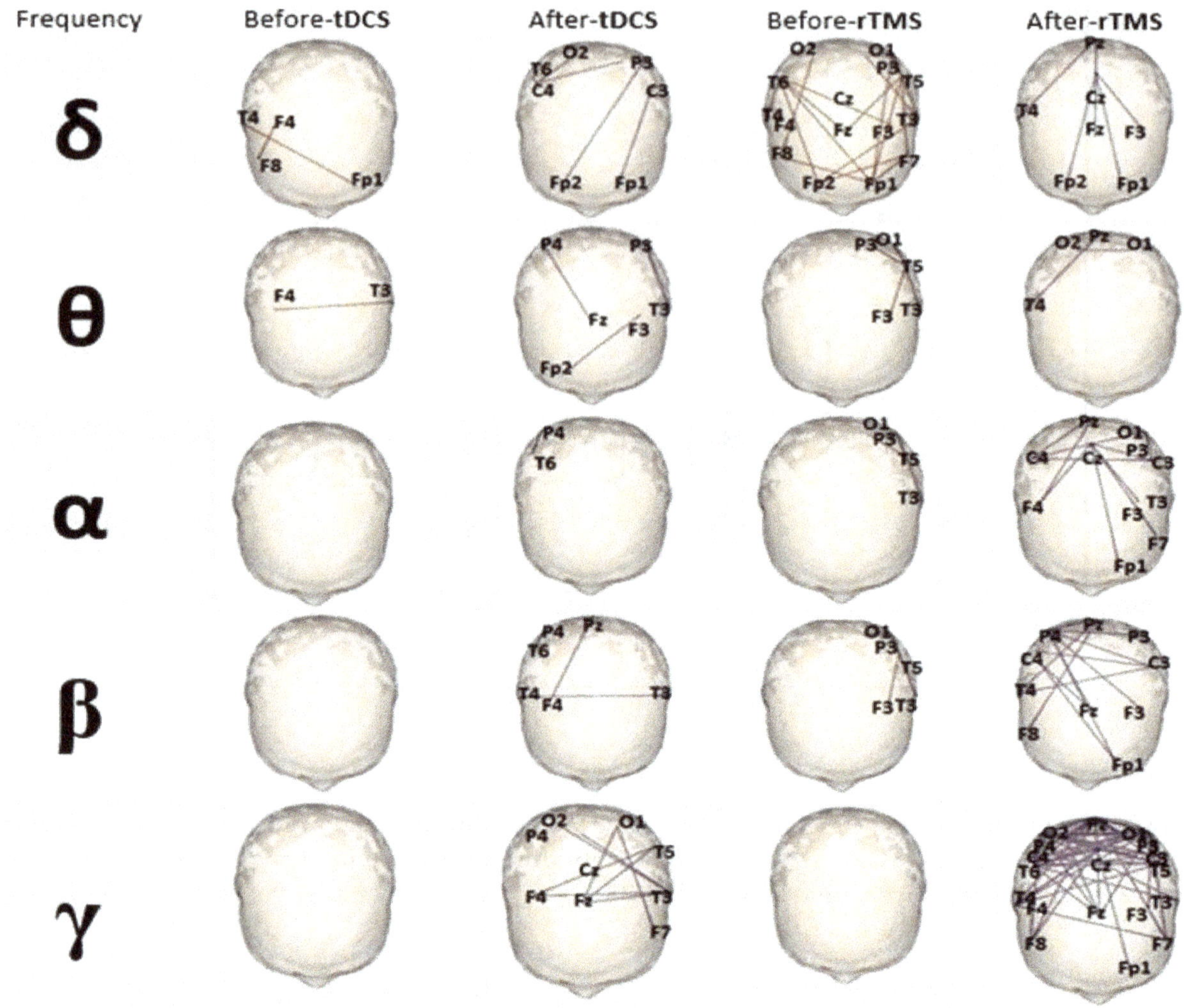

Figure 3. EEG-based analysis of brain functional connectivity. Note the positive change in all frequency bands after the intervention, but mainly in the γ band for both tDCS and rTMS, especially in the group that received rTMS (all electrodes' locations are statistically significant, $p < 0.05$).

3.4. ERP Analysis

Recordings were possible in only six patients in the initial evaluation; thus, after the intervention, only activity in those patients who collaborated during the task was recorded. All patients had a normal auditory brainstem response according to the normative laboratory data, but one patient had no ERP response. The P300 component showed a scalp distribution in the frontal and central regions, maximal in Fz. There was a shortening of P300 latency after treatment, with statistically significant differences with respect to the basal response (Wilcoxon matched pairs test, $p = 0.043$). P300 amplitude did not show statistically significant differences after treatment, even though the average value in the group was higher after the intervention (see Figure 4). The prolonged latency and low amplitude may be in agreement with the abnormal connectivity of the frontal lobes seen in ASD subjects [25], and engaged with attention circuits. The improvement of these parameters after NIBS might be a consequence of the improvement in functional connectivity and probably correlated with positive clinical changes in attentiveness, concentration, and speed of answering questions from a parent.

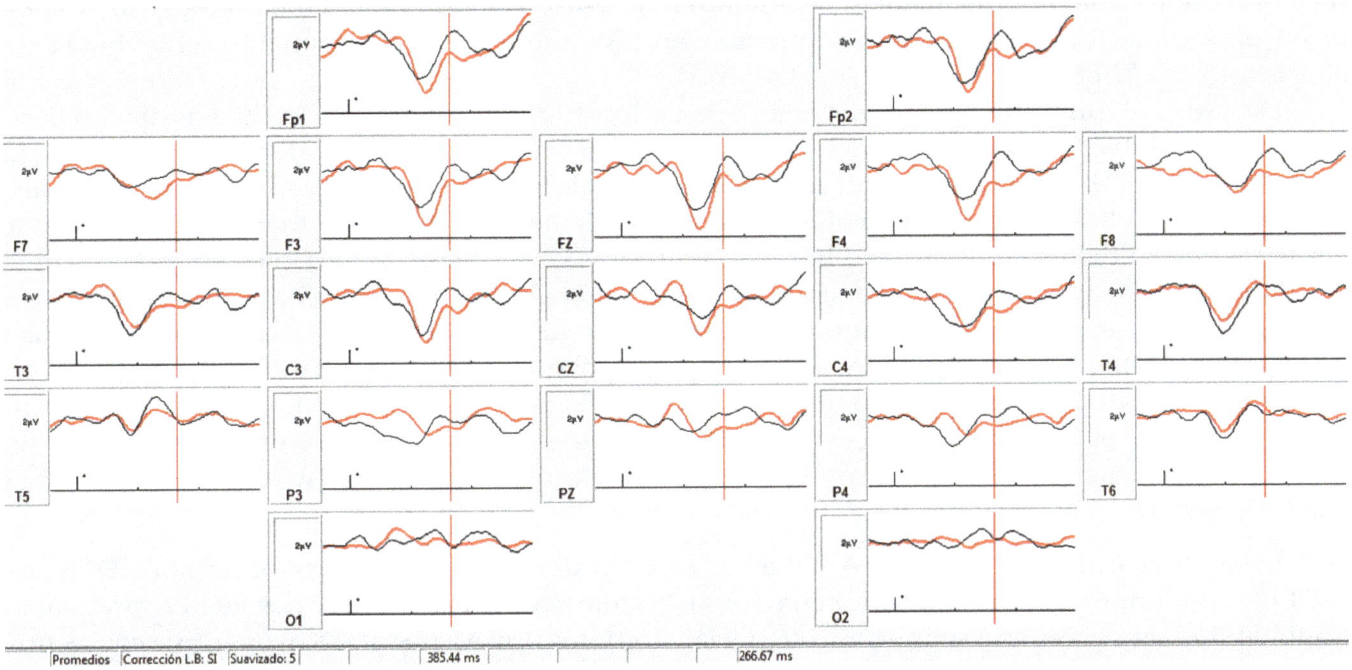

Figure 4. Grand averaged infrequent target. Black trace: pre-intervention (Amplitude and latency at Fz: 3.09 μV, 410 ms); red trace: post-intervention (Amplitude and latency at Fz: 3.28 μV, 371 ms).

4. Discussion

Our results reproduce similar neuromodulatory effects to those reported previously by two other research groups who used the same target (L-DLPFC), applying either rTMS or tDCS [9,11,26]. Casanova et al. pioneered the use of therapeutic NIBS in autism and described the effects of one weekly low-frequency rTMS (1 Hz) during 12 weeks in 25 ASD children and adolescents. In that study they reported a significant reduction in repetitive and restricted behavior patterns and irritability, but no changes in social awareness or hyperactivity. They also described an increase in the amount of gamma activity in the EEG, shortening of the P300 component of ERP, and an increase of amplitude in the group receiving the intervention [9]. They used 150 TMS pulses per session, one session per week, and 12 sessions in total. In our study, the number of stimuli per session and the total number of sessions were considerably higher; this is in correspondence with recommended practical aspects for conventional use of NIBS in other diseases such as depression, obsessive compulsive disorder, chronic pain, etc., in order to obtain a sustained effect [27,28]. This could likely explain the significant clinical improvement in our group, not only in the abovementioned domains, but also in social aspects and communication. We also were able to establish that NIBS' effects persisted into the sixth month after completion of treatment, a result that, as far as we know, has never been reported by any other group; this is a very important finding because it would probably indicate that patients would need a new treatment cycle (e.g., a second cycle of NIBS) six months after the previous intervention to maintain clinical improvement. Of course, it would also be interesting to know how the behavior of our patients will develop over the next six months and the forthcoming years (long-term outcome).

Another interesting double-blind and randomized trial in adult ASD patients was published by Enticott et al. using the dorsomedial prefrontal cortex as the target, and stimulating with the HAUT coil, which makes it possible to reach deep structures in the brain [12]. They applied 10 daily sessions of 5 Hz, 1500 pulses at resting motor threshold intensity. The clinical response was evaluated immediately after the intervention and one month later, and they reported a significant reduction in social relating symptoms (relative to sham participants) for both post-treatment assessments. Those in the active condition also showed a reduction in self-oriented anxiety during difficult and emotional social situations from pre-treatment to one-month follow-up. They suggested the need to use extended protocols such as those used to treat depression, and we agree that it is essential to achieving lasting effects for both NIBS methods, rTMS or tDCS [28].

D'Urso et al. published the results of an open pilot study using cathodic tDCS over the L-DLPFC in 10 young adults (18–25 years old) with 10 daily sessions of 1.5 mA, with evaluation two weeks after the intervention. They reported an improvement in autistic behavior of 26.7% according to the change observed in the clinical scale they applied; only two patients did not change their initial scale values, while the rest of the group improved in their symptoms [11]. There are two main differences in the tDCS protocol we applied in younger children (5–10 years old): first, again we used a higher number of sessions and second, the stimulation intensity in our case was 1 mA. NIBS in children seems to be as safe as in the adult population, so the same safety guidelines are indicated for its use in any population [29,30]. It is important to mention that in the case of tDCS, there is not enough evidence about the safety of 2 mA in young people (<18 years old), and most research has been done using 1 mA; however, there are also a few papers describing the absence of adverse effects with the use of 2 mA in pediatric patients [13].

In another interesting article, Amatachaya et al. described the effects of anodal tDCS over L-DLPF, with improvement in autistic behavior in 20 children with ASD. They designed a randomized, double-blind crossover and sham-controlled trial, applying 1 mA anodal tDCS over five consecutive days, and a washout period of four weeks This result reactivates the essential research question as to whether the clinical, biochemical, and physiological effects are polarity-dependent or not [10,31–35].

There are results from clinical trials with other diseases and physiological studies in which the opposite effects of cathodic and anodic tDCS have been well documented [35,36]. Our results using cathodic tDCS or low-frequency rTMS over the L-DLPFC share the same theoretical basis developed by Casanova et al. and D'Urso et al., though we studied a low sample number (24 patients), and by design we employed an open trial without the use of placebo stimulation. Nevertheless, the results are reproducible in G1 and G2, with patients being their own controls from the start of the intervention. We also had the opportunity to compare the effects of low-frequency rTMS and cathodic tDCS at the same time, but in ASD patients of different ages and with our experimental design we demonstrated that there are no differences, at least not in their clinical effects. Certainly, there was an important effect achieved by increasing functional connectivity with the use of both the stimulating methods, rTMS and tDCS, with a clear superiority of rTMS-induced changes. Of course, more research is needed to draw well-documented conclusions. Other authors have described improvements in particular aspects of adult ASD patients such as working memory and better syntax acquisition following single-dose anodal tDCS over the left and right dorsolateral prefrontal cortex (first case) or exclusively over the left dorsolateral prefrontal cortex [13,37] There were also positive changes in P300 ERP, but due to the low number of subjects in whom it was possible to carry out the passive oddball paradigm, we cannot make any comparison between the two different stimulating methods. Unfortunately, sample sizes for EEG-based connectivity analysis and ERP paradigm could not include all the patients, because, in close relationship with the complexity of the used method, when we carried out their initial electrophysiological evaluation (before intervention), not all recordings had a high enough quality for analysis.

5. Conclusions

Twenty sessions of NIBS over L-DLPFC improves autistic symptoms in ASD children, with a lasting effect of six months.

Acknowledgments: The authors appreciate the contribution of all parents of and children participating in the study. We also thank Tlalli Mota and Jim Clifford for helping with the review of the manuscript.

Author Contributions: All authors contributed substantially to the work reported. Lázaro Gómez participated in the design of the research, NIBS sessions, analysis, and discussion of the results, and wrote the manuscript. Belkis Vidal and Maribel Serguera participated in the diagnosis of patients and clinical evaluation of all the scales. Hector Vera Cuesta and Carlos Maragoto Rizo contributed to the diagnosis and clinical data of patients. Lilia Maria Morales and Sheyla Berrillo contributed to the analysis of the EEG traces and functional connectivity calculations. Margarita Báez carried out ERP recordings and analysis. Abel Sánchez and Celia Alarcón performed the technical work for recordings of EEG and ERP. Tairí Marín, Marlén Denis, Yaumara Cabrera, Yaima LLanez, and Lucila Duiéguez participated in the NIBS sessions. Maria de los Angeles Robinson Agramonte participated in the analysis and discussion of the results and review of the manuscript.

References

1. Casanova, M.F.; Buxhoeveden, D.P.; Switala, A.E.; Roy, E. Minicolumnar pathology in autism. *Neurology* **2002**, *58*, 428–432. [CrossRef] [PubMed]
2. Freitag, C.M.; Luders, E.; Hulst, H.E.; Narr, K.L.; Thompson, P.M.; Toga, A.W.; Krick, C.; Konrad, C. Total brain volume and corpus callosum size in medication-naive adolescents and young adults with autism spectrum disorder. *Biol. Psychiatry* **2009**, *66*, 316–319. [CrossRef] [PubMed]
3. Kumar, A.; Sundaram, S.K.; Sivaswamy, L.; Behen, M.E.; Makki, M.I.; Ager, J.; Janisse, J.; Chugani, H.T.; Chugani, D.C. Alterations in frontal lobe tracts and corpus callosum in young children with autism spectrum disorder. *Cereb. Cortex* **2010**, *20*, 2103–2113. [CrossRef] [PubMed]
4. Casanova, M.F.; El-Baz, A.; Vanbogaert, E.; Narahari, P.; Switala, A. A topographic study of minicolumnar core width by lamina comparison between autistic subjects and controls: Possible minicolumnar disruption due to an anatomical element in-common to multiple laminae. *Brain Pathol.* **2010**, *20*, 451–458. [CrossRef] [PubMed]
5. Fatemi, S.H.; Reutiman, T.J.; Folsom, T.D.; Rustan, O.G.; Rooney, R.J.; Thuras, P.D. Downregulation of GABAA receptor protein subunits alpha6, beta2, delta, epsilon, gamma2, theta, and rho2 in superior frontal cortex of subjects with autism. *J. Autism Dev. Disord.* **2014**, *44*, 1833–1845. [CrossRef] [PubMed]
6. Enticott, P.G.; Kennedy, H.A.; Rinehart, N.J.; Tonge, B.J.; Bradshaw, J.L.; Fitzgerald, P.B. GABAergic activity in autism spectrum disorders: An investigation of cortical inhibition via transcranial magnetic stimulation. *Neuropharmacology* **2013**, *68*, 202–209. [CrossRef] [PubMed]
7. Oberman, L.M.; Pascual-Leone, A.; Rotenberg, A. Modulation of corticospinal excitability by transcranial magnetic stimulation in children and adolescents with autism spectrum disorder. *Front. Hum Neurosci.* **2014**, *8*. [CrossRef] [PubMed]
8. Baruth, J.M.; Casanova, M.F.; El-Baz, A.; Horrell, T.; Mathai, G.; Sears, L.; Sokhadze, E. Low-frequency repetitive transcranial magnetic stimulation (rTMS) modulates evoked-gamma frequency oscillations in autism spectrum disorder (ASD). *J. Neurother.* **2010**, *14*, 179–194. [CrossRef] [PubMed]
9. Casanova, M.F.; Baruth, J.M.; El-Baz, A.; Tasman, A.; Sears, L.; Sokhadze, E. Repetitive transcranial magnetic stimulation (rTMS) modulates event-related potential (ERP) indices of attention in autism. *Transl. Neurosci.* **2012**, *3*, 170–180. [CrossRef] [PubMed]
10. Amatachaya, A.; Auvichayapat, N.; Patjanasoontorn, N.; Suphakunpinyo, C.; Ngernyam, N.; Aree-uea, B.; Keeratitanont, K.; Auvichayapat, P. Effect of anodal transcranial direct current stimulation on autism: A randomized double-blind crossover trial. *Behav. Neurol.* **2014**, *2014*. [CrossRef] [PubMed]
11. D'Urso, G.; Bruzzese, D.; Ferrucci, R.; Priori, A.; Pascotto, A.; Galderisi, S.; Altamura, A.C.; Bravaccio, C. Transcranial direct current stimulation for hyperactivity and noncompliance in autistic disorder. *World J. Biol. Psychiatry* **2015**, *16*, 361–366. [CrossRef] [PubMed]
12. Enticott, P.G.; Fitzgibbon, B.M.; Kennedy, H.A.; Arnold, S.L.; Elliot, D.; Peachey, A.; Zangen, A.; Fitzgerald, P.B. A double-blind, randomized trial of deep repetitive transcranial magnetic stimulation (rTMS) for autism spectrum disorder. *Brain Stimul.* **2014**, *7*, 206–211. [CrossRef] [PubMed]
13. Schneider, H.D.; Hopp, J.P. The use of the Bilingual Aphasia Test for assessment and transcranial direct current stimulation to modulate language acquisition in minimally verbal children with autism. *Clin. Linguist. Phon.* **2011**, *25*, 640–654. [CrossRef] [PubMed]
14. Downar, J.; Daskalakis, Z.J. New targets for rTMS in depression: A review of convergent evidence. *Brain Stimul.* **2013**, *6*, 231–240. [CrossRef] [PubMed]

15. Gómez, L.; Denis, M.; Marín, T.; Vidal, B.; Maragoto, C.; Vera, C.; Serguera, M.; Morales, L.; Báez, M.; Sánchez, A.; et al. Estudio piloto sobre el efecto de la Estimulación Cerebral No Invasiva en el Trastorno del Espectro Autista. *Rev. Mex. Neurocienc.* **2016**, *17*, 51.
16. Gómez, L.; Denis, M.; Marín, T.; Vidal, B.; Maragoto, C.; Vera, H.; Serguera, M.; Morales, L.; Báez, M.; Sánchez, A.; et al. Non invasive brain stimulation in children with autism spectrum disorder. *Brain Stimul.* **2017**, *10*, 347. [CrossRef]
17. Schopler, E.; Reichler, R.; DeVellis, R.; Daly, K. Toward objective classification of childhood autism: Childhood Autism Rating Scale (CARS). *J. Autism Dev. Disord.* **1980**, *10*, 91–103. [CrossRef] [PubMed]
18. Lord, C.; Rutter, M.; Le Couteur, A. Autism diagnostic interview-revised: A revised version of a diagnostic interview for caregivers of individuals with possible pervasive developmental disorders. *J. Autism Dev. Disord.* **1994**, *24*, 659–685. [CrossRef] [PubMed]
19. Krug, D.; Arisk, J.; Almond, P. Behavior checklist for identifying severely handicapped individuals with high levels of autistic behavior. *J. Child Psychol. Psychiatry* **1980**, *21*, 221–229. [CrossRef] [PubMed]
20. Magiati, I.; Moss, J.; Yates, R.; Charman, T.; Howlin, P. Is the Autism Treatment Evaluation Checklist a useful tool for monitoring progress in children with autism spectrum disorders? *J. Intellect. Disabil. Res.* **2011**, *55*, 302–312. [CrossRef] [PubMed]
21. Busner, J.; Targum, S. The clinical global impressions scale: Applying a research tool in clinical practice. *Psychiatry* **2007**, *4*, 28–37. [PubMed]
22. Stam, J.C.; van Dijk, B.W. Synchronization likelihood: An unbiased measure of generalized synchronization in multivariate data sets. *Phys. D Nonlinear Phenom.* **2002**, *163*, 236–251. [CrossRef]
23. Näätänen, R. The role of attention in auditory information processing as revealed by event-related potentials and other brain measures of cognitive function. *Behav. Brain Sci.* **1990**, *13*, 201–233. [CrossRef]
24. Rossi, S.; Hallet, M.; Rossini, P.M.; Pascual-Leone, A. Safety, ethical considerations, and application guidelines for the use of transcranial magnetic stimulation in clinical practice and research. *Clin. Neurophysiol.* **2009**, *120*, 2008–2039. [CrossRef] [PubMed]
25. Catani, M.; Dell'Acqua, F.; Budisavljevic, S.; Howells, H.; Thiebaut de Schotten, M.; Froudist-Walsh, S.; D'Anna, L.; Thompson, A.; Sandrone, S.; Bullmore, E.; et al. Frontal networks in adults with autism spectrum disorder. *Brain* **2016**, *139*, 616–630. [CrossRef] [PubMed]
26. Baruth, J.M.; Wall, C.A.; Patterson, M.C.; Port, J.D. Proton magnetic resonance spectroscopy as a probe into the pathophysiology of autism spectrum disorders (ASD): A review. *Autism Res.* **2013**, *6*, 119–133. [CrossRef] [PubMed]
27. Lefaucheur, J.P.; Andre-Obadia, N.; Poulet, E.; Devanne, H.; Haffen, E.; Londero, A.; Cretin, B.; Leroi, A.M.; Radtchenko, A.; Saba, G.; et al. French guidelines on the use of repetitive transcranial magnetic stimulation (rTMS): Safety and therapeutic indications. *Neurophysiol. Clin.* **2011**, *41*, 221–295. [CrossRef] [PubMed]
28. Perera, T.; George, M.; Grammer, G.; Janicak, P.; Pascual-Leone, A.; Wirecki, T. The clinical TMS society consensus review and treatment recommendations for TMS therapy for major depressive disorder. *Brain Stimul.* **2016**, *9*, 336–346. [CrossRef] [PubMed]
29. Hameed, M.Q.; Dhamne, S.C.; Gersner, R.; Kaye, H.L.; Oberman, L.M.; Pascual-Leone, A.; Rotenberg, A. Transcranial magnetic and direct current stimulation in children. *Curr. Neurol. Neurosci. Rep.* **2017**, *17*. [CrossRef] [PubMed]
30. Krishnan, C.; Santos, L.; Peterson, M.; Ehinger, M. Safety of noninvasive brain stimulation in children and adolescents. *Brain Stimul.* **2015**, *8*, 76–87. [CrossRef] [PubMed]
31. Jacobson, L.; Koslowsky, M.; Lavidor, M. tDCS polarity effects in motor and cognitive domains: A meta-analytical review. *Exp. Brain Res.* **2012**, *216*, 1–10. [CrossRef] [PubMed]
32. Joos, K.; De, R.D.; Van de Heyning, P.; Vanneste, S. Polarity specific suppression effects of transcranial direct current stimulation for tinnitus. *Neural Plast.* **2014**, *2014*. [CrossRef] [PubMed]
33. Ladeira, A.; Fregni, F.; Campanha, C.; Valasek, C.A.; De, R.D.; Brunoni, A.R.; Boggio, P.S. Polarity-dependent transcranial direct current stimulation effects on central auditory processing. *PLoS ONE* **2011**, *6*, e25399. [CrossRef] [PubMed]
34. Sohn, M.K.; Jee, S.J.; Kim, Y.W. Effect of transcranial direct current stimulation on postural stability and lower extremity strength in hemiplegic stroke patients. *Ann. Rehabil. Med.* **2013**, *37*, 759–765. [CrossRef] [PubMed]

35. Stagg, C.J.; Best, J.G.; Stephenson, M.C.; O'Shea, J.; Wylezinska, M.; Kincses, Z.T.; Morris, P.G.; Matthews, P.M.; Johansen-Berg, H. Polarity-sensitive modulation of cortical neurotransmitters by transcranial stimulation. *J. Neurosci.* **2009**, *29*, 5202–5206. [CrossRef] [PubMed]
36. D'Urso, G.; Brunoni, A.R.; Anastasia, A.; Micillo, M.; Mantovani, A. Polarity-dependent effects of transcranial direct current stimulation in obsessive-compulsive disorder. *Neurocase* **2016**, *22*, 60–64. [CrossRef] [PubMed]
37. Van Steenburgh, J.J.; Varvaris, M.; Schretlen, J.; Vannorsdall, T.J.; Gordon, B. Balanced bifrontal transcranial direct current stimulation enhaces working memory in adults with high-functioning autism: A sham-controlled crossover study. *Mol. Autism* **2017**, *8*, 40. [CrossRef] [PubMed]

6

The Effects of Hypoxia and Inflammation on Synaptic Signaling in the NS

Gatambwa Mukandala, Ronan Tynan, Sinead Lanigan and John J. O'Connor *

UCD School of Biomolecular and Biomedical Science, UCD Conway Institute of Biomolecular and Biomedical Research, Belfield, Dublin 4, Ireland; Gatambwa.mukandala@ucdconnect.ie (G.M.); ronan.tynan@ucdconnect.ie (R.T.); sinead.lanigan@ucdconnect.ie (S.L.)

* Correspondence: john.oconnor@ucd.ie

Academic Editor: Donna Gruol

Abstract: Normal brain function is highly dependent on oxygen and nutrient supply and when the demand for oxygen exceeds its supply, hypoxia is induced. Acute episodes of hypoxia may cause a depression in synaptic activity in many brain regions, whilst prolonged exposure to hypoxia leads to neuronal cell loss and death. Acute inadequate oxygen supply may cause anaerobic metabolism and increased respiration in an attempt to increase oxygen intake whilst chronic hypoxia may give rise to angiogenesis and erythropoiesis in order to promote oxygen delivery to peripheral tissues. The effects of hypoxia on neuronal tissue are exacerbated by the release of many inflammatory agents from glia and neuronal cells. Cytokines, such as TNF-α, and IL-1β are known to be released during the early stages of hypoxia, causing either local or systemic inflammation, which can result in cell death. Another growing body of evidence suggests that inflammation can result in neuroprotection, such as preconditioning to cerebral ischemia, causing ischemic tolerance. In the following review we discuss the effects of acute and chronic hypoxia and the release of pro-inflammatory cytokines on synaptic transmission and plasticity in the central nervous system. Specifically we discuss the effects of the pro-inflammatory agent TNF-α during a hypoxic event.

Keywords: hypoxia; TNF-α; adenosine; HIF-1α; hippocampus; long-term potentiation; prolyl hydroxylase inhibitor

1. Introduction

In the central nervous system, hypoxia occurs when there is an inadequate supply of oxygen to neuronal tissue. During acute hypoxia multiple oxygen sensors are deployed allowing neurons to adapt to the response. These responses to hypoxia include synaptic signaling decreases usually as a result of anerobic metabolism changes whilst chronic hypoxia may give rise to more severe perturbations of synaptic transmission and the activation of transcription factors that regulate oxygen homoestasis [1]. Different neurons adapt to a decreased oxygen supply to the brain in many ways, reflecting the diverse role of neuronal functions and also the extent of the hypoxia experienced. It is now known that an hypoxic event in brain tissue can cause ATP to drop by as much as 90% in less than 5 min. Additionally, oxygen-sensitive ion channals including Na^+ and K^+ are activated bringing about changes in excitation and inhibition of neuronal and glial cells [2]. Depolarisation of cells may also take place causing the uptake of Na^+ and Cl^- into cells followed by passive influx of water, resulting in swelling and oedema [2]. Hypoxic insults may also activate voltage-gated Ca^{2+} and K^+ ion channels and glutamate transporters, eventually causing excess glutamate to spill into the synaptic regions causing excitotoxicity. On the other hand, many of the long-term hypoxic responses are mediated by hypoxia inducible factors (HIF), such as HIF-1α [3,4]. HIF-1α is a universally expressed transcriptional mediator of the hypoxic response that is degraded in an oxygen-dependent manner. Under normoxic conditions, HIF-1α has a half-life of approximately 8 min due to hydroxylation by prolyl hydroxyl domains (PHDs) [5]. These PHDs exist in three different isoforms, PHD1, PHD2, and PHD3 and all require oxygen, iron, ascorbate and 2-oxoglutarate, a product of the oxygen dependent Kreb cycle, to hydroxylate HIF-1α. Under hypoxic conditions the Kreb cycle is inhbited leading to a reduction in 2-oxoglutarate, preventing the binding of PHDs to the targeting proline domains [4,6]. During hypoxia, the HIF-1α protein stabilizes allowing it to recruit transcriptional co-activators, which are blocked during normal conditions via factor inhibiting HIF (FIH) [7]. This complex then permits for the transcription of hypoxia-related proteins through binding of the hypoxic responsive element (HRE). HRE binding induces the expression of genes, such as erythropoietin, vascular endothelial growth factor and insulin growth factor. These all play a neuroprotetive role in response to the hypoxic insult.

These acute and chronic responses to hypoxia are clearly manifested during ischemic events in the brain. An example of one such event with a hypoxic component is stroke, which is caused by a reduction in blood flow as a result of an obstruction or rupture of blood vessels within the brain and may cause both acute and chronic episodes of hypoxia. This leads to complex pathological changes taking place, which may lead to tissue necrosis through increased inflammation and oxygen deprivation [8]. During an ischemic stroke the eventual restriction of oxygen in the brain due to an obstruction leads to a cascade of events including hypoxia, increased expression of pro-inflammatory cytokines like tumor necrosis factor alpha (TNF-α) and interleukin-1beta (IL-1β), as well as increased release of the excitatory neurotransmitter glutamate [9]. In this review we will discuss how hypoxia and the release of pro-inflammatory cytokines can effect synaptic transmission and plasticity in the central nervous system (CNS).

2. Hypoxia and Synaptic Signaling

Synaptic transmission in the CNS requires approximately 30% to 50% of cerebral oxygen. Therefore many of the changes in the CNS related to acute hypoxia stem from modifications of synaptic excitation and depression. The responses to hypoxia, which occur within seconds, most likely do not involve a role for HIF-1α stabilization. Additionally, upon re-oxygenation after a short period, synaptic transmission can recover to 100% in many brain regions [10]. This decrease in synaptic signaling during acute hypoxia is thought to protect some neurons during ischemic events. Adenosine is one of many neurotransmitters, which plays a vital role in the neuroprotective response to hypoxia [11]. Adenosine A_1 receptors (A_1Rs), in particular, play a part in altering neurotransmitter release [12] and have wide expression levels throughout the CNS [13]. This inhibitory neuromodulation by A_1Rs is coupled to inhibitory G_i or G_o containing G-proteins [14]. Activation of the receptor stimulates adenylyl cyclase, activates inwardly rectifying K^+ channels, thus inhibiting Ca^{2+} channels and activation of phospholipase C. This inhibits the release of a number of neurotransmitters including glutamate, dopamine, serotonin and acetylcholine thus making it the primary neuroprotective receptor. Adenosine forms through the enzymatic catabolism of adenosine triphosphate (ATP) into adenosine monophosphate (AMP), which then is broken down by ecto'5 nucelotidases into adenosine (see Figure 1). Adenosine kinase is mainly responsible for the removal of adenosine via phosphorylation to AMP [15]. Under hypoxic conditions when there is a build-up of adenosine in the extracellular space, hypoxia induced factors such as HIF-1α also cause an increase in the ecto'5 nucelotidases CD73, allowing for a breakdown of extracellular ATP into adenosine [16,17].

It is now known that during hypoxia, HIF-1α inhibits the equilibrative nucleoside transporters ent-1/2 located on the membranes of neurons and glia preventing adenosine reuptake into the neuronal cell [18]. Extracellular adenosine binds to A_1Rs located on both the postsynaptic and presynaptic membranes. Postsynaptic A_1R activation inhibits the activation of glutamatergic *N*-methyl-D-aspartate receptors (NMDARs) and adenosine binding to A_1Rs located presynaptically [14]. Inhibition of neurotransmitter release can be suppressed by the addition of an A_1R selective inhibitor, such as 8-cyclopentyl-1,3-dipropylxanthine (DPCPX), suggesting that adenosine binding is necessary for the reduction of post synaptic potentials [19]. It has also been shown that the A_1R binding of adenosine inhibits NMDA receptor activation [20]. Creation of knockout mice with the deletion of presynaptic A_1Rs, uncovered the neuroprotective role that adenosine receptor binding plays in the hypoxic response [21]. Synaptic depression of the excitatory post-synaptic potential (EPSP) was attenuated allowing activation of glutamatergic NMDA receptors and increasing the likelihood for excitotoxicity. More importantly decreased extracellular levels of adenosine have been shown to lead to a loss of hypoxia-induced neuroprotection after repeated exposure to hypoxia [22].

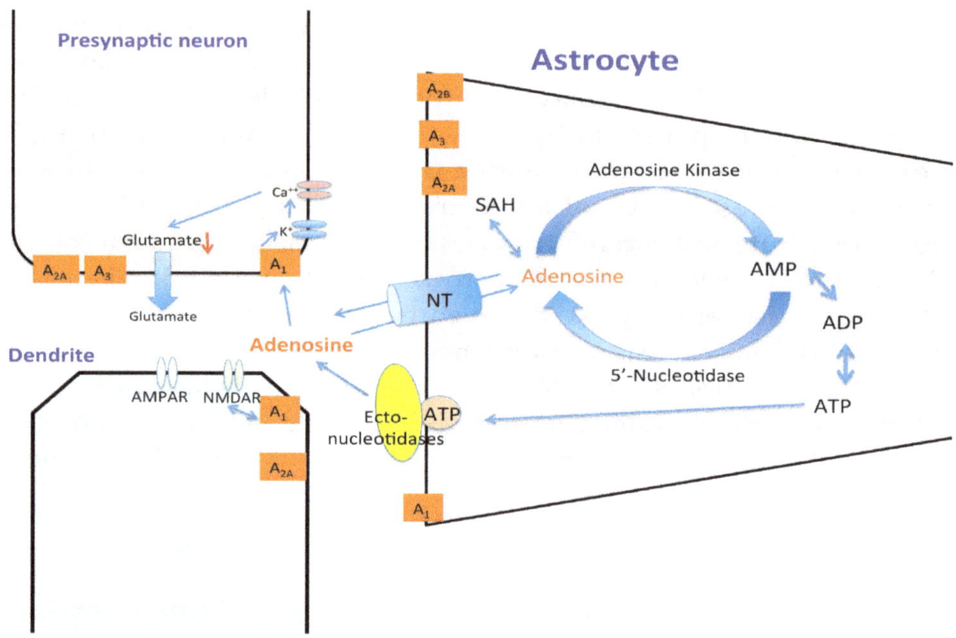

Figure 1. The effects of hypoxia on adenosine release in the CNS. Hypoxia causes a breakdown of extracellular ATP and AMP along with activation of membrane-bound transporters such as ectonucleotidases, leading to a build-up of extracellular adenosine. Adenosine binds presynaptically to A_1Rs attenuating voltage dependent calcium channel (VDCC) function and thus neurotransmitter release and also binds postsynaptically to A_1Rs receptors inactivating glutamatergic NMDARs. Adenosine is released from astrocytes in response to chronic hypoxia.

The depression of synaptic transmission in longer term hypoxia goes beyond a neuroprotective role. For example during longer duration hypoxia, nicotinamide adenine dinucleotide phosphate-oxidase oxidase production of reactive oxygen species (ROS) such as superoxides by microglial complement receptor 3 can activate protein phosphatase 2A (PP2A), which causes the internalization of postsynaptic α-amino-3-hydroxy-5-methyl-4-isoxazolepropionic acid receptors (AMPARs) through serine-threonine dephosphorlation [23]. This is similar to the discovery that the oxygen sensing *C-elegans* protein *egl-9*, which regulates HIF in an oxygen-dependent manner can also regulate C. *elegans* glutamate receptor-1 (GLR-1) trafficking through the generation of isoform-specific transgenes which interact with the GLR-1 promoter [24,25]. In normoxic conditions, egl-9 binds to Lin-10 preventing its phosphorylation, this complex then allows for the movement of glutamate receptors to the synapse. Under hypoxic conditions, Lin-10 is phosphorylated, thus preventing the formation of the EGL9/Lin-10 complex leading to a lack of synaptic GluR1 receptors [26].

One particular form of hypoxia, chronic intermittent hypoxia (CIH) may have specific detrimental effects on CNS function. CIH can lead to the over-activation of NMDARs, leading to an overload of intracellular Ca^{2+} and a dephosphorylation of extracellular signal-regulated kinases (ERK) [27]. The CA1 region of the hippocampus is thought to be selectively vulnerable to CIH damage due to the high density of glutamate receptors located on its pyramidal neurons [28]. CIH also leads to a reduction in the levels of the transcription factor cAMP response element-binding protein (CREB) in its phosphorylated form [29]. This reduction in activated CREB leads to a lowering of CREB transcriptional targets, such as brain-derived neurotrophic factor (BDNF), causing cognitive dysfunction [30]. The CIH-induced cognitive dysfunction was shown to be repaired through exogenous application of BDNF to the hypoxic cell [30]. Perinatal hypoxic events may also lead to increases in excitability in hippocampal regions. These events usually occur after asphyxia events just after birth and can lead to long term synaptic changes. Changes in excitability in some local brain regions such as the CA1 region have also been noted [31]. The pursuant neonatal seizures may be related to the phosphorylation of the AMPA GLUA1 receptors on serine 183 and serine 845. This may enhance AMPA receptor excitatory post synaptic currents (EPSCs) which allows for a decrease in the percentage of silent synapses and an increase in AMPA receptor function [32]. This loss of silent synapses is thought to be the mechanism, which attenuates synaptic plasticity in adult life [33]. In critical cases of hypoxia-re-oxygenation the brain loses the ability to form new memories. This anterograde amnesia is decoupled from the hippocampus and its primarily caused by adenosine up-regulation of caspase 1 and then IL-1β in the amygdala [34]. These effects were shown to last up to five hours after re-oxygenation with caspase inhibitors, such as YVAD-CMK, able to shorten the recovery time [34]. The links of hypoxia to cognitive disorders, as well as ability to cause neuronal apoptosis through hyper-excitability, displays the importance of understanding hypoxia and preventing its long-term effects.

3. Hypoxia and Synaptic Plasticity

As previously mentioned, hippocampal neuron exposure to hypoxia may lead to cognitive deficits due to synaptic plasticity impairments [35]. Many studies have investigated the relationship between oxygen deprivation and synaptic plasticity. Early studies indicated that brief periods of hypoxia could disrupt long-term potentiation (LTP) in the CA1 hippocampus and that this effect could be reproduced with brief application of adenosine prior to the induction of LTP [36–38]. It was later discovered that a brief anoxic episode, as opposed to hypoxia, applied to brain slices, could generate a new type of LTP although still voltage-, NMDA- [39], protein kinase C (PKC)- and NO-dependent [40–42]. It is proposed that it is the re-oxygenation and not initial de-oxygenation of neurons and the subsequent high concentration of glutamate that in fact causes the excessive activation of NMDARs and subsequent large influx of Ca^{2+} [43]. It has also been shown that chemically-induced hypoxia with the use of PHD inhibitors, and thus hypoxia mimetics, whilst having no effect on synaptic signaling at low concentrations *per se*, could inhibit LTP in the hippocampus [44,45]. Application of the iron chelator deferoxamine mesylate (DFO) or dimethyloxaloglycine (DMOG), both non-specific pharmacological inhibitors of PHD, and thus increasers of HIF-1α expression [46] could impair LTP in the CA1 hippocampus [4,44,45,47]. Interestingly the application of DMOG to the dentate gyrus region of hippocampal slices did not impair LTP [29]. It is believed that these effects of PHD inhibitors are not HIF-dependent. There is also increasing evidence for a role for CIH in synaptic plasticity and specifically LTP. Initial reports in early 2000 demonstrated that CIH treated animals demonstrated impaired LTP in isolated rat hippocampal slices [48,49]. More recently two reports have put forward evidence for a role for BDNF in this impairment [30,50]. They found that application of BDNF reversed the IH-induced impairment of LTP. In our own laboratories we have implicated a role for PHDs in this inhibition of LTP by intermittent hypoxia [29].

4. Hypoxia and Neuroinflammation in the CNS

During an ischemic stroke and resulting hypoxia, inflammatory cytokines are released by microglia, neurons and astrocytes with glutamate largely released by neurons. The up-regulation of pro-inflammatory cytokines through the activation of microglia and astrocytes in the brain contribute a great deal to ischemic brain damage [51]. During hypoxia, HIF-1α binds to HRE like binding sites allowing for the up-regulation of cytokines, such as IL-β, IL-6, IL-8, and TNF-α. Mutations in either the HIF-1α gene or its binding site at the promoter inhibit this cytokine up-regulation [46].

Up-regulation of IL-1β is related to hypoxic hyperexcitability due to the fact that IL-1β can activate tyrosine kinases, which then phosphorylate the NMDAR subunits, NR2A and NR2. This increase in NMDAR potentiation leads to excessive flow of Ca^{2+} leading to hyperexcitability and neuronal injury [52]. Hypoxia also leads to activation of nuclear factor κB (NFκB) signaling pathways whereby HIF-1α has a molecular interaction with the inflammatory mediator NFκB. HRE binding, as seen in Figure 2, allows for the expression of NFκB, which then activates the transcription of inflammatory genes and HIF proteins [53]. NFκB expression is increased when hypoxia is followed by a period of re-oxygenation [54]. Reactive oxygen species (ROS) have been shown to both activate and inactivate NFκB, which could explain the importance of the re-oxygenation period. ROS can trigger both apoptotic and necrotic cell death depending on the severity of the oxidative stress [55–57]. Another form of hypoxia, CIH, such as seen in sleep apnea can lead to neuronal cell death and one of the mechanisms involved may be inflammation. Neural inflammation caused by CIH can be region specific with the expression of microglial toll-like receptor-4 (TLR4) increased differentially across areas of the CNS [58]. Hypoxia-re-oxygenation increases microglial levels of inducible nitric oxide synthase (iNOS) leading to neuronal cell loss through apoptosis and memory impairment [59] Many other insults such as bacterial, viral, cytokines and neurodegenerative insults induce iNOS in microglia [60]. This increase in iNOS raises the levels of NO allowing for the inhibition of neuronal respiration causing glutamate release [61]. Rho-associated protein kinase (ROCK) is thought to play a vital role in this pathway as the introduction of the ROCK inhibitor, fasudil, attenuates the neuronal apoptosis [62]. Thus inflammatory pathways and microglial activation are key components to the hypoxic response whereby their activation allows for formation of ROS as well as having the ability to modulate glutamatergic receptors. The important role they play in causing neuronal cell damage as well their potential to be neuroprotective through hypoxic preconditioning makes the inflammatory response a vital therapeutic target in hypoxia. Only recently has it been reported that patients with obstructive sleep apnea (involving episodes of IH) were 1.37 times more likely to have Parkinson's disease than patients without the disease [63].

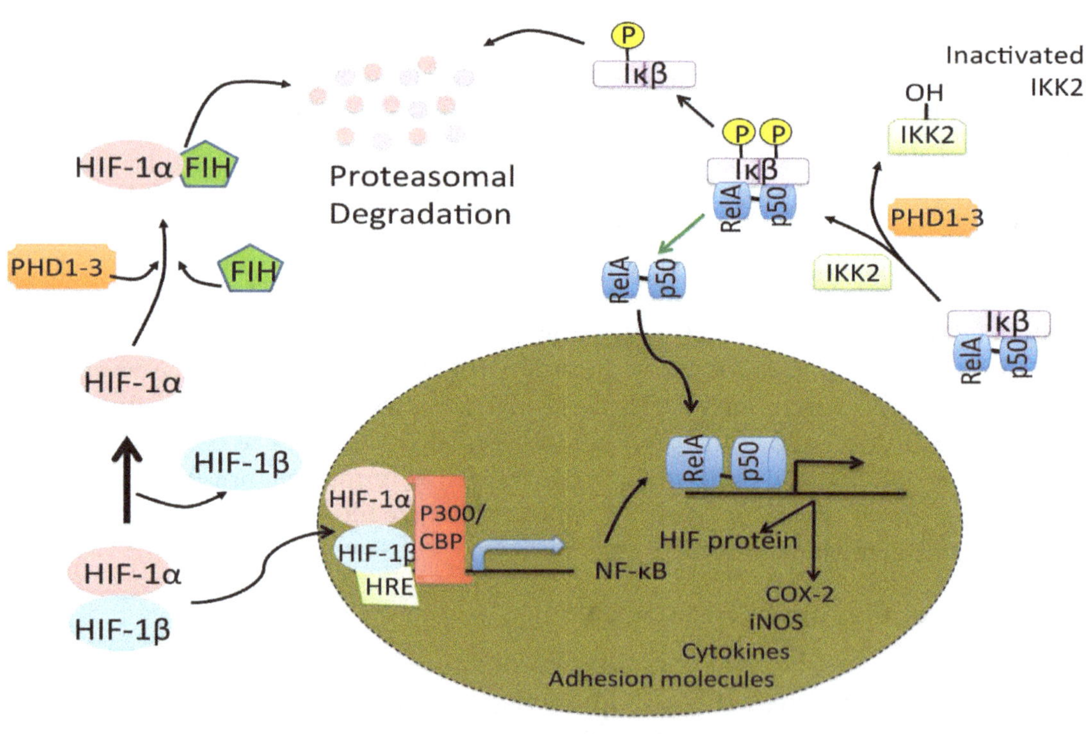

Figure 2. Hypoxia and NFκB activation. During hypoxic HIF-1α binding to the HRE induces the expression of NFκB (**left**). NFκB p50 p65 dimer is able to freely activate the transcription of inflammatory and HIF proteins (**right**).

5. TNF-α and Hypoxia

TNF-α, a pro-inflammatory cytokine produced primarily by monocytes and macrophages in the periphery and microglia and neurons in the CNS, is involved in the promotion of the inflammatory response and cognitive dysfunction [64,65]. TNF-α is initially produced as a 212-amino acid-long type II transmembrane that is stable as a homotrimer. The cleavage of the membrane-integrated form by TNF-α converting enzyme produces a soluble homotrimer, which binds to either of two receptors, TNF receptor type 1 (TNFR1) or TNF receptor type 2 (TNFR2). TNFR1 is constitutively expressed throughout most tissues and is thought to be the main TNF signaling receptor. The activation of TNF-R1 leads to either apoptotic cell death or the activation of either the caspase-8 pathway or c-Jun NH2-terminal kinase (JNK) pathways, or neuroprotection through the binding of IκB kinase (IKK) complex and the subsequent activation of the NFκB pathway [66]. The signaling network in TNF-R1 is interesting due to the extensive crosstalk between the NFκB, and JNK signaling pathways. The cells susceptibility to apoptosis increases in the absence of NFκB. The activation of TNFR2 leads to the activation of the NFκB pathway, phosphatidyl-inositol-3 kinase (PI3K) and subsequent transcription of neuroprotective mediators like calbindin and manganese superoxide dismutase [67,68]. Specifically in microglia activation of TNFR2 anti-inflammatory pathways may be induced [69]. A putative role for TNF-α has been shown in rats infused with lipopolysaccharide (LPS may promote the secretion of pro-inflammatory cytokines including TNF-α and IL-1β) into the fourth ventricle to induce chronic neuroinflammation [70]. TNF-α synthesis inhibition was found to restore the neuronal function as well as reverse cognitive deficits induced by the chronic neuroinflammation [70].

It is becoming apparent that TNF-α is one of the most important inflammatory cytokines to be studied in relation to neuronal damage caused by the absence of oxygen due to the fact that it actively participates in the immune-mediated inflammation of stroke and other neurodegenerative diseases with an hypoxia component [71]. The release of TNF-α is a result of the pathogenesis of disorders such as stroke [72], Alzheimer's disease [73], Parkinson's disease [74] and severe infections such as meningitis [75], yet its role during hypoxia is not fully understood. In severe ischemia TNF-α levels appear to be elevated in affected brain tissue after 24 h [76]. One such critical role in neuroinflammation has been illustrated whereby TNF-α can damage dopaminergic neurons and thus anti-TNF agents may ameliorate Parkinson's disease [74]. Despite many research papers in this field few laboratories have investigated the effects of acute hypoxia and inflammatory mediators on synaptic transmission [77,78]. Recently our laboratory reported that recovery of synaptic transmission in CA1 neurons was impaired post-hypoxia in the presence of TNF-α [77]. It also been shown that HIF-1α has a binding site for the Fas Associated Death Domain promoter, which is an adapter molecule in TNFR1 mediated cell death. Therefore it has a direct role in TNF-α mediated apoptosis which may help explain the poor recovery of EPSPs following a hypoxic insult [79].

A growing body of evidence indicates that TNF-α may play a role in the regulation of tolerance to chronic hypoxia such as occurs in ischemia yet it has a deleterious effect in ischemic brain injury after stroke [80]. It seems that administration of a high dose of lipopolysaccharide (LPS) may induce a robust inflammatory response that can result in lethal septic shock whereas administration of a low dose of LPS may induce a protective state of tolerance to subsequent exposure to LPS at doses that might cause serious injury [81,82]. In fact LPS preconditioning is known to exert neuroprotection from cerebral ischemia [83,84]. In cerebellar granule neurons the neuroprotective effects of LPS preconditioning were said to be independent of endogenous IL-1β but dependent on endogenous TNF-α and also IL-6 [85]. Our laboratories have recently provided evidence that TNF-α has a preconditioning effect following a glutamate toxic insult 24 h later in the CA1 region of rat organotypic slices [65]. We suggested that the preconditioning effects may be as a result of changing resting Ca^{2+} levels and Ca^{2+} influx in the presence of TNF-α.

6. TNF-α and Synaptic Plasticity

A growing body of evidence has highlighted the role of TNF-α in glutamatergic synaptic plasticity and scaling. It has been shown that TNF-α has an inhibitory effect on LTP in both the CA1 and dentate gyrus [76,86–89]. Studies initially carried out by Tancredi *et al.* (1992) [90] showed an inhibitory effect of TNF-α on LTP induction in the CA1 region, which was concentration-dependent. However, they demonstrated that short-term application of TNF-α (>50 min) did not affect LTP. These findings and others highlight the various parameters involved in the regulatory role that this cytokine plays in synaptic plasticity. The inhibitory actions of TNF-α on LTP have been shown to be mediated through the signaling pathways, P38 MAP kinase and JNK [91]. Butler *et al.* (2004) [88] reported that the inhibition of LTP by TNF-α was in fact a biphasic response. SB203580, a P38 MAPK inhibitor, blocked the early inhibition of LTP by TNF-α but did not reverse its late inhibition (3 h following induction), possibly due to the requirement for new protein synthesis. Using antagonists for metabotropic glutamate receptor 5 (mGluR5) and ryanodine, a potential role for metabotropic glutamate receptors and ryanodine sensitive intracellular Ca^{2+} stores in TNF-α mediated inhibition of LTP have also been proposed [87].

Other studies have provided evidence that exogenous application of TNF-α whilst not inhibiting LTP in the CA1 region of the hippocampus may alter homeostatic plasticity (synaptic scaling) rather than synaptic plasticity [92]. These studies have shown that glia released TNF-α is required for synaptic scaling through AMPAR trafficking to the membrane [92–94]. Others have reported that the increase in AMPAR expression on the cell surface is mediated through the P13 kinase pathway and the AMPARs trafficked were lacking the GLR-2 subunit. Since LTP is dependent on synaptic glutamate it is also interesting to note that TNF-α has been shown to increase glutamate release from astrocytes [95], block glutamate transporters [96], and also may have a modulatory effect on the expression of GLT-1 and GLT-2. These effects combined may result in increased glutamate concentrations in the synaptic cleft [97,98]. TNFR1, but not TNFR2, may play an important role in AMPAR localization on the membrane of cortical neurons. Deletion of TNFR1 resulted in a decrease of AMPAR clustering on the synaptic membrane, which was not rescued by exogenous application of TNF-α [99]. These observations indicate a potential therapeutic approach for TNF-α via TNFR1 in mediating AMPAR excitotoxicity. Glutamatergic gliotransmission is an important stimulatory input to excitatory synapses and it has been shown that TNF-α is a modulator of this process in the dentate gyrus [100]. Many of the discrepancies observed with regard to the effects of TNF-α on LTP may be region specific or indeed depend on the induction protocol used to induce LTP. There are many factors regulating the magnitude of LTP induced by different parameters such as high frequency stimulation and theta burst stimulation [101] (Figure 3). Recently, we have shown that the stimulation parameters used to induce LTP may have an influence on TNF-α's ability to inhibit LTP [102]. TNF-α has no inhibitory effect on LTP when induced with prolonged high frequency stimulation (HFS) whereas full inhibition was observed when LTP was induced by theta burst stimulation (TBS). Figure 3 illustrates a potential mechanism that might explain this discrepancy whereby TBS may trigger alternative signaling cascades to HFS that can be modulated by TNF-α.

7. TNF-α, Hypoxia and Synaptic Plasticity

Hippocampal slices exposed to acute hypoxia may recover when oxygen is re-introduced. Recently it has been shown that in the presence of TNF-α there is an impairment in the recovery of synaptic transmission in the CA1 region post-hypoxia [77]. Conversely, hypoxia has also been shown to increase intercellular Ca^{2+} levels and activate calmodulin-dependent protein kinase II (CaMKII) through a TNF-α independent mechanism [103]. However CaMKII is also capable of activating the PI3K-PKCλ-AMPAR signaling pathway. TNF-α has been found to play roles in cell adhesion up-regulation, disruption of the blood brain barrier and is a key component for the participation of glial cells in the physiological control of synaptic transmission and plasticity through the release of glutamate, a process known as glutamatergic gliotranmission [100,104]. TNF-α has been shown to increase the release of glutamate from astrocytes, maintain glutamate levels through the blocking of glutamate transporters [96] and modulate the expression of Glut-1 and Glut-2. All these effects by TNF-α result in the increase in the concentration of glutamate in the synaptic cleft, which may have an influence on the magnitude of LTP post-hypoxia. Using a robust LTP-inducing stimulus protocol we have been able to demonstrate a significant enhancing effect of TNF-α on LTP post hypoxia but only in the dentate gyrus of the hippocampus [102]. In the presence of DMOG (a non-specific PHD inhibitor) this enhancement of LTP was still evident perhaps indicating a novel HIF/PHD-independent effect of TNF-α [102].

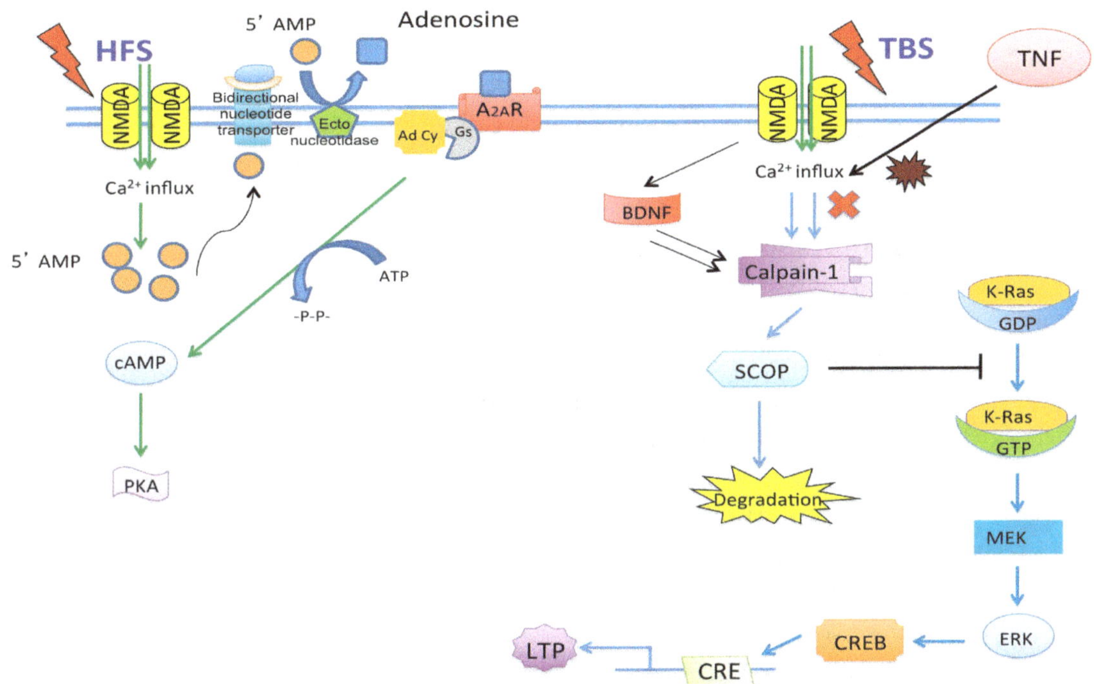

Figure 3. Putative signaling pathways activated after HFS- and TBS-induced LTP. HFS-induced LTP may be dependent on the breakdown of 5′ AMP into adenosine. Adenosine activates the $A_{2A}R$ receptor leading to cAMP and PKA activation. TBS-induced LTP involves the influx of Ca^{2+} and subsequent activation of calpain-1. The activation of calpain-1 leads to a calapin-1-mediated suprachiasmatic nucleus circadian oscillatory protein degradation and ERK activation. Exogenous TNF-α inhibits LTP induced by TBS only. During hypoxia, TNF-α may have potentiating effect on HFS-induced LTP but not TBS.

8. Conclusions

Hypoxia is one of the key components, which can arise from neuropathological conditions such as stroke, Parkinson's or Alzheimer's disease. Hypoxic events can cause the release of pro-inflammatory cytokines from neurons and glial cells, such as TNF-α, which can lead to further neurotoxicity or indeed neuroprotection in the brain. However, the effects of TNF-α on neurons during de- and re-oxygenation of neurons is largely unknown. Many studies have now shown that pro-inflammatory cytokines, such as TNF-α, play a key role in the regulation of synaptic transmission and plasticity in the absence and presence of acute hypoxia, especially within the hippocampus. The mechanisms by which elevated levels of TNF-α have an enhancing or detrimental effect on synaptic signaling and synaptic plasticity in the presence or after a hypoxic event remains to be elucidated.

Acknowledgments: We would like to thank Irish Aid and University College Dublin for financial support.

Author Contributions: Gatambwa Mukandala wrote the sections on TNF- and hypoxia and hypoxia and neuroinflammation in the CNS and conceived and designed experiments referred to in the review. Ronan Tynan wrote the sections on hypoxia and synaptic signaling and hypoxia and synaptic plasticity. Sinead Lanigan wrote the introduction and edited the final version of the manuscript and figures. John J. O'Connor conceived and designed the experiments referred to in the review, contributed reagents/materials/analysis tools and wrote the paper.

Abbreviations

A_1Rs	Adenosine A_1 receptors
AMP	adenosine monophosphate
AMPARs	α-amino-3-hydroxy-5-methyl-4-isoxazolepropionic acid receptors
ATP	adenosine triphosphate
BDNF	brain-derived neurotrophic factor
CaMKII	calmodulin-dependent protein kinase II
CIH	chronic intermittent hypoxia
CNS	central nervous system
CREB	cAMP response element-binding protein
DMOG	dimethyloxaloglycine
DPCPX	8-cyclopentyl-1,3-dipropylxanthine
EPSP	excitatory post-synaptic potential
ERK	extracellular signal-regulated kinases
HIF	hypoxia inducible factors
HRE	hypoxic responsive element
IL-1β	interleukin-1beta
iNOS	inducible nitric oxide synthase
LPS	lipopolysaccharide
LTP	long-term potentiation
NFkB	nuclear factor kB
NMDAR	*N*-methyl-D-aspartate receptors
PHDs	prolyl hydroxyl domains
PI3K	phosphatidyl-inositol-3 kinase
ROCK	Rho-associated protein kinase
ROS	reactive oxygen species
TNF-α	tumor necrosis factor alpha

References

1. Sharp, F.R.; Bernaudin, M. HIF1 and oxygen sensing in the brain. *Nat. Rev. Neurosci.* **2004**, *5*, 437–448. [CrossRef] [PubMed]
2. Bickler, P.E.; Donohoe, P.H. Adaptive responses of vertebrate neurons to hypoxia. *J. Exp. Biol.* **2002**, *205*, 3579–3586.
3. Eltzschig, H.K.; Bratton, D.L.; Colgan, S.P. Targeting hypoxia signaling for the treatment of ischaemic and inflammatory diseases. *Nat. Rev. Drug Discov.* **2014**, *13*, 852–869. [CrossRef] [PubMed]
4. Corcoran, A.; O'Connor, J.J. Hypoxia-inducible factor signaling mechanisms in the central nervous system. *Acta Physiol.* **2013**, *208*, 298–310. [CrossRef] [PubMed]
5. Moroz, E.; Carlin, S.; Dyomina, K.; Burke, S.; Thaler, H.T.; Blasberg, R.; Serganova, I. Real-time imaging of HIF-1α stabilization and degradation. *PLoS ONE* **2009**, *4*, e5077. [CrossRef] [PubMed]
6. Webb, J.D.; Coleman, M.L.; Pugh, C.W. Hypoxia, hypoxia-inducible factors (HIF), HIF hydroxylases and oxygen sensing. *Cell. Mol. Life Sci.* **2009**, *66*, 3539–3554. [CrossRef] [PubMed]
7. Semenza, G.L. Oxygen sensing, hypoxia-inducible factors, and disease pathophysiology. *Annu. Rev. Pathol.* **2014**, *9*, 47–71. [CrossRef] [PubMed]

8. Kamel, H.; Iadecola, C. Brain-immune interactions and ischemic stroke: Clinical implications. *Arch Neurol.* **2012**, *69*, 576–581. [PubMed]
9. Amantea, D.; Micieli, G.; Tassorelli, C.; Cuartero, M.I.; Ballesteros, I.; Certo, M.; Moro, M.A.; Lizasoain, I.; Bagetta, G. Rational modulation of the innate immune system for neuroprotection in ischemic stroke. *Front. Neurosci.* **2015**, *9*, 147. [CrossRef] [PubMed]
10. Lipton, P.; Whittingham, T.S. The effect of hypoxia on evoked potentials in the *in vitro* hippocampus. *J. Physiol.* **1979**, *287*, 427–438. [CrossRef] [PubMed]
11. Björklund, O.; Shang, M.; Tonazzini, I.; Daré, E.; Fredholm, B.B. Adenosine A1 and A3 receptors protect astrocytes from hypoxic damage. *Eur. J. Pharmacol.* **2008**, *596*, 6–13. [CrossRef] [PubMed]
12. Palmer, T.M.; Stiles, G.L. Adenosine receptors. *Neuropharmacology* **1995**, *34*, 683–694. [CrossRef]
13. Reppert, S.M.; Weaver, D.R.; Stehle, J.H.; Rivkees, S.A. Molecular cloning and characterization of a rat A1-adenosine receptor that is widely expressed in brain and spinal cord. *Mol. Endocrinol.* **1991**, *5*, 1037–1048. [CrossRef] [PubMed]
14. McCool, B.A.; Farroni, J.S. A1 adenosine receptors inhibit multiple voltage-gated Ca^{2+} channel subtypes in acutely isolated rat basolateral amygdala neurons. *Br. J. Pharmacol.* **2001**, *132*, 879–888. [CrossRef] [PubMed]
15. Boison, D. Adenosine kinase, epilepsy and stroke: Mechanisms and therapies. *Trends Pharmacol. Sci.* **2006**, *27*, 652–658. [CrossRef] [PubMed]
16. Görlach, A. Control of adenosine transport by hypoxia. *Circ. Res.* **2005**, *97*, 1–3. [CrossRef] [PubMed]
17. Takahashi, T.; Otsuguro, K.; Ohta, T.; Ito, S. Adenosine and inosine release during hypoxia in the isolated spinal cord of neonatal rats. *Br. J. Pharmacol.* **2010**, *161*, 1806–1816. [CrossRef] [PubMed]
18. Morote-Garcia, J.C.; Rosenberger, P.; Nivillac, N.M.; Coe, I.R.; Eltzschig, H.K. Hypoxia-inducible factor-dependent repression of equilibrative nucleoside transporter 2 attenuates mucosal inflammation during intestinal hypoxia. *Gastroenterology* **2009**, *136*, 607–618. [CrossRef] [PubMed]
19. Choi, I.S.; Cho, J.H.; Lee, M.G.; Jang, I.S. Enzymatic conversion of ATP to adenosine contributes to ATP-induced inhibition of glutamate release in rat medullary dorsal horn neurons. *Neuropharmacology* **2015**, *93*, 94–102. [CrossRef] [PubMed]
20. De Mendonça, A.; Sebastião, A.M.; Ribeiro, J.A. Inhibition of NMDA receptor-mediated currents in isolated rat hippocampal neurones by adenosine A1 receptor activation. *Neuroreport* **1995**, *6*, 1097–1100. [CrossRef] [PubMed]
21. Arrigoni, E.; Crocker, A.J.; Saper, C.B.; Greene, R.W.; Scammell, T.E. Deletion of presynaptic adenosine A1 receptors impairs the recovery of synaptic transmission after hypoxia. *Neuroscience* **2005**, *132*, 575–580. [CrossRef] [PubMed]
22. Cui, M.; Bai, X.; Li, T.; Chen, F.; Dong, Q.; Zhao, Y.; Liu, X. Decreased extracellular adenosine levels lead to loss of hypoxia-induced neuroprotection after repeated episodes of exposure to hypoxia. *PLoS ONE* **2013**, *8*, e57065. [CrossRef] [PubMed]
23. Zhang, J.; Malik, A.; Choi, H.B.; Ko, R.W.; Dissing-Olesen, L.; MacVicar, B.A. Microglial CR3 activation triggers long-term synaptic depression in the hippocampus via NADPH oxidase. *Neuron* **2014**, *82*, 195–207. [CrossRef] [PubMed]
24. Ma, D.K.; Vozdek, R.; Bhatla, N.; Horvitz, H.R. CYSL-1 interacts with the O_2-sensing hydroxylase EGL-9 to promote H_2S-modulated hypoxia-induced behavioral plasticity in C. elegans. *Neuron* **2012**, *73*, 925–940. [CrossRef] [PubMed]
25. Park, E.C.; Ghose, P.; Shao, Z.; Ye, Q.; Kang, L.; Xu, X.Z.; Powell-Coffman, J.A.; Rongo, C. Hypoxia regulates glutamate receptor trafficking through an HIF-independent mechanism. *EMBO J.* **2012**, *31*, 1379–1393. [CrossRef] [PubMed]
26. Epstein, A.C.; Gleadle, J.M.; McNeill, L.A.; Hewitson, K.S.; O'Rourke, J.; Mole, D.R.; Mukherji, M.; Metzen, E.; Wilson, M.I.; Dhanda, A.; *et al.* C. elegans EGL-9 and mammalian homologs define a family of dioxygenases that regulate HIF by prolyl hydroxylation. *Cell* **2001**, *107*, 43–54. [CrossRef]
27. Wang, J.; Ming, H.; Chen, R.; Ju, J.M.; Peng, W.D.; Zhang, G.X.; Liu, C.F. CIH-induced neurocognitive impairments are associated with hippocampal Ca^{2+} overload, apoptosis, and dephosphorylation of ERK1/2 and CREB that are mediated by overactivation of NMDARs. *Brain Res.* **2015**, *1625*, 64–72. [CrossRef] [PubMed]
28. McDonald, J.W.; Johnston, M.V. Physiological and pathophysiological roles of excitatory amino acids during central nervous system development. *Brain Res. Brain Res. Rev.* **1990**, *15*, 41–70. [CrossRef]

29. Wall, A.M.; Corcoran, A.E.; O'Halloran, K.D.; O'Connor, J.J. Effects of prolyl-hydroxylase inhibition and chronic intermittent hypoxia on synaptic transmission and plasticity in the rat CA1 and dentate gyrus. *Neurobiol. Dis.* **2014**, *62*, 8–17. [CrossRef] [PubMed]
30. Xie, H.; Leung, K.L.; Chen, L.; Chan, Y.S.; Ng, P.C.; Fok, T.F.; Wing, Y.K.; Ke, Y.; Li, A.M.; Yung, W.H. Brain-derived neurotrophic factor rescues and prevents chronic intermittent hypoxia-induced impairment of hippocampal long-term synaptic plasticity. *Neurobiol. Dis.* **2010**, *40*, 155–162. [CrossRef] [PubMed]
31. Jensen, F.E.; Wang, C.; Stafstrom, C.E.; Liu, Z.; Geary, C.; Stevens, M.C. Acute and chronic increases in excitability in rat hippocampal slices after perinatal hypoxia *in vivo*. *J. Neurophysiol.* **1998**, *79*, 73–81. [PubMed]
32. Zhou, C.; Lippman, J.J.; Sun, H.; Jensen, F.E. Hypoxia-induced neonatal seizures diminish silent synapses and long-term potentiation in hippocampal CA1 neurons. *J. Neurosci.* **2011**, *31*, 18211–18222. [CrossRef] [PubMed]
33. Kerchner, G.A.; Nicoll, R.A. Silent synapses and the emergence of a postsynaptic mechanism for LTP. *Nat. Rev. Neurosci.* **2008**, *9*, 813–825. [CrossRef] [PubMed]
34. Chiu, G.S.; Chatterjee, D.; Darmody, P.T.; Walsh, J.P.; Meling, D.D.; Johnson, R.W.; Freund, G.G. Hypoxia/reoxygenation impairs memory formation via adenosine-dependent activation of caspase 1. *J. Neurosci.* **2012**, *32*, 13945–13955. [CrossRef] [PubMed]
35. Row, B.W.; Liu, R.; Xu, W.; Kheirandish, L.; Gozal, D. Intermittent hypoxia is associated with oxidative stress and spatial learning deficits in the rat. *Am. J. Respir. Crit. Care Med.* **2003**, *167*, 1548–1553. [CrossRef] [PubMed]
36. Arai, A.; Kessler, M.; Lynch, G. The effects of adenosine on the development of long-term potentiation. *Neurosci. Lett.* **1990**, *119*, 41–44. [CrossRef]
37. Arai, A.; Vanderklish, P.; Kessler, M.; Lee, K.; Lynch, G. A brief period of hypoxia causes proteolysis of cytoskeletal proteins in hippocampal slices. *Brain Res.* **1990**, *555*, 276–280. [CrossRef]
38. Lyubkin, M.; Durand, D.M.; Haxhiu, M.A. Interaction between tetanus long-term potentiation and hypoxia-induced potentiation in the rat hippocampus. *J. Neurophysiol.* **1997**, *78*, 2475–2482. [PubMed]
39. Hammond, C.; Crépel, V.; Gozlan, H.; Ben-Ari, Y. Anoxic LTP sheds light on the multiple facets of NMDA receptors. *Trends Neurosci.* **1994**, *17*, 497–503. [CrossRef]
40. Hsu, K.S.; Huang, C.C. Characterization of the anoxia-induced long-term synaptic potentiation in area CA1 of the rat hippocampus. *Br. J. Pharmacol.* **1997**, *122*, 671–681. [CrossRef] [PubMed]
41. Huang, C.C.; Hsu, K.S. Nitric oxide signaling is required for the generation of anoxia-induced long-term potentiation in the hippocampus. *Eur. J. Neurosci.* **1997**, *9*, 2202–2206. [CrossRef] [PubMed]
42. Weilinger, N.L.; Tang, P.L.; Thompson, R.J. Anoxia-induced NMDA receptor activation opens pannexin channels via Src family kinases. *J. Neurosci.* **2012**, *32*, 12579–12588. [CrossRef] [PubMed]
43. Kass, I.S.; Lipton, T.P. Calcium and Long-term transmission damage following anoxia in dentate gyrus and CA1 regions of the rat hippocampal slice. *J. Physiol.* **1986**, *378*, 313–334. [CrossRef] [PubMed]
44. Muñoz, P.; Humeres, A.; Elgueta, C.; Kirkwood, A.; Hidalgo, C.; Núñez, M.T. Iron mediates *N*-methyl-D-aspartate receptor-dependent stimulation of calcium-induced pathways and hippocampal synaptic plasticity. *J. Biol. Chem.* **2011**, *286*, 13382–13392. [CrossRef] [PubMed]
45. Corcoran, A.; Kunze, R.; Harney, S.C.; Breier, G.; Marti, H.H.; O'Connor, J.J. A role for prolyl hydroxylase domain proteins in hippocampal synaptic plasticity. *Hippocampus* **2013**, *872*, 861–872. [CrossRef] [PubMed]
46. Zhang, W.; Petrovic, J.M.; Callaghan, D.; Jones, A.; Cui, H.; Howlett, C.; Stanimirovic, D. Evidence that hypoxia-inducible factor-1 (HIF-1) mediates transcriptional activation of interleukin-1beta (IL-1β) in astrocyte cultures. *J. Neuroimmunol.* **2006**, *174*, 63–73. [CrossRef] [PubMed]
47. Batti, L.; Taylor, C.T.; O'Connor, J.J. Hydroxylase inhibition reduces synaptic transmission and protects against a glutamate-induced ischemia in the CA1 region of the rat hippocampus. *Neuroscience* **2010**, *167*, 1014–1024. [CrossRef] [PubMed]
48. Wang, X.R.; Ma, Q.; Ding, A.S.; Zeng, B.X.; Wang, F.Z. Effects of intermittent hypoxia on long-term potentiation in hippocampal dentate gyrus of rat. *Zhongguo Ying Yong Sheng Li Xue Za Zhi* **2001**, *17*, 18–20. [PubMed]
49. Payne, R.S.; Goldbart, A.; Gozal, D.; Schurr, A. Effect of intermittent hypoxia on long-term potentiation in rat hippocampal slices. *Brain Res.* **2004**, *1029*, 195–199. [CrossRef] [PubMed]

50. Xie, H.; Yung, W. Chronic intermittent hypoxia-induced deficits in synaptic plasticity and neurocognitive functions: A role for brain-derived neurotrophic factor. *Acta Pharmacol. Sin.* **2012**, *33*, 5–10. [CrossRef] [PubMed]
51. Domac, F.M.; Somay, G.; Misirli, H.; Erenoglu, N.Y. Tumor necrosis factor alpha serum levels and inflammatory response in acute ischemic stroke. *Neurosciences* **2007**, *12*, 25–30. [PubMed]
52. Viviani, B.; Bartesaghi, S.; Gardoni, F.; Vezzani, A.; Behrens, M.M.; Bartfai, T.; Binaglia, M.; Corsini, E.; Di Luca, M.; Galli, C.L.; Marinovich, M. Interleukin-1beta enhances NMDA receptor-mediated intracellular calcium increase through activation of the Src family of kinases. *J. Neurosci.* **2003**, *23*, 8692–8700. [PubMed]
53. Eltzschig, H.K.; Carmeliet, P. Hypoxia and inflammation. *N. Engl. J. Med.* **2011**, *364*, 656–665. [PubMed]
54. Stanimirovic, D.; Zhang, W.; Howlett, C.; Lemieux, P.; Smith, C. Inflammatory gene transcription in human astrocytes exposed to hypoxia: Roles of the nuclear factor-kappaB and autocrine stimulation. *J. Neuroimmunol.* **2001**, *119*, 365–376. [CrossRef]
55. Morgan, M.J.; Liu, Z.-G. Crosstalk of reactive oxygen species and NF-κB signaling. *Cell Res.* **2011**, *21*, 103–115. [CrossRef] [PubMed]
56. Saito, Y.; Nishio, K.; Ogawa, Y.; Kimata, J.; Kinumi, T.; Yoshida, Y.; Noguchi, N.; Niki, E. Turning point in apoptosis/necrosis induced by hydrogen peroxide. *Free Radic. Res.* **2006**, *40*, 619–630. [CrossRef] [PubMed]
57. Takeda, M.; Shirato, I.; Kobayashi, M.; Endou, H. Hydrogen peroxide induces necrosis, apoptosis, oncosis and apoptotic oncosis of mouse terminal proximal straight tubule cells. *Nephron* **1999**, *81*, 234–238. [CrossRef] [PubMed]
58. Smith, S.M.; Friedle, S.A.; Watters, J.J. Chronic intermittent hypoxia exerts CNS region-specific effects on rat microglial inflammatory and TLR4 gene expression. *PLoS ONE* **2013**, *8*, e81584. [CrossRef] [PubMed]
59. Udayabanu, M.; Kumaran, D.; Nair, R.U.; Srinivas, P.; Bhagat, N.; Aneja, R.; Katyal, A. Nitric oxide associated with iNOS expression inhibits acetylcholinesterase activity and induces memory impairment during acute hypobaric hypoxia. *Brain Res.* **2008**, *1230*, 138–149. [CrossRef] [PubMed]
60. Saha, R.N.; Pahan, K. Regulation of Inducible Nitric Oxide Synthase Gene in Glial Cells. *Antioxid. Redox Signal.* **2006**, *8*, 929–947. [CrossRef] [PubMed]
61. Yang, Q.; Wang, Y.; Feng, J.; Cao, J.; Chen, B. Intermittent hypoxia from obstructive sleep apnea may cause neuronal impairment and dysfunction in central nervous system: The potential roles played by microglia. *Neuropsychiatr. Dis. Treat.* **2013**, *9*, 1077–1086. [PubMed]
62. Ding, J.; Li, Q.Y.; Wang, X.; Sun, C.H.; Lu, C.Z.; Xiao, B.G. Fasudil protects hippocampal neurons against hypoxia-reoxygenation injury by suppressing microglial inflammatory responses in mice. *J. Neurochem.* **2010**, *114*, 1619–1629. [CrossRef] [PubMed]
63. Yeh, N.C.; Tien, K.J.; Yang, C.M.; Wang, J.J.; Weng, S.F. Increased risk of Parkinson's disease in patients with obstructive sleep apnea: A population-based, propensity score-matched, longitudinal follow-up study. *Medicine* **2016**, *95*, e2293. [CrossRef] [PubMed]
64. Baune, B.T.; Camara, M.-L.; Eyre, H.; Jawahar, C.; Anscomb, H.; Körner, H. Tumour necrosis factor—Alpha mediated mechanisms of cognitive dysfunction. *Transl. Neurosci.* **2012**, *3*, 263–277. [CrossRef]
65. Watters, O.; O'Connor, J.J. A role for tumor necrosis factor-α in ischemia and ischemic preconditioning. *J. Neuroinflamm.* **2011**, *8*, 1–8. [CrossRef] [PubMed]
66. Chen, G.; Goeddel, D.V. TNF-R1 signaling: A beautiful pathway. *Science* **2002**, *296*, 1634–1635. [CrossRef] [PubMed]
67. Glazner, G.W.; Mattson, M.P. Differential effects of BDNF, ADNF9, and TNFα on levels of NMDA receptor subunits, calcium homeostasis, and neuronal vulnerability to excitotoxicity. *Exp. Neurol.* **2000**, *161*, 442–452. [CrossRef] [PubMed]
68. Marchetti, L.; Klein, M.; Schlett, K.; Pfizenmaier, K.; Eisel, U.L. Tumor necrosis factor (TNF)-mediated neuroprotection against glutamate-induced excitotoxicity is enhanced by *N*-methyl-D-aspartate receptor activation. Essential role of a TNF receptor 2-mediated phosphatidylinositol 3-kinase-dependent NF-kappa B pathway. *J. Biol. Chem.* **2004**, *279*, 32869–32881. [CrossRef] [PubMed]
69. Veroni, C.; Gabriele, L.; Canini, I.; Castiello, L.; Coccia, E.; Remoli, M.E.; Columba-Cabezas, S.; Aricò, E.; Aloisi, F. Agresti, C. Activation of TNF receptor 2 in microglia promotes induction of anti-inflammatory pathways. *Mol. Cell. Neurosci.* **2010**, *45*, 234–244. [CrossRef] [PubMed]

70. Belarbi, K.; Jopson, T.; Tweedie, D.; Arellano, C.; Luo, W.; Greig, N.H.; Rosi, S. TNF-α protein synthesis inhibitor restores neuronal function and reverses cognitive deficits induced by chronic neuroinflammation. *J. Neuroinflamm.* **2012**, *9*, 23. [CrossRef] [PubMed]
71. Marousi, S.; Antonacopoulou, A.; Kalofonos, H.; Papathanasopoulos, P.; Karakantza, M.; Ellul, J. Functional inflammatory genotypes in ischemic stroke: Could we use them to predict age of onset and long-term outcome? *Stroke Res. Treat.* **2011**, *2011*, 792923. [CrossRef] [PubMed]
72. Klein, B.D.; White, H.S.; Callahan, K.S. Cytokine and intracellular signaling regulation of tissue factor expression in astrocytes. *Neurochem. Int.* **2000**, *36*, 441–449. [CrossRef]
73. Tsoi, L.-M.; Wong, K.-Y.; Liu, Y.-M.; Ho, Y.-Y. Apoprotein E isoform-dependent expression and secretion of pro-inflammatory cytokines TNF-alpha and IL-6 in macrophages. *Arch. Biochem. Biophys.* **2007**, *460*, 33–40. [CrossRef] [PubMed]
74. Lull, M.E.; Block, M.L. Microglial activation and chronic neurodegeneration. *Neurotherapeutics* **2010**, *7*, 354–365. [CrossRef] [PubMed]
75. Barichello, T.; dos Santos, I.; Savi, G.D.; Simões, L.R.; Silvestre, T.; Comim, C.M.; Sachs, D.; Teixeira, M.M.; Teixeira, A.L.; Quevedo, J. TNF-α, IL-1β, IL-6, and cinc-1 levels in rat brain after meningitis induced by Streptococcus pneumoniae. *J. Neuroimmunol.* **2010**, *221*, 42–45. [CrossRef] [PubMed]
76. Liu, T.; Clark, R.K.; McDonnell, P.C.; Young, P.R.; White, R.F.; Barone, F.C.; Feuerstein, G.Z. Tumor necrosis factor-alpha expression in ischemic neurons. *Stroke* **1994**, *25*, 1481–1488. [CrossRef] [PubMed]
77. Batti, L.; O'Connor, J.J. Tumor necrosis factor-alpha impairs the recovery of synaptic transmission from hypoxia in rat hippocampal slices. *J. Neuroimmunol.* **2010**, *218*, 21–27. [CrossRef] [PubMed]
78. O'Connor, J.J. Targeting tumour necrosis factor-α in hypoxia and synaptic signaling. *Ir. J. Med. Sci.* **2013**, *182*, 157–162. [CrossRef] [PubMed]
79. Hindryckx, P.; De Vos, M.; Jacques, P.; Ferdinande, L.; Peeters, H.; Olievier, K.; Bogaert, S.; Brinkman, B.; Vandenabeele, P.; Elewaut, D. Hydroxylase inhibition abrogates TNF-α-induced intestinal epithelial damage by hypoxia-inducible factor-1-dependent repression of FADD. *J. Immunol.* **2010**, *185*, 6306–6316. [CrossRef] [PubMed]
80. Rosenzweig, H.L.; Minami, M.; Lessov, N.S.; Coste, S.C.; Stevens, S.L.; Henshall, D.C.; Meller, R.; Simon, R.P.; Stenzel-Poore, M.P. Endotoxin preconditioning protects against the cytotoxic effects of TNFα after stroke: A novel role for TNFalpha in LPS-ischemic tolerance. *J. Cereb Blood Flow Metab.* **2007**, *27*, 1663–1674. [CrossRef] [PubMed]
81. Fan, H.; Cook, J.A. Molecular mechanisms of endotoxin tolerance. *J. Endotoxin Res.* **2004**, *10*, 71–84. [CrossRef] [PubMed]
82. Stetler, R.A.; Leak, R.K.; Gan, Y.; Li, P.; Zhang, F.; Hu, X.; Jing, Z.; Chen, J.; Zigmond, M.J.; Gao, Y. Preconditioning provides neuroprotection in models of CNS disease: Paradigms and clinical significance. *Prog. Neurobiol.* **2014**, *114*, 58–83. [CrossRef] [PubMed]
83. Bastide, M.; Gelé, P.; Pétrault, O.; Pu, Q.; Caliez, A.; Robin, E.; Deplanque, D.; Duriez, P.; Bordet, R. Delayed cerebrovascular protective effect of lipopolysaccharide in parallel to brain ischemic tolerance. *J. Cereb. Blood Flow Metab.* **2003**, *23*, 399–405. [CrossRef] [PubMed]
84. Karikó, K.; Weissman, D.; Welsh, F.A. Inhibition of toll-like receptor and cytokine signaling—A unifying theme in ischemic tolerance. *J. Cereb. Blood Flow Metab.* **2004**, *24*, 1288–1304. [CrossRef] [PubMed]
85. Lastres-Becker, I.; Cartmell, T.; Molina-Holgado, F. Endotoxin preconditioning protects neurones from *in vitro* ischemia: Role of endogenous IL-1beta and TNF-alpha. *J. Neuroimmunol.* **2006**, *173*, 108–116. [CrossRef] [PubMed]
86. Pickering, M.; O'Connor, J.J. Pro-inflammatory cytokines and their effects in the dentate gyrus. *Prog. Brain Res.* **2007**, *163*, 339–354. [PubMed]
87. Cumiskey, D.; Butler, M.P.; Moynagh, P.N.; O'Connor, J.J. Evidence for a role for the group I metabotropic glutamate receptor in the inhibitory effect of tumor necrosis factor-alpha on long-term potentiation. *Brain Res.* **2007**, *1136*, 13–19. [CrossRef] [PubMed]
88. Butler, M.P.; O'Connor, J.J.; Moynagh, P.N. Dissection of tumor-necrosis factor-alpha inhibition of long-term potentiation (LTP) reveals a p38 mitogen-activated protein kinase-dependent mechanism which maps to early-but not late-phase LTP. *Neuroscience* **2004**, *124*, 319–326. [CrossRef] [PubMed]

89. Cunningham, A.J.; Murray, C.A.; O'Neill, L.A.J.; Lynch, M.A.; O'Connor, J.J. Interleukin-1β (IL-1β) and tumour necrosis factor (TNF) inhibit long-term potentiation in the rat dentate gyrus *in vitro*. *Neurosci. Lett.* **1996**, *203*, 17–20. [CrossRef]
90. Tancredi, V.; D'Arcangelo, G.; Grassi, F.; Tarroni, P.; Palmieri, G.; Santoni, A.; Eusebi, F. Tumor necrosis factor alters synaptic transmission in rat hippocampal slices. *Neurosci. Lett.* **1992**, *146*, 176–178. [CrossRef]
91. Curran, B.; Murray, H.; O'Connor, J.J. A role for c-jun n-terminal kinase in the inhibition of long-term potentiation by interleukin-1β and long-term depression in the rat dentate gyrus *in vitro*. *Neuroscience* **2003**, *118*, 347–357. [CrossRef]
92. Stellwagen, D.; Malenka, R.C. Synaptic scaling mediated by glial TNF-alpha. *Nature* **2006**, *440*, 1054–1059. [CrossRef] [PubMed]
93. Beattie, E.C.; Stellwagen, D.; Morishita, W.; Bresnahan, J.C.; Ha, B.K.; Von Zastrow, M.; Beattie, M.S.; Malenka, R.C. Control of synaptic strength by glial TNFalpha. *Science* **2002**, *295*, 2282–2285. [CrossRef] [PubMed]
94. Stellwagen, D.; Beattie, E.C.; Seo, J.Y.; Malenka, R.C. Differential regulation of AMPA receptor and GABA receptor trafficking by tumor necrosis factor-alpha. *J. Neurosci.* **2005**, *25*, 3219–3228. [CrossRef] [PubMed]
95. Vesce, S.; Rossi, D.; Brambilla, L.; Volterra, A. Glutamate release from astrocytes in physiological conditions and in neurodegenerative disorders characterized by neuroinflammation. *Int. Rev. Neurobiol.* **2007**, *82*, 57–71. [PubMed]
96. Korn, T.; Magnus, T.; Jung, S. Autoantigen specific T cells inhibit glutamate uptake in astrocytes by decreasing expression of astrocytic glutamate transporter GLAST: A mechanism mediated by tumor necrosis factor-alpha. *FASEB J.* **2005**, *19*, 1878–1880. [CrossRef] [PubMed]
97. Boycott, H.E.; Wilkinson, J.A.; Boyle, J.P.; Pearson, H.A.; Peers, C. Differential involvement of TNF alpha in hypoxic suppression of astrocyte glutamate transporters. *Glia* **2008**, *56*, 998–1004. [CrossRef] [PubMed]
98. Carmen, J.; Rothstein, J.D.; Kerr, D.A. Tumor necrosis factor-alpha modulates glutamate transport in the CNS and is a critical determinant of outcome from viral encephalomyelitis. *Brain Res.* **2009**, *1263*, 143–154. [CrossRef] [PubMed]
99. He, P.; Liu, Q.; Wu, J.; Shen, Y. Genetic deletion of TNF receptor suppresses excitatory synaptic transmission via reducing AMPA receptor synaptic localization in cortical neurons. *FASEB J.* **2012**, *26*, 334–345. [CrossRef] [PubMed]
100. Santello, M.; Bezzi, P.; Volterra, A. TNF-α controls glutamatergic gliotransmission in the hippocampal dentate gyrus. *Neuron* **2011**, *69*, 988–1001. [CrossRef] [PubMed]
101. Arai, A.; Lynch, G. Factors regulating the magnitude of long-term potentiation induced by theta pattern stimulation. *Brain Res.* **1992**, *598*, 173–184. [CrossRef]
102. Wall, A.M.; Mukandala, G.; Nigel, H.; O'Connor, J.J. Tumor necrosis factor-α potentiates long-term potentiation in the rat dentate gyrus after acute hypoxia. *J. Neurosci. Res.* **2015**, *93*, 815–829. [CrossRef] [PubMed]
103. Culver, C.; Sundqvist, A.; Mudie, S.; Melvin, A.; Xirodimas, D.; Rocha, S. Mechanism of hypoxia-induced NF-kappaB. *Mol. Cell. Biol.* **2010**, *30*, 4901–4921. [CrossRef] [PubMed]
104. Pickering, M.; Cumiskey, D.; O'Connor, J.J. Actions of TNF-α on glutamatergic synaptic transmission in the central nervous system. *Exp. Physiol.* **2005**, *90*, 663–670. [CrossRef] [PubMed]

7

Prior Binge Ethanol Exposure Potentiates the Microglial Response in a Model of Alcohol-Induced Neurodegeneration

Simon Alex Marshall [1], Chelsea Rhea Geil [2] and Kimberly Nixon [2,*]

[1] Department of Psychology & Neuroscience; University of North Carolina-Chapel Hill, Chapel Hill, NC 27599, USA; simon.alexm@unc.edu

[2] Department of Pharmaceutical Sciences, College of Pharmacy, University of Kentucky, Lexington, KY 40536, USA; chelsea.geil@uky.edu

* Correspondence: kim-nixon@uky.edu

Academic Editor: Donna Gruol

Abstract: Excessive alcohol consumption results in neurodegeneration which some hypothesize is caused by neuroinflammation. One characteristic of neuroinflammation is microglial activation, but it is now well accepted that microglial activation may be pro- or anti-inflammatory. Recent work indicates that the Majchrowicz model of alcohol-induced neurodegeneration results in anti-inflammatory microglia, while intermittent exposure models with lower doses and blood alcohol levels produce microglia with a pro-inflammatory phenotype. To determine the effect of a repeated binge alcohol exposure, rats received two cycles of the four-day Majchrowicz model. One hemisphere was then used to assess microglia via immunohistochemistry and while the other was used for ELISAs of cytokines and growth factors. A single binge ethanol exposure resulted in low-level of microglial activation; however, a second binge potentiated the microglial response. Specifically, double binge rats had greater OX-42 immunoreactivity, increased ionized calcium-binding adapter molecule 1 (Iba-1+) cells, and upregulated tumor necrosis factor-α (TNF-α) compared with the single binge ethanol group. These data indicate that prior ethanol exposure potentiates a subsequent microglia response, which suggests that the initial exposure to alcohol primes microglia. In summary, repeated ethanol exposure, independent of other immune modulatory events, potentiates microglial activity.

Keywords: alcohol; ethanol; microglia; cytokines; TNF-alpha; alcoholism; microglial priming; neurodegeneration

---

1. Introduction

Nearly 14% of the United States population meets the diagnostic criteria for an alcohol use disorder (AUD) in any given year [1]. Excessive alcohol consumption produces neurodegeneration in humans [2–4], an effect that has been confirmed in various pre-clinical models [5–8]. Due to its preventable nature, alcoholism traditionally has not been defined as a neurodegenerative disorder, but chronic, excessive consumption may cause damage in the temporal lobe on par with diseases such as Alzheimer's [4]. Indeed, alcoholic-related dementia is the second leading cause of dementia in the United States only behind Alzheimer's disease [9,10]. Even in the absence of dementia, cognitive deficits such as increased impulsivity and impaired executive decision-making are found in many with AUDs [11,12]. Alcohol-induced neurodegeneration and the associated cognitive deficits are thought to be critical factors in the development of AUDs [13–15].

Despite the number of reports in human and preclinical models describing the neurotoxic effects of alcohol, the mechanism of how alcohol produces neurodegeneration is unclear [16]. One such mechanism that has recently gained attention is the impact of excessive alcohol consumption on the neuroimmune system, and particularly, microglia [17,18]. Analysis of the brains of human alcoholics suggests that excessive alcohol consumption leads to microglial activation [19–21], but whether this activation is the cause or consequence of alcohol-induced neurodegeneration is an active debate [22]. This discussion is due, in part, to a lack of understanding of the effect of alcohol on microglia coupled with the recent appreciation of the role of microglia in both neurodegenerative and regenerative processes [22–25]. Although microglia have historically been discussed as the phagocytes of the central nervous system (CNS), these cells are far more complex, existing in a continuum of phenotypes or stages of activation [26]. Microglia are constantly surveying the parenchyma in non-pathological conditions; where in response to even a subtle change in their environment, microglia alter their morphological and functional characteristics, a process termed microglial activation [27]. The nomenclature for these stages or phenotypes vary. Terms like M1 and classical activation are applied when microglia have an amoeboid morphology and secrete pro-inflammatory cytokines, whereas M2 and alternative activation are used to describe microglia with bushier ramifications that secrete anti-inflammatory cytokines [26,28]. In neurodegenerative diseases where microglial activation drives neuronal loss, microglia are generally fully or classically activated (*i.e.*, M1 phenotype), secreting pro-inflammatory factors and undergoing uncontrolled phagocytosis [25,29]. How alcohol affects microglia is not well described and appears to vary depending on the model. Most reports of alcohol-induced microglia activation assume that all activated microglia are pro-inflammatory [19,23,30]. However, in the one model with alcohol-induced neurodegeneration, the Majchrowicz four-day binge model, only a low level of activation or alternative (M2) phenotype has been observed [22,24,31].

The variability of microglial phenotypes observed across different AUD models may be due to the pattern of alcohol exposure, specifically intermittent *versus* sustained intoxication. Interestingly, the intermittent exposure models show stronger evidence of pro-inflammatory microglia even with lower doses of ethanol [22,30]. These disparate findings across models led us to question whether the initial hit of alcohol exposure "primes" microglia such that intermittent exposure leads to a potentiated response. Primed microglia have similar morphology and cytokine/growth factor profiles as the M2/alternative microglia, but primed microglial activation is potentiated when subsequent neuroimmunomodulators are applied [28,32,33]. Ethanol's ability to prime microglia and exacerbate the neuroimmune response to subsequent neuroimmune stimuli is suggested also by the enhanced microglia response to LPS following alcohol exposure [23,34,35]. However, the ability of a second "hit" or insult of ethanol to potentiate the neuroimmune response (independent of peripheral immunomodulators) has not been examined. Therefore, the current study determines whether a second binge ethanol exposure can potentiate the microglia response to binge alcohol exposure. Investigating whether repeated ethanol exposure differentially affects microglia is important considering that the majority of individuals suffering from an AUD drink in a binge pattern that produces periods of high BECs interspersed with periods of withdrawal and abstinence [36–38]. Specifically, this study examines both functional and morphological indices of microglial activation in the hippocampus and entorhinal cortex, regions consistently damaged in this model [7,8].

2. Materials and Methods

2.1. Alcohol Administration Model

A total of 33 adult male Sprague-Dawley rats (Table 1; Charles River Laboratories; Raleigh, NC, USA) were used in these experiments. Procedures performed were approved by the University of Kentucky Institutional Animal Care and Use Committee (protocol #2008-0321, approved 20/6/2008) and conformed to the Guidelines for the Care and Use of Laboratory Animals [39]. Animals weighed approximately 275–300 g at arrival and were pair-housed in a University of Kentucky AALAC accredited vivarium with a 12 h light:dark cycle. Rats were allowed to acclimate to the vivarium for two days followed by three days of handling before any experimentation. Except during the binge periods, animals had *ad libitum* food and water access. Following acclimation, rats underwent a modified version of the Majchrowicz AUD model similar to previously published reports [40–42]; however, animals used in this study underwent the Majchrowicz 4-day paradigm twice separated by seven days. Rats were divided into four groups of comparable weights as summarized in Table 1. Briefly, rats were gavaged intragastrically with either ethanol (25% *w/v*) or control diet (isocaloric dextrose) in Vanilla Ensure Plus® (Abbott Laboratories; Chicago, IL, USA) every 8 h. Initially, each rat in an ethanol group received 5 g/kg of ethanol, but subsequent doses were titrated using the individual rat's behavioral intoxication score on a six-point scale identical to previous reports [40]. Control rats received an average of the volume given to the ethanol group. All rats were then given seven days of recovery with *ad libitum* access to food and water. A seven-day recovery period was chosen because microglial activation is elevated for a week after ethanol exposure [22], and seven days allowed animals to recover from withdrawal and regain body mass lost during the prior binge. Thus, on the 11th day, the Majchrowicz binge model was repeated with rats receiving either ethanol or control diet (Table 1). A separate group had *ad libitum* access to food and water throughout all periods. For all groups, body weights were assessed daily during the binge procedures. The percent difference in weight at the start and end of the 15-day treatment period was calculated.

Table 1. Experimental Design.

Group	Binge 1 (4 Days)	Recovery (7 Days)	Binge 2 (4 Days)
Con/Con (n = 10)	Control Diet		Control Diet
Con/EtOH (n = 11)	Control Diet	*Ad libitum* chow	Ethanol Diet
EtOH/EtOH (n = 8)	Ethanol Diet		Ethanol Diet
Ad libitum (n = 4)	N/A		N/A

2.2. Blood Ethanol Concentration Determination

To determine blood ethanol concentrations (BECs), tail blood was collected ninety minutes after the seventh session of ethanol dosing during Binge 1 and/or at euthanasia (Binge 2). Bloods were centrifuged for 5 min at 1800 × g to separate plasma from red blood cells and immediately stored at −20 °C. BECs were determined from supernatant serum on an AM1 Alcohol Analyser (Analox; London, UK) calibrated against a 300 mg/dL external standard. Each sample was run in triplicate and the average of these runs was calculated and expressed in mg/dL ± SEM.

2.3. Tissue Processing

Rats were euthanized within 2–4 h of their final gavage by rapid decapitation. Brains were extracted and dissected into two hemispheres on ice. The left hemisphere was fixed by immersion in 4% paraformaldehyde in phosphate buffer (pH = 7.4) for 2 h, rinsed and stored in phosphate buffered saline at 4 °C until use in immunohistochemical experiments. The right hemisphere was further dissected to remove the hippocampus and entorhinal cortex. Extracted regions were snap frozen on dry ice and stored at −80 °C until use in enzyme linked immunosorbent assays (ELISAs).

2.4. Immunohistochemistry

Immunohistochemical procedures were similar to previous reports [22,31]. The left hemisphere was sectioned in a 1:12 series at 40 μm thickness with a vibrating microtome (Leica VT1000S; Wetzlar, Germany) and sections were stored in cryoprotectant at −20 °C. Adjacent series of every 12th section were processed for immunohistochemistry. Briefly, after a series of washes (TBS, pH = 7.5), quenching of endogenous peroxidases (0.6% H_2O_2 in TBS) and blocking of nonspecific antibody binding (TBS, 0.1% triton X-100, and 3% horse or goat serum as appropriate), tissue series was incubated overnight in one of the following primary antibodies at 4 °C: mouse anti-OX-42 (1:1000; Serotec MCA275; Raleigh, NC, USA), mouse anti-ED-1 (1:500; Serotec MCA341), mouse anti-OX-6 (1:500; Serotec, MC2687), or rabbit anti-Iba-1 (1:1000; Wako, 019-19741; Richmond, VA, USA). Primaries were chosen for their specificity for microglia phenotypes [26,43]. OX-42 was selected as a marker of microglial activation because it recognizes cluster of differentiation molecule 11b/c (CD11b/c) of complement receptor 3 (CR3), which is constitutively expressed in microglia; however, upregulation of CD11b/c is one of the first indications of microglial activation [44–46]. Both ED-1 and OX-6 are selective for more classical forms of microglial activation [26]. ED-1 recognizes the lysosomal membranes of microglia and is thought to be an indication of phagocytic activity [47]. OX-6, however, is an antibody against the major histocompatibility complex-II that elicits T-helper cell activation [26,48]. The Iba-1 antibody was selected because it recognizes a calcium binding protein expressed in all microglia [49]. Sections were incubated in secondary antibody (biotinylated horse anti-mouse, rat adsorbed, or biotinylated goat anti-rabbit, Vector Laboratories, Burlingame, CA, USA), avidin-biotin-peroxidase complex (ABC Elite Kit, Vector Laboratories) and the chromagen, nickel-enhanced 3,3′-diaminobenzidine tetrahydrochloride (Polysciences; Warrington, PA, USA), as previously described [22,31]. Following the final wash, all processed sections were mounted onto glass slides, dried and coverslipped with Cytoseal® (Stephens Scientific, Wayne, NJ, USA).

During quantification, slides were coded to ensure the experimenter was blind to treatment condition. To determine OX-42 immunoreactivity, images of the hippocampus (Bregma −2.50 and −4.00 mm) or entorhinal cortex (Bregma −3.00 and −6.00 mm) were obtained with a 10× objective on an Olympus BX-51 microscope (Olympus, Center Valley, PA, USA) linked to a motorized stage (Prior, Rockland, MA, USA), microcator and DP70 digital camera (Olympus) [50]. OX-42 immunoreactivity was determined by optical density with Visiomorph™ (Visiopharm, Hørsholm, Denmark). Subregions of the hippocampus (dentate gyrus (DG), cornu amonis (CA1 and CA2/3)) and the entorhinal cortex were traced separately and the percent area of OX-42 immunopositive pixels within each region of interest was determined. Immunoreactivity was then normalized to the *ad libitum* control group and expressed as percent of control.

For ED-1 or OX-6 immunohistochemistry, sections were qualitatively assessed in the hippocampus and entorhinal cortex as in past reports [22]. To determine the impact of ethanol on microglia number, Iba-1+ cells were counted within the hippocampus and the entorhinal cortex. Iba-1+ cells within the subregions of the hippocampus were estimated by unbiased stereological methods as previously reported [22,51]. NewCAST™ Stereology software (Visiopharm version 3.6.4.0) coupled to the same Olympus BX-51 microscope system above applied a 70 μm × 70 μm counting frame and cells were randomly sampled using a 20 μm dissector height with 2 μm guard zones within the CA1 (400 μm x,y step length), CA2/3 (250 μm x,y step length), and DG (250 μm x,y step length). Total Iba-1+ cells were calculated using the equation (1):

$$N = \sum Q \times 1/asf \times 1/tsf \times 1/ssf \quad (1)$$

where Q is the number of cells counted, asf is the area sampling fraction, tsf is the thickness sampling fraction, and ssf is the section sampling fraction [52]. Coefficients of error ranged from 0.011 to 0.039 and averaged 0.023 ± 0.001. For the entorhinal cortex, microglia number was determined using a profile counting method [53]. Images of the entorhinal cortex were collected with a 10× objective using a SPOT Advanced™ camera (SPOT Imaging Solutions, Sterling Heights, MI, USA). Iba-1+ cells were quantified in collected images by an automated counting system (Image Pro Plus 6.3; Media Cybernetics, Rockville, MD, USA) and expressed as mean Iba-1+ cells/section ± SEM as previously described [22].

2.5. Enzyme Linked Immunosorbent Assay

Hippocampus and entorhinal cortex from the right hemisphere were processed for ELISA as reported previously [22,54]. Briefly, tissues were homogenized in an ice-cold lysis buffer (1 mL of buffer/50 mg of tissue; pH = 7.4), then tumor necrosis factor-α (TNF-α; Invitrogen, #KRC3011C; Camarillo, CA, USA) and interleukin-10 (IL-10; Invitrogen, #KRC0101) cytokine protein was determined via ELISA according to the manufacturer's instructions. These two cytokines were used to assess pro or anti-inflammatory microglia, respectively [43]. Brain derived neurotrophic factor (BDNF) was measured in the hippocampus (Millipore, #CYT306; Billerica, MA, USA) as the hippocampus is more susceptible to alcohol-induced BDNF dysregulation [55,56]. All samples and standards were run in duplicate. Absorbance was measured at 450 nm on a DXT880 Multimode Detector plate reader (Beckman Coulter; Brea, CA, USA). Cytokine concentrations were normalized to the total protein content as determined by a Pierce BCA Protein Assay Kit (Thermo Scientific; Rockford, IL, USA) and reported as pg/mg of total protein $\pm$ SEM.

2.6. Statistical Analyses

Data were analyzed and graphed using Prism (version 5.04, GraphPad Software, Inc. La Jolla, CA, USA). Effects were considered significantly different if $p < 0.05$. Behavioral scores were analyzed with a Kruskal-Wallis test. All other analyses used a one-way ANOVA with *post-hoc* Tukey's test to compare groups if an effect of treatment was observed. Where appropriate, each region of the hippocampus or entorhinal cortex was considered independent and therefore analyzed separately. Correlations were conducted to examine the relationship of microglial markers of activation and the animal model data as well as microglial activation and cytokine concentration. Correlations were only run within the Con/EtOH or EtOH/EtOH group if *post-hoc* analyses showed a significant difference to control groups. Spearman analyses were used for intoxication behavior scores (nonparametric), while Pearson's analyses were used for all other factors (parametric).

3. Results

3.1. Animal Treatment Data

For animal model data, each binge period was analyzed independently. For example, BECs from Binge 1 and Binge 2 for the EtOH/EtOH group were analyzed separately. No differences were detected between any groups in either intoxication score (H(3) = 5.60, $p = 0.07$; grand mean = 1.6 $\pm$ 0.1) or in BECs ($F(2,24) = 0.78$, $p = 0.32$; grand mean = 399.8 $\pm$ 12.4 mg/dL) as shown in Table 2. However, one-way ANOVA revealed differences in the average dose per day ($F(2,24) = 4.235$, $p = 0.03$). A *post-hoc* Tukey's test indicated that ethanol doses of Binge 2 in the EtOH/EtOH rats were significantly higher than ethanol doses of the single binge (Con/EtOH) rats (Table 2). Body weights were also assessed to determine whether restricted caloric intake affected microglia activation [57,58]. One-way ANOVA indicated that treatment affected weight change ($F(2,24) = 4.235$, $p = 0.03$) (Table 2). A *post-hoc* Tukey's test showed that the weight change differed between all of the liquid diet groups (Con/Con, Con/EtOH, and EtOH/EtOH) compared with the *ad libitum* group. There was a significant effect of receiving ethanol on weight loss compared with the Con/Con group, but no difference between the Con/EtOH and EtOH/EtOH groups was observed (Table 3).

Table 2. Alcohol Model Data.

Group	Intoxication Behavior (0–5 Scale)	Dose (g/kg/day)	BEC (mg/dL)
Con/EtOH (15th Day)	1.8 $\pm$ 0.1	9.6 $\pm$ 0.2	422.2 $\pm$ 21.1
EtOH/EtOH Binge 1 (4th Day)	1.7 $\pm$ 0.1	9.9 $\pm$ 0.4	378.7 $\pm$ 17.7
EtOH/EtOH Binge 2 (15th Day)	1.3 $\pm$ 0.2	11.0 $\pm$ 0.5 #	390.3 $\pm$ 24.0

# $p < 0.05$ compared to Con/EtOH.

Table 3. Body Weight.

Group	% Difference
Con/Con ($n = 10$)	+1.0% ± 1.4% †
Con/EtOH ($n = 11$)	−6.6% ± 2.1% *
EtOH/EtOH ($n = 8$)	−8.7% ± 1.7% *
Ad libitum ($n = 4$)	+25.2% ± 1.7%

* $p < 0.05$ *vs.* Con/Con and *ad libitum*; † $p < 0.05$ *vs. ad libitum* only.

3.2. OX-42 Immunoreactivity Increased by EtOH Exposure

OX-42 expression was examined to determine whether microglia were further or differentially activated following a second binge exposure. OX-42 positive cells were apparent in all treatment groups, which is consistent with its constitutive expression in all types of microglia [59]; however, there was a visibly distinct increase in immunoreactivity in ethanol treated animals accompanied by an apparent morphological change. Microglia in ethanol animals appeared to have shorter but thickened ramifications compared with the control animals (Figures 1B,C and 2B,C). One-way ANOVAs indicated a significant effect of treatment in the CA1 ($F(3,29) = 16.81$, $p < 0.0001$), CA2/3 ($F(3,29) = 18.34$, $p < 0.0001$), and DG ($F(3,29) = 14.43$, $p < 0.0001$) fields (Figure 1), as well as in the entorhinal cortex ($F(3,28) = 19.01$, $p < 0.0001$) (Figure 2). As expected based on previous data [22], *post-hoc* Tukey's tests indicated a significant increase in OX-42 density in all ethanol treated groups in all subregions of the hippocampus compared with the control or *ad libitum* groups. Importantly, the EtOH/EtOH group showed greater immunoreactivity than Con/EtOH in all regions analyzed except the DG. Moreover, no difference in OX-42 was observed between *ad libitum* animals and the Con/Con group. Correlations between binge model parameters (intoxication behavior, dose per day, total dose, BEC, percent weight loss) and OX-42 immunoreactivity were run within the EtOH/EtOH and Con/EtOH group, but no significant correlations were observed (Table 4).

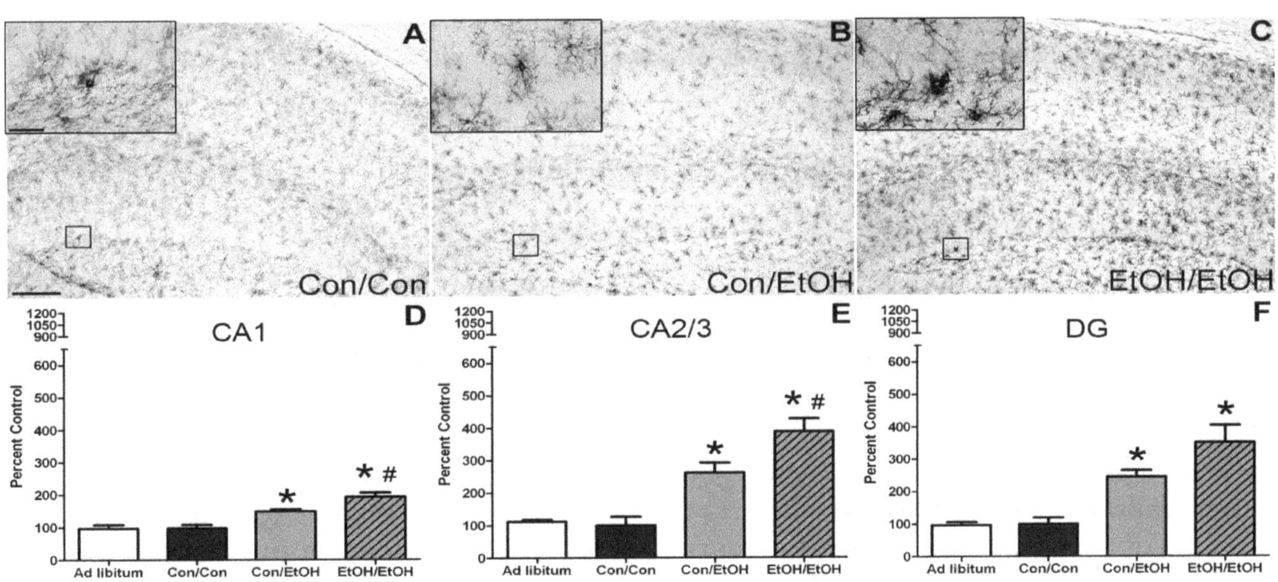

Figure 1. Potentiated Microglial Activation in the Hippocampus by Repeated Ethanol Exposure. OX-42 (CD11b/c) is upregulated in the hippocampus of ethanol-exposed rats as shown in representative photomicrographs of the (**A**–**C**) hippocampal dentate gyrus for (**B**) Con/EtOH and (**C**) EtOH/EtOH groups compared to (**A**) controls. Analysis of OX-42 immunoreactivity indicated that the EtOH/EtOH group had significantly more staining than the Con/EtOH group in the: (**D**) cornu amonis 1 (CA1) and (**E**) cornu amonis 2/3 (CA2/3) regions but not the (F) dentate gyrus (DG). Data expressed as a percentage of *ad libitum* control (not shown). Images were taken at 50× magnification with insets at 600× magnification. Scale bar = 200 μm; inset 30 μm. * $p < 0.05$ compared to *ad libitum* and Con/Con groups; # $p < 0.05$ compared to Con/EtOH.

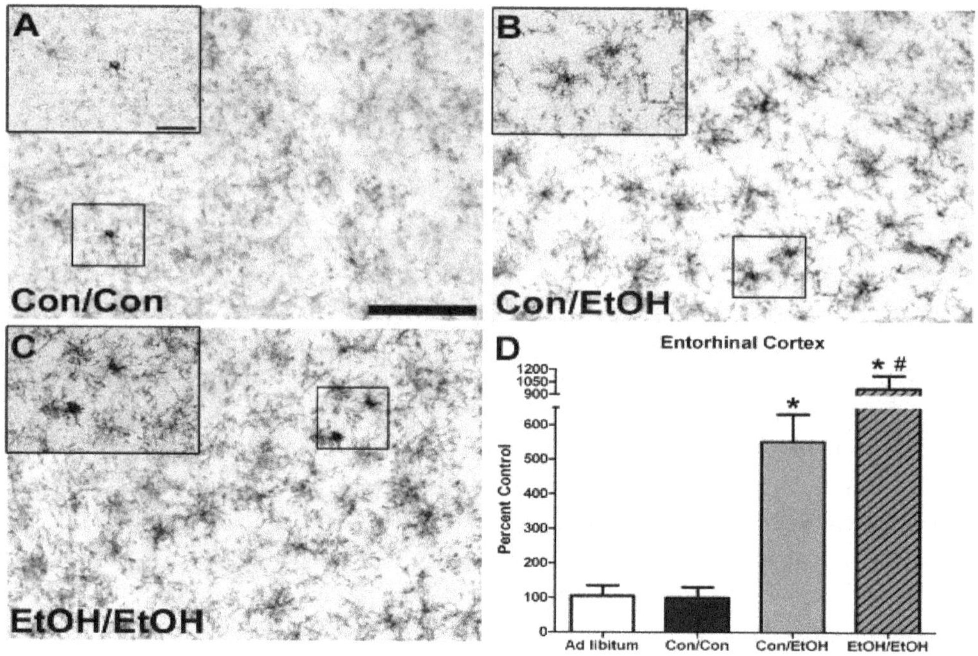

Figure 2. Potentiated Microglial Activation in the Entorhinal Cortex by Repeated Ethanol Exposure. OX-42 (CD11b) is upregulated in the entorhinal cortex of ethanol-exposed rats as shown in representative photomicrographs of the (**A–C**) entorhinal cortex for (**B**) Con/EtOH and (**C**) EtOH/EtOH groups compared to (**A**) controls. Analysis of OX-42 immunoreactivity indicated that the EtOH/EtOH group had significantly more positive pixels than the Con/EtOH group in the (**D**) entorhinal cortex. Data expressed as a percentage of *ad libitum* control (not shown). Images were taken at 200× magnification with insets at 600× magnification. Scale bar = 100 μm; inset 30 μm. * $p < 0.05$ compared to *ad libitum* and Con/Con groups; # $p < 0.05$ compared to Con/EtOH.

Table 4. No Correlation between OX-42 and Model Parameters or Microglia Number.

-	Hippocampus		Entorhinal Cortex	
Parameter	Con/EtOH	EtOH/EtOH	Con/EtOH	EtOH/EtOH
Intoxication Behavior	S = 0.433	S = 0.523	S = 0.628	S = 0.371
Dose/Day	$p = -0.321$	$p = -0.053$	$p = -0.488$	$p = -0.456$
Total Dose	$p = -0.303$	$p = -0.0267$	$p = -0.331$	$p = -0.575$
BEC	$p = 0.424$	$p = -0.572$	$p = -0.082$	$p = 0.032$
Percent Weight Loss	$p = -0.222$	$p = 0.249$	$p = 0.029$	$p = 0.319$
Iba-1+ Cells	$p = 0.161$	$p = 0.539$	$p = -0.136$	$p = 0.357$

3.3. Lack of ED-1 or OX-6 Positive Cells

The ED-1 antibody was used to identify phagocytic microglia, whereas OX-6 was used to visualize the upregulation of MHC-II [26,29]. No ED-1 (Figure 3) positive cells were observed within the parenchyma of the hippocampus or entorhinal cortex of any animal in any group. No OX-6 (Figure 4) positive cells were observed within the parenchyma of the hippocampus or entorhinal cortex of any group, except for one EtOH/EtOH treated animal. This animal had several OX-6 cells in the more posterior regions of the hippocampus and entorhinal cortex (Figure 4D,H) but was not an outlier for any intoxication parameter including BEC, intoxication behavior, or ethanol dose per day. Interestingly, the morphology of these cells still appeared to be characteristic of the low grade, partial activation state of microglia as they are ramified and not amoeboid [26]. ED-1 and OX-6 positive cells were visible in blood vessels, the hippocampal fissure, and along the meninges in all treatment groups (Figures 3 and 4) similar to that observed previously following binge ethanol exposure [22,60]. Thus, repeated exposure to four-day binge ethanol treatment failed to significantly induce microglia to a phagocytic phenotype or state that expressed MHC-II in the brain parenchyma.

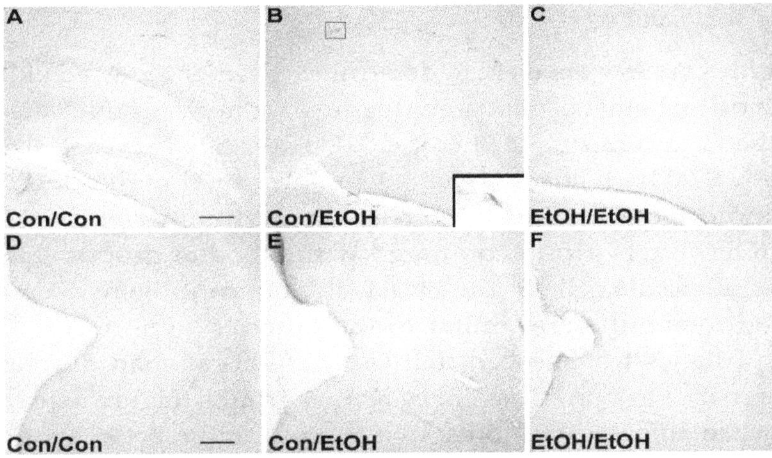

Figure 3. Lack of ED-1 Positive Cells. ED-1 was not visible in the parenchyma of the (**A–C**) hippocampus or (**D–F**) entorhinal cortex as seen in representative photomicrographs in (**A**,**D**) controls, (**B**,**E**) Con/EtOH (**C**,**F**) or EtOH/EtOH groups. ED-1 positive cells could be seen along the hippocampal fissure and blood vessels as shown in the inset of B. Scale bars = 200 μm.

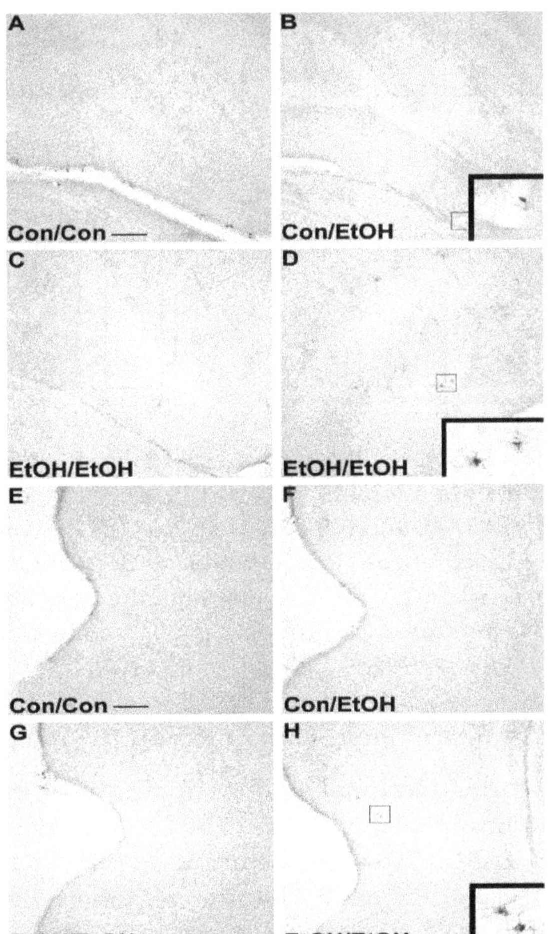

Figure 4. Lack of OX-6 Positive Cells. No OX-6 positive cells were observed regardless of treatment, except in one EtOH/EtOH rat as shown in representative photomicrographs of the (**A–C**) hippocampus or (**E–H**) entorhinal cortex in (**A**,**E**) controls, (**B**,**F**) Con/EtOH (**C**,**G**) or EtOH/EtOH groups. OX-6 positive cells could be seen along blood vessels as shown in the inset of B. One EtOH/EtOH animal showed upregulation of OX-6 in both the (**D**) hippocampus and (**H**) entorhinal cortex. Scale bars = 200 μm.

3.4. Differential Effects of Treatment on Number of Microglia

Stereology and profile counts were used to determine whether repeated ethanol exposure affected the number of microglia during ethanol exposure (Figure 5). One-way ANOVAs indicated a significant effect of treatment in the CA1 ($F(3,29) = 161.6$, $p < 0.0001$), CA2/3 ($F(3,29) = 17.99$, $p < 0.0001$), and DG ($F(3,29) = 69.98$, $p < 0.0001$) fields, as well as in entorhinal cortex ($F(3,28) = 6.78$, $p = 0.001$). *Post-hoc* Tukey's tests indicated a significant increase in the number of Iba-1+ cells throughout the hippocampus in the EtOH/EtOH group compared with all other groups (Figure 5A–C). However, in the entorhinal cortex microglia cells in the EtOH/EtOH group were decreased compared to the *ad libitum* and control groups but were similar to the number seen in Con/EtOH treated animals (Figure 5D). A *post-hoc* Tukey's test showed that Con/EtOH rats had decreased Iba-1+ cells in all regions measured as compared to Con/Con and *ad libitum* groups (Figure 5) [61]. Importantly, because the number of microglia can affect immunoreactivity, a correlation between the number of microglia *versus* OX-42 immunoreactivity was run, but no significant relationship was observed.

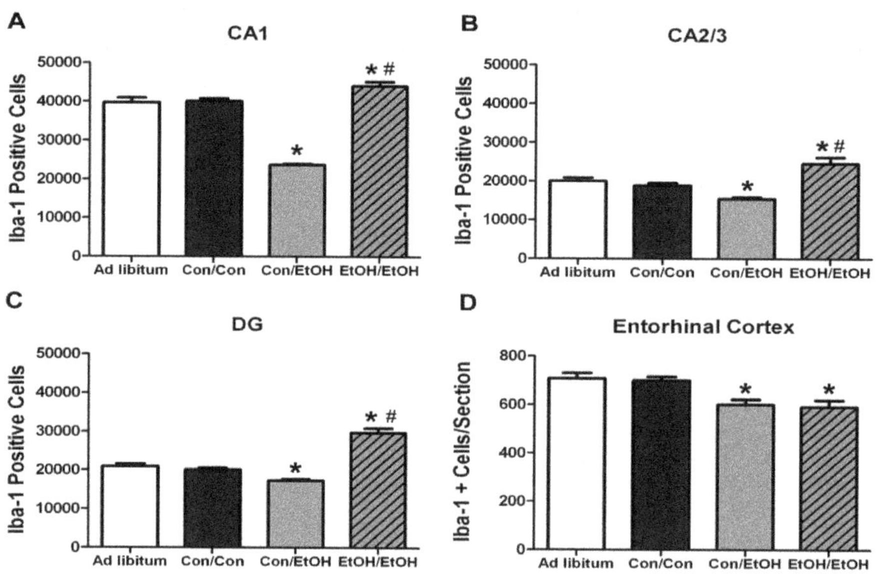

Figure 5. Microglial Cell Counts Differentially Altered by Ethanol Experience. Stereological estimates indicate an increase in the number of microglia in the EtOH/EtOH group in the (**A**) cornu amonis 1 (CA1), (**B**) cornu amonis 2/3 (CA2/3), and (**C**) dentate gyrus (DG) compared with all other groups. However, the number of microglia in the Con/EtOH group was decreased throughout the hippocampus. In the (**D**) entorhinal cortex, microglia were decreased in both the Con/EtOH and EtOH/EtOH groups compared to both the *ad libitum* and Con/Con groups. * $p < 0.05$ compared to *ad libitum* and Con/Con group; # $p < 0.05$ *versus* Con/EtOH.

3.5. Increased Pro-Inflammatory Cytokine Expression in EtOH/EtOH Group

ELISAs were used to assess the functional state of microglia, specifically the anti-inflammatory cytokine, IL-10, and the pro-inflammatory cytokine, TNF-α. No changes were seen in IL-10 during intoxication among any groups in either the hippocampus ($F(3,28) = 0.57$, $p = 0.64$) or the entorhinal cortex ($F(3,24) = 0.50$, $p = 0.69$; Figure 6A,B). However, one-way ANOVAs of TNF-α protein concentrations indicated a significant effect of treatment in the hippocampus ($F(3,28) = 4.658$, $p = 0.009$) but not the entorhinal cortex ($F(3,24) = 0.99$, $p = 0.41$). *Post-hoc* Tukey's tests indicated a significant increase in TNF-α in the hippocampus in the EtOH/EtOH group compared to all other groups (Figure 6C). Correlations of binge parameters *versus* immunohistochemical results were run within the EtOH/EtOH group to further probe the distribution of TNF-α concentrations (Table 5). BECs correlated with TNF-α concentration ($P(8) = 0.807$, $p = 0.016$; Figure 7).

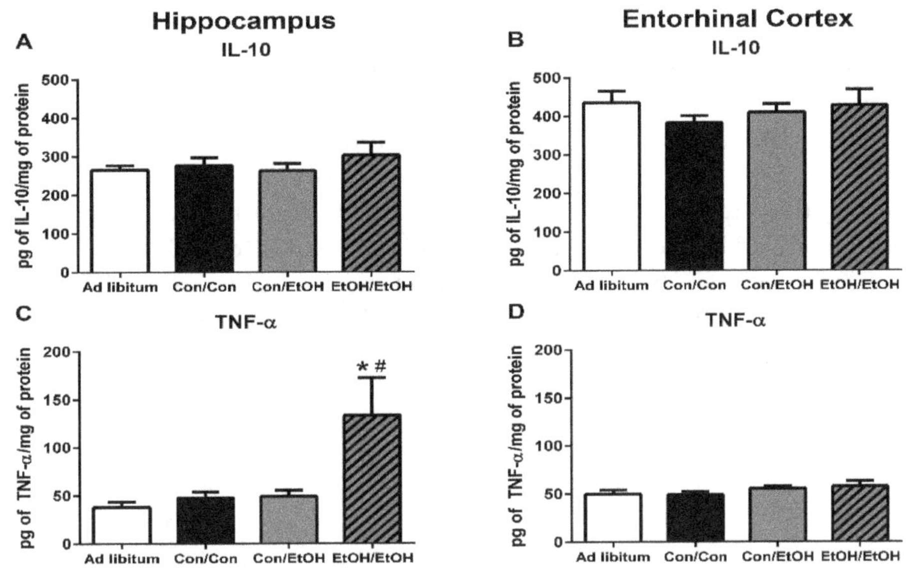

Figure 6. Increased TNF-α in EtOH/EtOH Group. Concentrations of (**A**,**B**) interleukin-10 (IL-10) and (**C**,**D**) tumor necrosis factor-α (TNF-α) were determined by ELISA in both the hippocampus (**A**,**C**) and entorhinal cortex (**B**,**D**). No change in IL-10 was measured in either the hippocampus or the entorhinal cortex, but at least a 2.7-fold increase in TNF-α was measured in the (**C**) hippocampus in the EtOH/EtOH group compared with all other groups. However, no change in TNF-α was seen in the (**D**) entorhinal cortex. * $p < 0.05$ compared to *ad libitum* and Con/Con groups; # $p < 0.05$ compared to Con/EtOH.

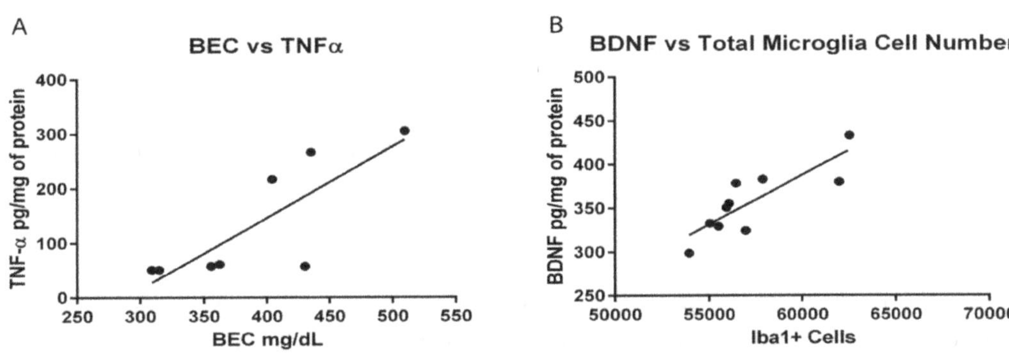

Figure 7. Correlations of Cytokines: (**A**) A positive correlation between blood ethanol concentration (BEC) and tumor necrosis factor-α (TNF-α) concentration. Animals with BECs over 400 mg/dL appear to have an increase in TNF-α. (**B**) A positive correlation between hippocampal estimates of microglia number and brain derived neurotrophic factor (BDNF) concentrations in the Con/EtOH group. A decline in the number of microglia cells correlated with decreases in BDNF concentrations.

Table 5. Select Hippocampal Cytokine and Growth Factor Correlations.

-	TNF-α		BDNF	
Parameter	Con/EtOH	EtOH/EtOH	Con/EtOH	EtOH/EtOH
Intoxication Behavior	S = 0.451	S = 0.371	S = −0.421	S = 0.216
Dose/Day	$p = -0.525$	$p = -0.544$	$p = 0.166$	$p = -0.149$
Total Dose	$p = -0.496$	$p = -0.355$	$p = 0.160$	$p = -0.144$
BEC	$p = -0.081$	$p = 0.807$ *	$p = 0.166$	$p = 0.298$
Percent Weight Loss	$p = 0.117$	$p = 0.610$	$p = 0.395$	$p = -0.473$
OX-42+ Density	$p = 0.493$	$p = -0.139$	$p = 0.253$	$p = -0.254$
Iba-1+ Cells	$p = -0.225$	$p = -0.372$	$p = 0.835$ *	$p = 0.224$

* $p < 0.05$.

3.6. *Differential Effects of Treatment on BDNF Concentrations*

Hippocampal BDNF concentrations were assessed to see the potential impact of microglia activity because alternative microglia, observed herein, are associated with neurotrophic support [62]. A one-way ANOVA on BDNF concentrations indicated a significant effect of treatment in the hippocampus ($F(3,28) = 19.00$, $p < 0.0001$). *Post-hoc* Tukey's tests indicated a 20% increase in BDNF concentration in the hippocampus in the EtOH/EtOH compared with all other groups, but Con/EtOH rats had decreased concentrations of BDNF compared to both the Con/Con and *ad libitum* groups (Figure 8). Correlations between binge animal model data as well as markers of microglial activation were run *versus* BDNF concentrations for both the Con/EtOH and EtOH/EtOH groups (Table 5). The estimated total number of microglia (P(10) = 0.835, $p = 0.003$) was correlated to BDNF concentrations only in the Con/EtOH group (Figure 7).

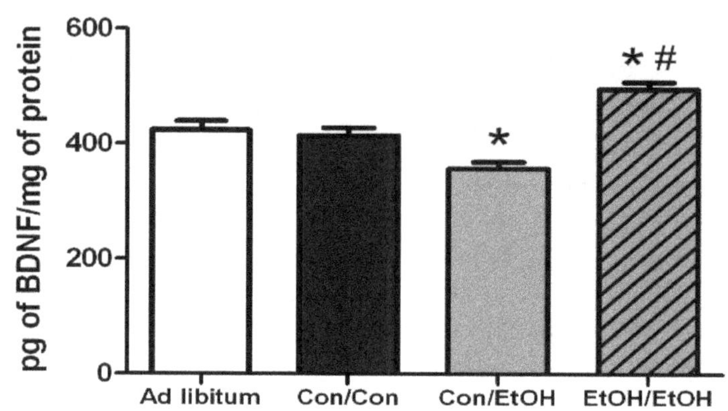

Figure 8. Ethanol Experience-Contingent Effects on BDNF. Concentrations of brain derived neurotrophic factor (BDNF) were determined by ELISA in the hippocampus. BDNF was decreased by approximately 15% in Con/EtOH treated animals compared with Con/Con or *ad libitum* groups but increased by 20% in the EtOH/EtOH group. * $p < 0.05$ *vs. ad libitum* and Con/Con groups; # $p < 0.05$ *vs.* to Con/EtOH.

4. Discussion

These data collectively indicate that microglia previously activated by alcohol exposure can be further exacerbated by a second alcohol binge. This point was demonstrated by: (a) potentiated OX-42 immunoreactivity; (b) increased microglial number; and (c) increased TNF-α concentration in EtOH/EtOH (double binge) rats compared with Con/EtOH (single binge) rats. The alcohol model used produces a low-grade microglial activation state that is similar to an M2 phenotype [22,31]. However, as the subsequent binge produced more pro-inflammatory-like effects, these alcohol-activated microglia may also be primed. This enhanced response to a second binge aligns with the definition of microglial priming, which is where a stimulus changes microglia to be more susceptible to and over-respond to a second insult [33,63,64]. Primed microglia and/or an exacerbated microglial response could lead to abnormally increased cell death and is a hypothesized etiology of neurodegenerative disorders [28]. Furthermore, given that the majority of individuals with an AUD drink in an episodic binge pattern [38,65], the repeated cycles of binge drinking with periods of withdrawal, and therefore repeated microglial insult, may lead to even more dynamic microglial activation over time.

The first evidence of this potentiated microglia response in the double binge group was increased immunoreactivity to the OX-42 antibody. Increased OX-42 immunoreactivity, which labels CR3, is one of the earliest signs of microglial activation [22,46]. CR3 is associated with cell adhesion necessary for removing pathogens or damaged/dying neurons [45,66,67]. Increased OX-42 staining has been reported in a number of animal models of ethanol exposure [22,68–70]. The current study confirms those findings; but furthers that work by showing that a second hit of binge ethanol exposure potentiates OX-42 immunoreactivity. A potentiated increase in OX-42 immunoreactivity, or CR3 density, by ethanol is particularly interesting because CR3 is intimately involved in microglial priming [33]. The increased upregulation of CR3 in the EtOH/EtOH (double binge) rats compared with Con/EtOH (single binge) rats suggests that binge ethanol exposure acts as a priming stimulus to microglia. Morphology, though not specifically quantified, appeared consistent with a low grade/phenotype of activation as cells were ramified and not amoeboid (e.g., Figure 1) [26]. A bushy, ramified microglial morphology is also consistent with that observed in other pathologies that report a primed microglia state [33,64,71]. Furthermore, despite the potentiation of CR3 receptor density, no changes in ED-1 or OX-6 expression were seen following the second binge. The lack of visible ED-1+ or OX-6+ cells concurs with other reports in this model that do not show signs of classical microglial activation following ethanol exposure [22,31,60].

Because multiple endpoints should be measured to understand the phenotype of microglia after insult, functional outputs such as hallmark pro- and anti-inflammatory cytokines were measured to better understand the type of microglial activation associated with a second "hit" of ethanol exposure. No change in the concentration of the hallmark anti-inflammatory cytokine, IL-10, was observed in either ethanol exposure group in the hippocampus or entorhinal cortex. The lack of IL-10 response during intoxication confirms previous findings in this model, although IL-10 is decreased in a mouse AUD model [22,23]. However, upregulation of TNF-α in the hippocampus in the EtOH/EtOH group compared with all other groups suggests that the second binge promoted a pro-inflammatory state. This finding is highly distinct from multiple previous reports using Majchrowicz-like models where no effect of ethanol was observed on TNF-α concentrations [22,24,31] and highlights the impact of repeated ethanol exposure on pro-inflammatory cytokine production and microglial activation. The potentiation of TNF-α expression by the second hit of ethanol, much like the morphological indices, is a common response for microglia that are primed and then hit with a secondary peripheral immune insult [28,64,72]. In fact, alcohol and other drugs of abuse have been shown to prime the TNF-α response to other immune stimulators [23,63], but these finding specifically suggest that alcohol exposure can act as both the priming and secondary stimulus resulting in an increase in TNF-α.

In the Majchrowicz model, microglia loss was observed during the last days of intoxication [61], whereas microglia proliferation occurs after the cessation of alcohol exposure, on the second day of abstinence [31,60]. Therefore, Iba-1+ cell number was assessed to determine how multiple cycles of ethanol affects microglia number. The single ethanol binge (Con/EtOH group) reduced the number of Iba-1+ microglia, in both the hippocampus and entorhinal cortex. Our recent work supports that this reduction is likely due to degeneration of microglia following 4-day binge exposure [61]. Interestingly, the second binge (EtOH/EtOH group) resulted in an increased number of Iba-1+ microglia in the hippocampus compared to either the control group or single binge (Con/EtOH) group. It is plausible that the increase in Iba-1+ cells in the EtOH/EtOH group observed in the hippocampus is due to microglial proliferation at two days following the first binge [22,31,60]. This effect also suggests that ethanol does not significantly reduce these newly proliferated microglial cells. It is of note that the effect of ethanol on microglia number varied by region: in the entorhinal cortex, both the single and double binge resulted in a decrease in the number of microglia consistent with our recent report [61]. The lack of increased Iba-1+ cells in the entorhinal cortex of EtOH/EtOH group is likely related to the finding that microglia neither proliferate dramatically at two days post-binge in the entorhinal cortex nor is there a significant increase in microglia number after seven days;, however, both proliferation and increased Iba-1+ cells have been observed in the hippocampus at this same time point [22,60]. Why microglia proliferate in the hippocampus but not entorhinal cortex after binge ethanol exposure is puzzling. Neurons in the entorhinal cortex degenerate more robustly, peaking at four days of exposure [5,7,8], which is followed by other signs of reactive microgliosis [22]. More studies are necessary to fully understand the dynamic effects of alcohol on microglia number, especially considering the recent discoveries that microglia contribute to synapse refinement and plasticity [25]. These data support the hypothesis that a second binge alcohol exposure exacerbates the microglial response, since an increase in the number of activated microglia would likely result in a potentiated neuroimmune response during the second binge.

Hippocampal BDNF concentrations were determined in order to assess the impact of microglia reactivity and changes in microglia number on the surrounding environment. BDNF plays a pivotal role in neuronal integrity and its dysregulation is associated with neurodegeneration [73]. In the Con/EtOH group, BDNF was decreased, the number of microglia were decreased and there was a significant correlation between the number of microglia and BDNF protein expression. However, in the EtOH/EtOH treated animals, where microglia were more activated and their numbers were increased, a significantly higher BDNF concentration was observed, though this value did not correlate significantly to microglia number. It is possible that the increase in BDNF concentrations is due to cells other than microglia, such as astrocytes, neurons, and other CNS cells secreting BDNF [74]. In addition, the effect of ethanol on BDNF expression is quite complex [75]. Nevertheless, the interplay between the increased cytokine and neurotrophin production observed in the EtOH/EtOH group requires further study to understand its functional implications.

The experimental design to use the same animals for both immunohistochemical and ELISA experiments allowed for a series of correlations to help determine what aspect of ethanol exposure, in this AUD model, was associated with microglial reactivity. OX-42 immunoreactivity did not correlate to average dose per day or to the total dose of ethanol in either the Con/EtOH or EtOH/EtOH groups. This lack of correlation is important as immune modulators such as LPS have dose-dependent responses in microglia reactivity [76]. The lack of correlation between OX-42 and total dose of ethanol suggests that ethanol potentiates the OX-42 response by acting as a secondary stimulus rather than an additive effect of the accumulative dose. Moreover, no relationship between the number of Iba-1+ cells and OX-42 immunoreactivity were observed, supporting that increased OX-42 immunoreactivity was a result of microglial activation and not an artifact of the change in cell number [77]. Correlations were also used to examine the relationship between OX-42 immunoreactivity or Iba-1 cell number and functional indices (cytokine/neurotrophin production). However, neither CR3 receptor (OX-42) upregulation nor Iba-1+ cell number was significantly correlated with TNF-α expression. Interestingly, the bimodal distribution of TNF-α production observed in the EtOH/EtOH group did map on to BECs. Although the mechanism by which BECs are related to TNF-α were not measured, at minimum, this correlation suggests that as BECs increase with repeated exposure, a primed microglial state may cause increased pro-inflammatory cytokines. Finally, in relation to BDNF, only microglia cell number in the Con/EtOH group showed a significant correlation with BDNF concentrations supporting the idea that microglial dysfunction and subsequent loss of trophic factors may contribute to neurodegeneration, especially alcoholic brain damage [61]. Correlations are not being interpreted as causation, but they do provide direction for what aspects of alcohol-exposure impact microglia reactivity leading to a primed microglial state.

Some evidence of classical activation has been observed in other AUD models, an effect that may be attributable to species differences and/or variations in the duration and pattern of exposure [30,69]. While previous reports suggested that the difference in microglia reactivity was due to these aforementioned variations in AUD models, the current data in this report more definitively indicates that it is the repeated insult that may drive the greater microglial response. For example, a model of alcohol exposure with lower total doses of alcohol dispersed over a longer period of time produced more OX-6 positive cells than the exposure used herein, where OX-6 expression may have been an anomaly in a single animal [30]. The appearance of the OX-6+ cells, however, in both models still appeared to be the bushy, ramified morphology associated with a low-level or M2-like activation. Indeed, the only alcohol study, human or animal, where ED-1+ microglia have been observed, is from a study in which rats underwent four cycles of a Majchrowicz-like model with three days between binges. However, the high mortality rate and severe weight loss of rats in that report make interpretations difficult. One interpretation is that microglial activation may have occurred due to the stress of repetitive gavage and/or weight loss [57,78–80]. Thus, the current study specifically used a seven day abstinence period to allow rats to recover from four days of intoxication and the significant withdrawal sequelae that occurs in this model [40]. Moreover, because some weight loss is observed in the Majchrowicz model [40], repetitive gavage may be stressful [81], and both of these aspects modulate microglial reactivity [78,82], a group with *ad libitum* access to food and water was included. None of the measures of microglia activation were different between the *ad libitum* group and the Con/Con group despite their slight weight loss and experience with gavage. Moreover, weight loss did not correlate with any measure of microglial activation in animals receiving ethanol.

The potentiated microglia activation seen in this double binge AUD model suggests that the microglial response can be altered by ethanol alone and supports the idea that chronic ethanol exposure can elicit a more pro-inflammatory state than a single bout of binge exposure. The lack of expression of ED-1 and morphology of OX-42+ and Iba-1+ cells support that even with the two binges, cells are not fully or classically activated. However, microglia are "further" down the spectrum towards classical activation than a single binge alone. These data coupled with the lack of evidence for classically activated microglia in human alcoholic brain—whether the markers are not expressed or no one has examined those particular markers—supports that initially microglia activation is likely a consequence of alcoholic neuropathology and not a cause. Whether this increased response causes microglia to over-respond to insult or if it makes the brain more susceptible to ongoing neuroinflammation should be considered in future experiments. In addition, how these effects relate to changes in neurodegeneration, specifically neuronal or volume loss, is an important area for future study. Because microglia have the capacity to maintain low grade activation or a primed state for extensive periods following insult, including alcohol exposure [22,83], the episodic nature of binge drinking would lead to a cycle of repeated priming and over-response in individuals suffering from an AUD [18,38,65]. Understanding the mechanisms that underlie or contribute to alcohol-induced neurodegeneration may provide a novel therapeutic target to ameliorate damage and prevent the downward spiral into an AUD [14,84].

5. Conclusions

In summary, these studies present a novel view of the impact of alcohol abuse on microglial activity. Specifically, data presented herein indicate that alcohol causes a shift in microglial phenotypes to a primed state. Although this study focuses on how later bouts of alcohol can exacerbate the microglial response, the implications of an alcohol-induced primed microglial state also extend to how the microglia of alcoholics may respond to infections or other alcohol related immune responses in the peripheral system. This research provides a context in which to consider the implications of microglia on alcohol-induced neurodegeneration and further indicates that targeting the neuroimmune system may alleviate deficits caused by excessive alcohol consumption.

Acknowledgments: The authors gratefully acknowledge support from NIAAA (R01AA016959; F31AA023459), NIDA (T32DA016176), and NIGMS (K12GM000678).

Author Contributions: Alex Marshall and Kimberly Nixon conceived and designed the experiments; Alex Marshall and Chelsea Geil performed the experiments; Alex Marshall analyzed the data; and all authors contributed to the interpretation of the data, writing and editing the manuscript.

Abbreviations

The following abbreviations are used in this manuscript:

AALAC	Association for the Assessment and Accreditation of Laboratory Animal Care
ANOVA	Analysis of Variance
AUD	Alcohol Use Disorder
BBB	Blood Brain Barrier
BEC	Blood Ethanol Concentration

BDNF	Brain Derived Neurotrophic Factor
CA	Cornu Amonis
CNS	Central Nervous System
Con	Control
CR3	Complement Receptor 3
DG	Dentate Gyrus
ELISA	Enzyme-Linked ImmunoSorbent Assay
EtOH	Ethanol
Iba-1	Ionized calcium-Binding Adapter molecule 1
IL-10	InterLeukin-10
ip	Intraperitoneal
TBS	Tris-Buffered Saline
TNF-α	Tumor Necrosis Factor alpha

References

1. Grant, B.F.; Saha, T.D.; Ruan, W.J.; Goldstein, R.B.; Chou, S.P.; Jung, J.; Zhang, H.; Smith, S.M.; Pickering, R.P.; Huang, B.; *et al.* Epidemiology of DSM-5 drug use disorder: Results from the national epidemiologic survey on alcohol and related conditions-III. *JAMA Psychiatry* **2016**, *73*, 39–47. [CrossRef] [PubMed]
2. Zahr, N.M.; Kaufman, K.L.; Harper, C.G. Clinical and pathological features of alcohol-related brain damage. *Nat. Rev. Neurol.* **2011**, *7*, 284–294. [CrossRef] [PubMed]
3. Sullivan, E.V.; Marsh, L.; Mathalon, D.H.; Lim, K.O.; Pfefferbaum, A. Age-related decline in MRI volumes of temporal lobe gray matter but not hippocampus. *Neurobiol. Aging* **1995**, *16*, 591–606. [CrossRef]
4. Pfefferbaum, A.; Lim, K.O.; Zipursky, R.B.; Mathalon, D.H.; Rosenbloom, M.J.; Lane, B.; Ha, C.N.; Sullivan, E.V. Brain gray and white matter volume loss accelerates with aging in chronic alcoholics: A quantitative MRI study. *Alcohol Clin. Exp. Res.* **1992**, *16*, 1078–1089. [CrossRef] [PubMed]
5. Obernier, J.A.; Bouldin, T.W.; Crews, F.T. Binge ethanol exposure in adult rats causes necrotic cell death. *Alcohol Clin. Exp. Res.* **2002**, *26*, 547–557. [CrossRef] [PubMed]
6. Pascual, M.; Blanco, A.M.; Cauli, O.; Minarro, J.; Guerri, C. Intermittent ethanol exposure induces inflammatory brain damage and causes long-term behavioural alterations in adolescent rats. *Eur. J. Neurosci.* **2007**, *25*, 541–550. [CrossRef] [PubMed]
7. Collins, M.A.; Corse, T.D.; Neafsey, E.J. Neuronal degeneration in rat cerebrocortical and olfactory regions during subchronic "binge" intoxication with ethanol: Possible explanation for olfactory deficits in alcoholics. *Alcohol Clin. Exp. Res.* **1996**, *20*, 284–292. [CrossRef] [PubMed]
8. Kelso, M.L.; Liput, D.J.; Eaves, D.W.; Nixon, K. Upregulated vimentin suggests new areas of neurodegeneration in a model of an alcohol use disorder. *Neuroscience* **2011**, *197*, 381–393. [CrossRef] [PubMed]
9. Gupta, S.; Warner, J. Alcohol-related dementia: A 21st-century silent epidemic? *Br. J. Psychiatry* **2008**, *193*, 351–353. [CrossRef] [PubMed]
10. Smith, D.M.; Atkinson, R.M. Alcoholism and dementia. *Int. J. Addict.* **1995**, *30*, 1843–1869. [CrossRef] [PubMed]
11. Petry, N.M. Delay discounting of money and alcohol in actively using alcoholics, currently abstinent alcoholics, and controls. *Psychopharmacology* **2001**, *154*, 243–250. [CrossRef] [PubMed]
12. Nixon, S.J.; Prather, R.; Lewis, B. Sex differences in alcohol-related neurobehavioral consequences. *Handb. Clin. Neurol.* **2014**, *125*, 253–272. [PubMed]
13. Crews, F.T.; Boettiger, C.A. Impulsivity, frontal lobes and risk for addiction. *Pharm. Biochem. Behav.* **2009**, *93*, 237–247. [CrossRef] [PubMed]
14. Koob, G.F.; Le Moal, M. Drug abuse: Hedonic homeostatic dysregulation. *Science* **1997**, *278*, 52–58. [CrossRef] [PubMed]
15. Crews, F.T. Alcohol and neurodegeneration. *CNS Drug Rev.* **1999**, *5*, 379–394. [CrossRef]
16. Crews, F.T.; Nixon, K. Mechanisms of neurodegeneration and regeneration in alcoholism. *Alcohol Alcohol* **2009**, *44*, 115–127. [CrossRef] [PubMed]

17. Crews, F.T.; Vetreno, R.P. Neuroimmune basis of alcoholic brain damage. *Int. Rev. Neurobiol.* **2014**, *118*, 315–357. [PubMed]
18. Crews, F.T.; Zou, J.; Qin, L. Induction of innate immune genes in brain create the neurobiology of addiction. *Brain Behav. Immun.* **2011**, *25*, S4–S12. [CrossRef] [PubMed]
19. Qin, L.; Crews, F.T. Nadph oxidase and reactive oxygen species contribute to alcohol-induced microglial activation and neurodegeneration. *J. Neuroinflamm.* **2012**, *9*, 5. [CrossRef] [PubMed]
20. He, J.; Crews, F.T. Increased MCP-1 and microglia in various regions of the human alcoholic brain. *Exp. Neurol.* **2008**, *210*, 349–358. [CrossRef] [PubMed]
21. Dennis, C.V.; Sheahan, P.J.; Graeber, M.B.; Sheedy, D.L.; Kril, J.J.; Sutherland, G.T. Microglial proliferation in the brain of chronic alcoholics with hepatic encephalopathy. *Metab. Brain Dis.* **2014**, *29*, 1027–1039. [CrossRef] [PubMed]
22. Marshall, S.A.; McClain, J.A.; Kelso, M.L.; Hopkins, D.M.; Pauly, J.R.; Nixon, K. Microglial activation is not equivalent to neuroinflammation in alcohol-induced neurodegeneration: The importance of microglia phenotype. *Neurobiol. Dis.* **2013**, *54*, 239–251. [CrossRef] [PubMed]
23. Qin, L.; He, J.; Hanes, R.N.; Pluzarev, O.; Hong, J.S.; Crews, F.T. Increased systemic and brain cytokine production and neuroinflammation by endotoxin following ethanol treatment. *J. Neuroinflamm.* **2008**, *5*, 10. [CrossRef] [PubMed]
24. Zahr, N.M.; Luong, R.; Sullivan, E.V.; Pfefferbaum, A. Measurement of serum, liver, and brain cytokine induction, thiamine levels, and hepatopathology in rats exposed to a 4-day alcohol binge protocol. *Alcohol Clin. Exp. Res.* **2010**, *34*, 1858–1870. [CrossRef] [PubMed]
25. Tremblay, M.E.; Stevens, B.; Sierra, A.; Wake, H.; Bessis, A.; Nimmerjahn, A. The role of microglia in the healthy brain. *J. Neurosci.* **2013**, *31*, 16064–16069. [CrossRef] [PubMed]
26. Raivich, G.; Bohatschek, M.; Kloss, C.U.; Werner, A.; Jones, L.L.; Kreutzberg, G.W. Neuroglial activation repertoire in the injured brain: Graded response, molecular mechanisms and cues to physiological function. *Brain Res. Rev.* **1999**, *30*, 77–105. [CrossRef]
27. Nimmerjahn, A.; Kirchhoff, F.; Helmchen, F. Resting microglial cells are highly dynamic surveillants of brain parenchyma *in vivo*. *Science* **2005**, *308*, 1314–1318. [CrossRef] [PubMed]
28. Perry, V.H.; Holmes, C. Microglial priming in neurodegenerative disease. *Nat. Rev. Neurol.* **2014**, *10*, 217–224. [CrossRef] [PubMed]
29. Graeber, M.B.; Streit, W.J. Microglia: Biology and pathology. *Acta Neuropathol.* **2009**, *119*, 89–105. [CrossRef] [PubMed]
30. Ward, R.J.; Colivicchi, M.A.; Allen, R.; Schol, F.; Lallemand, F.; de Witte, P.; Ballini, C.; Corte, L.D.; Dexter, D. Neuro-inflammation induced in the hippocampus of 'binge drinking' rats may be mediated by elevated extracellular glutamate content. *J. Neurochem.* **2009**, *111*, 1119–1128. [CrossRef] [PubMed]
31. McClain, J.A.; Morris, S.A.; Deeny, M.A.; Marshall, S.A.; Hayes, D.M.; Kiser, Z.M.; Nixon, K. Adolescent binge alcohol exposure induces long-lasting partial activation of microglia. *Brain Behav. Immun.* **2011**, *25*, S120–S128. [CrossRef] [PubMed]
32. Bilbo, S.D.; Schwarz, J.M. Early-life programming of later-life brain and behavior: A critical role for the immune system. *Front. Behav. Neurosci.* **2009**, *3*, 14. [CrossRef] [PubMed]
33. Ramaglia, V.; Hughes, T.R.; Donev, R.M.; Ruseva, M.M.; Wu, X.; Huitinga, I.; Baas, F.; Neal, J.W.; Morgan, B.P. C3-dependent mechanism of microglial priming relevant to multiple sclerosis. *Proc. Natl. Acad. Sci. USA* **2012**, *109*, 965–970. [CrossRef] [PubMed]
34. Qin, L.; Crews, F.T. Chronic ethanol increases systemic TLR3 agonist-induced neuroinflammation and neurodegeneration. *J. Neuroinflamm.* **2012**, *9*, 130. [CrossRef] [PubMed]
35. Qin, L.; Liu, Y.; Hong, J.S.; Crews, F.T. Nadph oxidase and aging drive microglial activation, oxidative stress, and dopaminergic neurodegeneration following systemic LPS administration. *Glia* **2013**, *61*, 855–868. [CrossRef] [PubMed]
36. Harford, T.C.; Grant, B.F.; Yi, H.Y.; Chen, C.M. Patterns of DSM-IV alcohol abuse and dependence criteria among adolescents and adults: Results from the 2001 national household survey on drug abuse. *Alcohol Clin. Exp. Res.* **2005**, *29*, 810–828. [CrossRef] [PubMed]
37. White, A.M.; Kraus, C.L.; Swartzwelder, H. Many college freshmen drink at levels far beyond the binge threshold. *Alcohol Clin. Exp. Res.* **2006**, *30*, 1006–1010. [CrossRef] [PubMed]

38. Hunt, W.A. Are binge drinkers more at risk of developing brain damage? *Alcohol* **1993**, *10*, 559–561. [CrossRef]
39. NRC. *Guide for the Care and Use of Laboratory Animals*; The National Academies Press: Washington, DC, USA, 1996.
40. Morris, S.A.; Kelso, M.L.; Liput, D.J.; Marshall, S.A.; Nixon, K. Similar withdrawal severity in adolescents and adults in a rat model of alcohol dependence. *Alcohol* **2010**, *44*, 89–98. [CrossRef] [PubMed]
41. McClain, J.A.; Morris, S.A.; Marshall, S.A.; Nixon, K. Ectopic hippocampal neurogenesis in adolescent male rats following alcohol dependence. *Addict. Biol.* **2014**, *19*, 687–699. [CrossRef] [PubMed]
42. Majchrowicz, E. Induction of physical dependence upon ethanol and the associated behavioral changes in rats. *Psychopharmacologia* **1975**, *43*, 245–254. [CrossRef] [PubMed]
43. Raivich, G.; Jones, L.L.; Werner, A.; Bluthmann, H.; Doetschmann, T.; Kreutzberg, G.W. Molecular signals for glial activation: Pro- and anti-inflammatory cytokines in the injured brain. *Acta Neurochir. Suppl.* **1999**, *73*, 21–30. [PubMed]
44. Hynes, R.O. Integrins: Versatility, modulation, and signaling in cell adhesion. *Cell* **1992**, *69*, 11–25. [CrossRef]
45. Morioka, T.; Kalehua, A.N.; Streit, W.J. Progressive expression of immunomolecules on microglial cells in rat dorsal hippocampus following transient forebrain ischemia. *Acta Neuropathol.* **1992**, *83*, 149–157. [CrossRef] [PubMed]
46. Robinson, A.P.; White, T.M.; Mason, D.W. Macrophage heterogeneity in the rat as delineated by two monoclonal antibodies MRC OX-41 and MRC OX-42, the latter recognizing complement receptor type 3. *Immunology* **1986**, *57*, 239–247. [PubMed]
47. Bauer, J.; Sminia, T.; Wouterlood, F.G.; Dijkstra, C.D. Phagocytic activity of macrophages and microglial cells during the course of acute and chronic relapsing experimental autoimmune encephalomyelitis. *J. Neurosci. Res.* **1994**, *38*, 365–375. [CrossRef] [PubMed]
48. O'Keefe, G.M.; Nguyen, V.T.; Benveniste, E.N. Regulation and function of class ii major histocompatibility complex, CD40, and B7 expression in macrophages and microglia: Implications in neurological diseases. *J. Neurovirol.* **2002**, *8*, 496–512. [CrossRef] [PubMed]
49. Ito, D.; Imai, Y.; Ohsawa, K.; Nakajima, K.; Fukuuchi, Y.; Kohsaka, S. Microglia-specific localisation of a novel calcium binding protein, iba1. *Mol. Brain Res.* **1998**, *57*, 1–9. [CrossRef]
50. Paxinos, G.; Watson, C. *The Rat Brain in Stereotaxic Coordinates/George Paxinos, Charles Watson, Compact*, 6th ed.; Elsevier Academic: London, UK, 2009.
51. Long, J.M.; Kalehua, A.N.; Muth, N.J.; Hengemihle, J.M.; Jucker, M.; Calhoun, M.E.; Ingram, D.K.; Mouton, P.R. Stereological estimation of total microglia number in mouse hippocampus. *J. Neurosci. Methods* **1998**, *84*, 101–108. [CrossRef]
52. West, M.J.; Slomianka, L.; Gundersen, H.J.G. Unbiased stereological estimation of the total number of neurons in the subdivisions of the rat hippocampus using the optical fractionator. *Anat. Rec.* **1991**, *231*, 482–497. [CrossRef] [PubMed]
53. Francisco, J.S.; Moraes, H.P.; Dias, E.P. Evaluation of the image-pro plus 4.5 software for automatic counting of labeled nuclei by PCNA immunohistochemistry. *Braz. Oral Res.* **2004**, *18*, 100–104. [CrossRef] [PubMed]
54. Rabuffetti, M.; Sciorati, C.; Tarozzo, G.; Clementi, E.; Manfredi, A.A.; Beltramo, M. Inhibition of caspase-1-like activity by Ac-Tyr-Val-Ala-Asp-chloromethyl ketone induces long-lasting neuroprotection in cerebral ischemia through apoptosis reduction and decrease of proinflammatory cytokines. *J. Neurosci.* **2000**, *20*, 4398–4404. [PubMed]
55. Miller, M.W.; Mooney, S.M. Chronic exposure to ethanol alters neurotrophin content in the basal forebrain-cortex system in the mature rat: Effects on autocrine-paracrine mechanisms. *J. Neurobiol.* **2004**, *60*, 490–498. [CrossRef] [PubMed]
56. Miller, M.W. Repeated episodic exposure to ethanol affects neurotrophin content in the forebrain of the mature rat. *Exp. Neurol.* **2004**, *189*, 173–181. [CrossRef] [PubMed]
57. Loncarevic-Vasiljkovic, N.; Pesic, V.; Todorovic, S.; Popic, J.; Smiljanic, K.; Milanovic, D.; Ruzdijic, S.; Kanazir, S. Caloric restriction suppresses microglial activation and prevents neuroapoptosis following cortical injury in rats. *PLoS ONE* **2012**, *7*, e37215. [CrossRef] [PubMed]
58. Tu, Y.F.; Lu, P.J.; Huang, C.C.; Ho, C.J.; Chou, Y.P. Moderate dietary restriction reduces p53-mediated neurovascular damage and microglia activation after hypoxic ischemia in neonatal brain. *Stroke* **2012**, *43*, 491–498. [CrossRef] [PubMed]

59. Akiyama, H.; McGeer, P.L. Brain microglia constitutively express beta-2 integrins. *J. Neuroimmunol.* **1990**, *30*, 81–93. [CrossRef]
60. Nixon, K.; Kim, D.H.; Potts, E.N.; He, J.; Crews, F.T. Distinct cell proliferation events during abstinence after alcohol dependence: Microglia proliferation precedes neurogenesis. *Neurobiol. Dis.* **2008**, *31*, 218–229. [CrossRef] [PubMed]
61. Marshall, S.A.; McClain, J.A.; Nixon, K. Microglial dystrophy following binge-like alcohol exposure in adolescent and adult rats. *Eur. J. Neurosci.* **2016**. submitted for publication.
62. Lai, A.Y.; Todd, K.G. Differential regulation of trophic and proinflammatory microglial effectors is dependent on severity of neuronal injury. *Glia* **2008**, *56*, 259–270. [CrossRef] [PubMed]
63. Chao, C.C.; Gekker, G.; Sheng, W.S.; Hu, S.; Tsang, M.; Peterson, P.K. Priming effect of morphine on the production of tumor necrosis factor-alpha by microglia: Implications in respiratory burst activity and human immunodeficiency virus-1 expression. *J. Pharmacol. Exp. Ther.* **1994**, *269*, 198–203. [PubMed]
64. Dilger, R.N.; Johnson, R.W. Aging, microglial cell priming, and the discordant central inflammatory response to signals from the peripheral immune system. *J. Leukoc. Biol.* **2008**, *84*, 932–939. [CrossRef] [PubMed]
65. McMahon, R.C.; Davidson, R.S.; Gersh, D.; Flynn, P. A comparison of continuous and episodic drinkers using the MCMI, MMPI, and alceval-r. *J. Clin. Psychol.* **1991**, *47*, 148–159. [CrossRef]
66. Relman, D.; Tuomanen, E.; Falkow, S.; Golenbock, D.T.; Saukkonen, K.; Wright, S.D. Recognition of a bacterial adhesion by an integrin: Macrophage CR3 ($\alpha_M\beta_2$, CD11b/CD18) binds filamentous hemagglutinin of Bordetella pertussis. *Cell* **1990**, *61*, 1375–1382. [CrossRef]
67. Tyler, C.M.; Boulanger, L.M. Complement-mediated microglial clearance of developing retinal ganglion cell axons. *Neuron* **2012**, *74*, 597–599. [CrossRef] [PubMed]
68. Fernandez-Lizarbe, S.; Pascual, M.; Guerri, C. Critical role of TLR4 response in the activation of microglia induced by ethanol. *J. Immunol.* **2009**, *183*, 4733–4744. [CrossRef] [PubMed]
69. Zhao, Y.N.; Wang, F.; Fan, Y.X.; Ping, G.F.; Yang, J.Y.; Wu, C.F. Activated microglia are implicated in cognitive deficits, neuronal death, and successful recovery following intermittent ethanol exposure. *Behav. Brain Res.* **2013**, *236*, 270–282. [CrossRef] [PubMed]
70. Crews, F.; Nixon, K.; Kim, D.; Joseph, J.; Shukitt-Hale, B.; Qin, L.; Zou, J. BHT blocks NF-κB activation and ethanol-induced brain damage. *Alcohol Clin. Exp. Res.* **2006**, *30*, 1938–1949. [CrossRef] [PubMed]
71. Sierra, A.; Gottfried-Blackmore, A.C.; McEwen, B.S.; Bulloch, K. Microglia derived from aging mice exhibit an altered inflammatory profile. *Glia* **2007**, *55*, 412–424. [CrossRef] [PubMed]
72. Perry, V.H.; Cunningham, C.; Holmes, C. Systemic infections and inflammation affect chronic neurodegeneration. *Nat. Rev. Immunol.* **2007**, *7*, 161–167. [CrossRef] [PubMed]
73. Lipsky, R.H.; Marini, A.M. Brain-derived neurotrophic factor in neuronal survival and behavior-related plasticity. *Ann. N. Y. Acad. Sci.* **2007**, *1122*, 130–143. [CrossRef] [PubMed]
74. Bejot, Y.; Prigent-Tessier, A.; Cachia, C.; Giroud, M.; Mossiat, C.; Bertrand, N.; Garnier, P.; Marie, C. Time-dependent contribution of non neuronal cells to BDNF production after ischemic stroke in rats. *Neurochem. Int.* **2011**, *58*, 102–111. [CrossRef] [PubMed]
75. Davis, M.I. Ethanol-BDNF interactions: Still more questions than answers. *Pharmacol. Ther.* **2008**, *118*, 36–57. [CrossRef] [PubMed]
76. Houdek, H.M.; Larson, J.; Watt, J.A.; Rosenberger, T.A. Bacterial lipopolysaccharide induces a dose-dependent activation of neuroglia and loss of basal forebrain cholinergic cells in the rat brain. *Inflamm. Cell Signal.* **2014**, *1*, e47. [PubMed]
77. Matos, L.L.; Trufelli, D.C.; de Matos, M.G.; da Silva Pinhal, M.A. Immunohistochemistry as an important tool in biomarkers detection and clinical practice. *Biomark Insights* **2010**, *5*, 9–20. [CrossRef] [PubMed]
78. Radler, M.E.; Wright, B.J.; Walker, F.R.; Hale, M.W.; Kent, S. Calorie restriction increases lipopolysaccharide-induced neuropeptide y immunolabeling and reduces microglial cell area in the arcuate hypothalamic nucleus. *Neuroscience* **2015**, *285*, 236–247. [CrossRef] [PubMed]
79. Sharrett-Field, L.; Butler, T.R.; Berry, J.N.; Reynolds, A.R.; Prendergast, M.A. Mifepristone pretreatment reduces ethanol withdrawal severity *in vivo*. *Alcohol Clin. Exp. Res.* **2013**, *37*, 1417–1423. [CrossRef] [PubMed]
80. Frank, M.G.; Baratta, M.V.; Sprunger, D.B.; Watkins, L.R.; Maier, S.F. Microglia serve as a neuroimmune substrate for stress-induced potentiation of CNS pro-inflammatory cytokine responses. *Brain Behav. Immun.* **2007**, *21*, 47–59. [CrossRef] [PubMed]

81. Arantes-Rodrigues, R.; Henriques, A.; Pinto-Leite, R.; Faustino-Rocha, A.; Pinho-Oliveira, J.; Teixeira-Guedes, C.; Seixas, F.; Gama, A.; Colaco, B.; Colaco, A.; *et al.* The effects of repeated oral gavage on the health of male CD-1 mice. *Lab. Anim.* **2012**, *41*, 129–134. [CrossRef] [PubMed]
82. Sugama, S. Stress-induced microglial activation may facilitate the progression of neurodegenerative disorders. *Med. Hypotheses* **2009**, *73*, 1031–1034. [CrossRef] [PubMed]
83. Obernier, J.A.; White, A.M.; Swartzwelder, H.S.; Crews, F.T. Cognitive deficits and CNS damage after a 4-day binge ethanol exposure in rats. *Pharmacol. Biochem. Behav.* **2002**, *72*, 521–532. [CrossRef]
84. Vetreno, R.P.; Crews, F.T. Current hypotheses on the mechanisms of alcoholism. *Handb. Clin. Neurol.* **2014**, *125*, 477–497. [PubMed]

8

Atypical Processing of Novel Distracters in a Visual Oddball Task in Autism Spectrum Disorder

Estate M. Sokhadze [1,2], Eva V. Lamina [1], Emily L. Casanova [1,2], Desmond P. Kelly [1,2], Ioan Opris [3], Irma Khachidze [4] and Manuel F. Casanova [1,2,*]

1 Department of Biomedical Sciences, University of South Carolina School of Medicine-Greenville, 200 Patewood Dr., Ste A200, Greenville, SC 29615, USA; SOKHADZE@greenvillemed.sc.edu (E.M.S.); LAMINAE@mailbox.sc.edu (E.V.L.); ECasanova@ghs.org (E.L.C.); DKelly@ghs.org (D.P.K.)

2 Developmental Behavioral Unit, Department of Pediatrics, Children's Hospital, Greenville Health System, Greenville, SC 29615, USA

3 School of Medicine, University of Miami, Miami, FL 33136, USA; ioanopris.phd@gmail.com

4 Centre of Experimental Biomedicine, 14 Gotya str., Tbilisi 0160, Georgia; irmakha@yahoo.com

* Correspondence: MCasanova@ghs.org

Abstract: Several studies have shown that children with autism spectrum disorder (ASD) show abnormalities in P3b to targets in standard oddball tasks. The present study employed a three-stimulus visual oddball task with novel distracters that analyzed event-related potentials (ERP) to both target and non-target items at frontal and parietal sites. The task tested the hypothesis that children with autism are abnormally orienting attention to distracters probably due to impaired habituation to novelty. We predicted a lower selectivity in early ERPs to target, frequent non-target, and rare distracters. We also expected delayed late ERPs in autism. The study enrolled 32 ASD and 24 typically developing (TD) children. Reaction time (RT) and accuracy were analyzed as behavioral measures, while ERPs were recorded with a dense-array EEG system. Children with ASD showed higher error rate without normative post-error RT slowing and had lower error-related negativity. Parietal P1, frontal N1, as well as P3a and P3b components were higher to novels in ASD. Augmented exogenous ERPs suggest low selectivity in pre-processing of stimuli resulting in their excessive processing at later stages. The results suggest an impaired habituation to unattended stimuli that incurs a high load at the later stages of perceptual and cognitive processing and response selection when novel distracter stimuli are differentiated from targets.

Keywords: event-related potential; autism spectrum disorder; attention; cognitive processes; reaction time

1. Introduction

Autism Spectrum Disorder (ASD) is characterized by severe disturbances in reciprocal social relations, varying degrees of language and communication difficulties, and behavioral patterns which are restricted, repetitive, and stereotyped [1]. Additionally, individuals with autism usually present excessive reactions to change in their environment such as aversive reactions to visual, auditory, and tactile stimuli. These perception and sensory reactivity abnormalities, found in a majority of subjects with ASD, affect their ability to effectively process information [2]. In a series of electrophysiological studies conducted by our group we explored specifics of event-related potential (i.e., ERP) reflecting information processing during performance on reaction time (RT) tasks in children with ASD [3–9]. Our prior studies explored the manifestations of excessive local connectivity and impaired distal functional connectivity, excessive cortical excitation/inhibition ratio, and deficient executive functioning in ASD by analyzing behavioral performance on attention tasks with concurrent dense-array ERP recording. More detailed theoretical considerations related to the results of these studies were discussed in our reviews on this topic [9–11].

The current study explored atypicality of reactivity to novel stimuli in autism during performance on a three-stimulus visual oddball task as reflected in RT and ERP. Elicitation of ERP waves related to novelty processing can be readily achieved through this type of oddball paradigm, in which subjects are exposed to continuous succession of three types of stimuli, one presented frequently (standard), while the two other types of stimuli are rare. One of the rare stimuli is designated as a target, whereas the second type rare stimuli has some distinction from target and is usually referred to as a novel, or novel distracter. Analysis of ERP components using this test paradigm is a useful way of investigating task-relevant and -irrelevant information processing stages as well as selective attention. Amplitude and latency characteristics of negative and positive ERP components at selected scalp topographic regions-of-interest (ROI) can provide valuable information about the early sensory perception processes and the higher-level processes including attention, cortical inhibition, response selection, error monitoring, memory update, and other cognitive activity related to working memory [11–15].

Event-related potentials reflect the activation of neural structures in primary sensory cortex, and in associative cortical areas related to higher order cognitive processes. ERP components can be categorized as short-latency (exogenous, e.g., N1) or long-latency (endogenous, e.g., P3) ERPs, which reflect early-stage, modality-specific and late-stage polymodal associative processing respectively. The early ERP components (e.g., P1, N1) reflect exogenous processes modulated by the physical attributes of the stimulus (i.e., brightness for visual stimuli; loudness of auditory stimuli, etc.), rather than by endogenous cognitive processes [16]. However, it has been noted that attention processes may operate even at the early stages of information intake and influence stimulus processing at the later stage [17]. Two endogenous components of the ERP, namely the N2 and P3, are thought to be directly associated with the cognitive processes of perception and selective attention [18]. The posterior visual N2 (labeled as N2b) is enhanced if the presented stimulus contains a perceptual feature or attributes defining the target in the task. In majority of oddball tasks, the N2b is related to the cognitive processes of stimulus identification and distinction [18,19]. In a modification of the oddball task, when rare distracters are presented along with standard and rare target stimuli, these distracters elicit a fronto-central P3a, whereas the targets elicit a parietally distributed P3b [20,21]. In a three stimulus oddball task the P3a is interpreted as "orienting" of attention to novelty, and the P3b as an index of ability to sustain attention to target. Error sensitivity can be examined by measuring response-locked ERP components associated with cortical responses to committed errors. Two ERP components relevant in this context are the error-related negativity (ERN) and the error-related positivity (Pe).

This study employed a visual novelty oddball task with simultaneous recording of motor responses and brain potentials in children with ASD and in typically developing (TD) children. Such an approach allowed us to analyze attentional and cognitive processing mechanisms recruited in typically developing subjects relative to children with autism. We proposed that early stages of the sensory visual signal processing in autism might be characterized by low selectivity and by reduced adaptation to task-irrelevant items. We predicted that in autism, as compared to TD controls, there would be a lower selectivity in early ERPs components in response to infrequent target, frequent non-target and rare novel distracters as well as delayed endogenous ERP components. In particular, we anticipated higher amplitudes of P1 and N1 not only to target but also to standard and novel stimuli reflective of deficits in stimulus category selectivity. Amplitude and latency of N2 and P3 components in ASD and TD children were expected to differ during later stages of information processing suggesting that a more effortful allocation was needed to sustain attention on target differentiation from the novel distracters. Differentiation of motor responses in terms of their correctness reflected in error-related potentials (ERN, Pe) was also expected to be deficient in children with ASD, and was predicted to negatively affect accuracy of motor responses.

2. Methods and Materials

2.1. Participants

Participants with autism spectrum disorder (ASD) (age range 9 to 18 years) were recruited through the Weisskopf Child Evaluation Center (WCEC). Diagnosis was made according to the Diagnostic and Statistical Manual of Mental Disorders (DSM-IV-TR) [22] or DSM-5 [1] and further ascertained with the Autism Diagnostic Interview—Revised (ADI-R) [23]. They also had a medical evaluation by a developmental pediatrician. All subjects had normal hearing based on past hearing screens. Participants either had normal vision or wore corrective lenses. Participants with a history of seizure disorder, significant hearing or visual impairment, a brain abnormality conclusive from imaging studies or an identified genetic disorder were excluded. All participants were high-functioning children with ASD with full scale IQ > 80 assessed using the Wechsler Intelligence Scale for Children, Fourth Edition (WISC-IV; [24]), the Stanford-Binet Intelligence Test [25], or the Wechsler Abbreviated Scale of Intelligence (WASI, [26]).

Typically developing (TD) children were recruited through advertisements in the local media. All TD participants were free of neurological or significant medical disorders, had normal hearing and vision, and were free of psychiatric, learning, or developmental disorders based on self- and parent reports. Subjects were screened for history of psychiatric or neurological diagnosis using the Structured Clinical Interview for DSM-IV Non-Patient Edition (SCID-NP, [27]). Participants within the control and autism groups were attempted to be matched for age, gender, and the socioeconomic status of their family.

The mean age of 32 participants enrolled in the ASD group was 13.09 ± 2.41 years (range 9–18 years, 29 males, 3 females), while the mean age of the TD group (N = 24) was 13.91 ± 2.91 years (9–20 years, 20 males, 4 females). The age difference between groups was not significant ($p = 0.38$, n.s.). All children with autism were high functioning individuals. Mean Full Scale IQ score for children with autism was 90.1 ± 14.9 and were collected from their most recent IQ evaluation records. Most of children in TD group did not have their IQ records available and their mean IQ data was not possible to report. Socioeconomic status of ASD and control groups was compared based on parent education and annual household income. The approximate household incomes did not reveal any statistically significant group differences. Participants in both groups had similar parent education levels.

The study complied with all relevant national regulations and institutional policies and was approved by the local Institutional Review Board (IRB). Participating subjects and their parents (or legal guardians) were provided with full information about the study including the purpose, requirements, responsibilities, reimbursement, risks, benefits, alternatives, and role of the local IRB. The consent and assent forms approved by the IRB were reviewed and explained to all subjects who expressed interest to participate. All questions were answered before consent signature was requested. If the individual agreed to participate, both she/he and parent/guardian signed and dated the consent form and/or assent form and received a copy countersigned by the investigator who obtained consent.

2.2. ERP Data Acquisition, and Signal Processing

Electroencephalographic (EEG) data was acquired with a 128 channel Electrical Geodesics Inc. (EGI) system (v. 200) consisting of Geodesic Sensor Net electrodes, Net Amps and Net Station software (Electrical Geodesics Inc., Eugene, OR, USA) running on a Macintosh G4 computer. EEG data were sampled at 500 Hz and 0.1–200 Hz analog filtered. Impedances were kept under 40 KΩ. According to the Technical Manual of EGI [28] this Net Sensor electrode impedance level is sufficient for quality recording of EEG with this system. The Geodesic Sensor Net is a lightweight elastic thread structure containing Ag/AgCl electrodes housed in a synthetic sponge on a pedestal. The sponges were soaked in a KCl solution to render them conductive. EEG data was recorded continuously. EEG channel with high impedance or with visually detectable artifacts (e.g., channel drift, gross movement, etc.) were marked as bad using the Net Station event marker tools in "on-line" mode for further removal in the "off-line" mode using the Net Station Waveform Tools (NSWT).

Stimulus-locked EEG recordings were segmented off-line into 1000 ms epochs spanning 200 ms pre-stimulus to 800 ms post-stimulus around the critical stimulus events: e.g., in an oddball task: (1) rare target, (2) rare non-target distracter (novel), (3) frequent non-target (standard). Data sets were digitally screened for artifacts (eye blinks, movements), and contaminated trials were removed using artifact rejection tools. The Net Station Waveform Tools' Artifact Detection module in "off-line" mode marks EEG channel bad if fast average amplitude exceeds 200 μV, differential average amplitude exceeds 100 μV or if channel has zero variance. Segments were marked bad if they contained more than 10 bad channels, or if eye blink or eye movement were detected (>70 μV). After detection of bad channels, the NSWT's "bad channel replacement" function was used for the replacement of data in bad channels with data interpolated from the remaining good channels (or segments) using spherical splines [29–32]. Response-locked ERPs were segmented off-line into 1000 ms epochs spanning 500 ms pre-error motor response to 500 ms post around the critical response event—commission error. Remaining data were digitally filtered using 60 Hz Notch and 0.3–20 Hz bandpass filters and then segmented by condition and averaged to create ERPs. Averaged ERP data were baseline corrected and re-referenced into an average reference frame. All stimuli and behavioral response collection was controlled by a PC computer running E-prime software (Psychology Software Tools Inc., Sharpsburg, PA, USA). Visual stimuli were presented on a 15 inch display. Manual responses were collected with a 5-button keypad (Serial Box, Psychology Software Tools Inc., Sharpsburg, PA, USA).

2.3. *Three Stimuli Visual Oddball Test with Novel Distracters*

This test represented a modification of traditional visual three-stimulus oddball task. Stimuli letters "X", "O", and novel distracters ("v", "^", ">" and "<" signs) were presented on the screen after fixation mark "+". One of the stimuli ("O") was presented on 50% of the trials (frequent standard); the novel stimuli stimulus (e.g., ">") was presented on 25% of the trials (rare distracter), whereas the third ("X") was presented on the remaining 25% of the trials and represented the target. Subjects were instructed to press a key when they see the target letter on the screen. Each stimulus was presented for 250 ms, with a variable (1000–1100 ms) inter-trial interval. There were 480 trials in total, with a break every 240 trials. The complete sequence took around 20 min.

2.4. *Behavioral Measures*

Behavioral response measures were mean reaction time (RT in ms) and response accuracy (percent of correct hits). Number and percent of commission and omission errors along with total number of errors was calculated for each participant. Post-error RT was calculated as RT to the first correct response after committed error (either omission of commission error). Difference between post-error RT and preceding correct RT to target was used to calculate normative post-error RT slowing values [5,8,33]. Analysis of distribution of RT in correct and error trials was conducted using sigmoid curve methodology from Opris et al. [34].

2.5. *Event-Related Potentials (ERP)*

2.5.1. Stimulus-Locked ERPs

ERP dependent measures were: adaptive mean amplitude and latency of ERP peak (e.g., P3a, P3b) within a temporal window across a region-of-interest (ROI) channel group. A list of ERP dependent variables included stimulus-averaged amplitude and latency of the frontal ERP components: N1 (80–180 ms post-stimulus), N2 (200–320 ms), and P3a (300–520 ms); and the posterior (parietal ROIs) ERP components P1 (80–180 ms), N2 (N2b, 180–320 ms) and P3b (320–560 ms). The frontal ROIs for N1, N2 and P3a components included following EGI channels: left ROI—EGI channel 12 (between FC1 and FCz), F1, F3 and FC1; midline ROI—FCz, Fz; right ROI—EGI channel 5 (between F2 and FCz),

F2, F4 and FC2. The parietal ROI for P1, N2 and P3b components included following EGI channels: left ROI—P1, P3, P7, PO3; midline—Pz; right ROI—EGI channel P2, P4, P8, PO8.

2.5.2. Response-Locked Dependent Variables (ERN/Pe)

Response locked dependent variables in this study were adaptive mean amplitude and latency of the Error-related Negativity (ERN peaking within 40–150 ms post-error) and Error-related Positivity (Pe, peaking within 100–300 ms post-error). The ROI for both ERN and Pe components included FCz, sites between FCz and FC3-C1, and between FCz and FC2-C2).

2.6. Statistical Data Analysis

Statistical analyses were performed on the subject-averaged behavioral (RT, error rate) and ERP data with the subject averages being the observations. The primary analysis model was the repeated measures ANOVA, with dependent variables being reaction time (RT), accuracy, commission and omission error rate, post-error RT slowing index, RT in correct and commission error trials, response locked ERN and Pe, and all the specific stimulus-locked ERP components' (N1, P1, N2, P3) amplitudes and latencies at the selected frontal and parietal ROIs. The data of each ERP dependent variable for each relevant ROI was analyzed using ANOVA with the following factors (all within-participants): *Stimulus* (target, novel, standard) and *Hemisphere* (left, right). The between subject factor was *Group* (ASD, CNT). Histograms with normal distribution curves along with skewness and kurtosis data were obtained for each dependent variable to determine normality of distribution and appropriateness of data for ANOVA test. In all ANOVAs, Greenhouse-Geisser corrected *p*-values were employed where appropriate. Since ASD group differences from TD group were the most important aspects of the study, the focus of analysis was on main effects of *Group* (ASD vs. TD) and their interactions with other variables. For the estimation of the effect size [35] we used Partial Eta Squared (η_p^2) measure. Statistical analysis was performed using SPSS v.22 and Sigma Stat 3.1 packages.

3. Results

3.1. Behavioral Responses

Reaction time to targets in autism group was not different from TD group (473.2 ± 93.5 vs. 465.6 ± 98.4, $F_{1,54} = 0.08$, $p = 0.78$, n.s.), but the difference in commission error rate was significant (5.57 ± 9.32 percent in ASD vs. 1.12 ± 1.20 percent in TD, $F_{1,54} = 4.48$, $p = 0.040$), being higher in the ASD group. The difference between mean RT in correct trials and post-error trials (i.e., post-error RT -minus-correct trial RT) was negative in autism but positive in controls, and this between-group difference was significant (−15.7 ± 50.1 ms in ASD vs. 19.4 ± 37.9 ms in TD, $F_{1,54} = 6.00$, $p = 0.019$, see Figure 1). Analysis of distribution of RT in correct and error trials using sigmoid curve method [34] did not show group differences, however in the ASD group distribution of RT in the error trials tended to be in the faster bin range (moda ~200 ms in error vs. ~400 ms in correct trials, see Figure 2.)

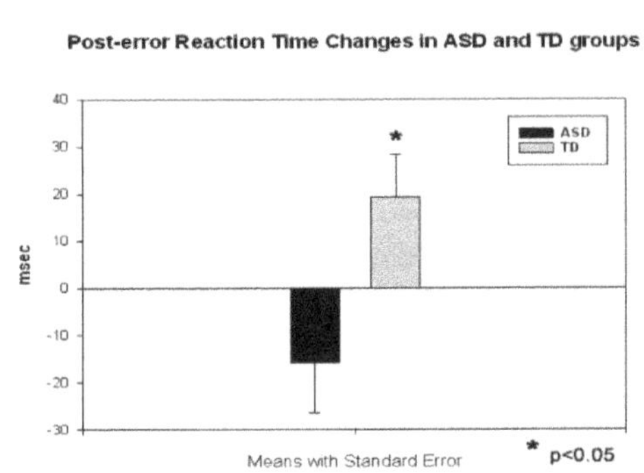

Figure 1. Post-error reaction time (RT) changes (calculated as a difference between the first post-error RT minus mean preceding RT) in ASD and TD children. Typical children show normative post-error RT slowing, conversely ASD children respond faster after having committed an error.

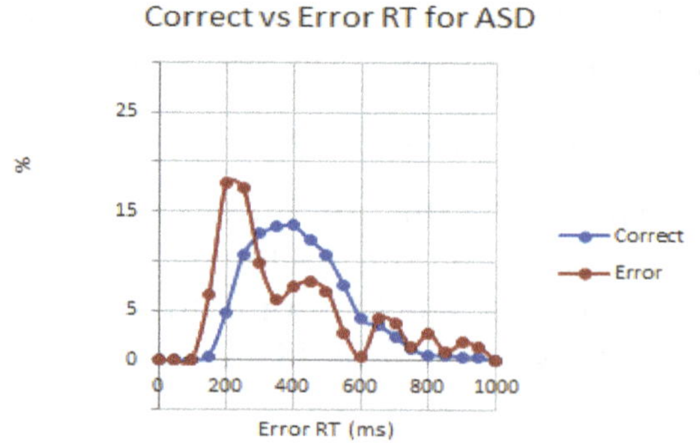

Figure 2. Distribution of RT in correct and error trials in children with ASD. Error trials had higher percentage in the faster bins of the histogram with moda around 200 ms vs. 400 ms in correct trials.

3.2. Motor Response-Locked Fronto-Central ERPs

ERN and Pe. One subject from the ASD group and 4 subjects from the TD group had no commission errors, therefore ERN/Pe datasets were comprised of 31 autistic children and 20 TD controls. Amplitude of the midline fronto-central ERN was significantly less negative in the ASD group as compared to the TD group (-2.69 ± 6.17 µV vs. -6.36 ± 4.43 µV, $F_{1,49} = 4.94$, $p = 0.031$). Latency of the ERN in the ASD group was delayed (107.5 ± 36.1 ms vs. 80.1 ± 20.7 ms, $F_{1,49} = 9.46$, $p = 0.003$). The only group difference in Pe measure was detected for the latency, though this difference barely reached minimal significance level and was featured by the tendency for prolonged latency in the ASD group (206.4 ± 44.9 ms vs. 183.3 ± 33.3 ms, $F_{1,49} = 4.05$, $p = 0.05$).

3.3. Stimulus-Locked Event-Related Potentials

3.3.1. Frontal ERPs

N1. *Stimulus* (target, standard, novel) factor had large main effect on N1 amplitude in both hemispheres ($F_{2,53} = 7.26$, $p = 0.002$, $\eta_p^2 = 0.22$). Amplitude of the frontal N1 to targets was bilaterally more negative in ASD group as compared to TD group (-3.68 ± 2.07 µV vs. -1.79 ± 2.29 µV, $F_{1,54} = 10.01$, $p = 0.003$). The ASD group showed as well more negative N100 amplitude to standards (-4.22 ± 1.71 µV vs. -2.39 ± 2.15 µV, $F_{1,54} = 12.05$, $p = 0.001$) and novels (-4.74 ± 2.02 µV vs. -2.61 ± 2.09 µV, $F_{1,54} = 13.87$, $p < 0.001$). Figure 3 illustrates group differences in response to target and novel stimuli. There were no interactions to report. Latency of the frontal N1 did not show any statistical group differences.

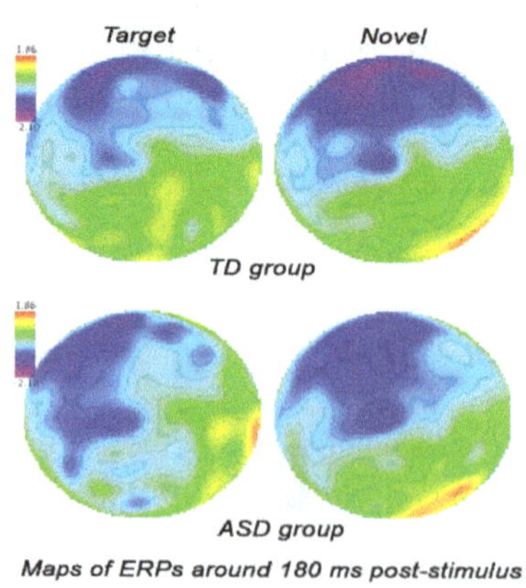

Figure 3. Grandaverage qEEG map of ERP to target and novel stimuli around 180 ms post-stimulus in ASD and TD children. Children with ASD showed comparable high negativity (N1 ERP component) to both targets and novels.

N2a. Most pronounced group differences resulted when target and novel stimuli effects were compared. Stimulus type had medium main effect on amplitude of the bifrontal N2 ($F_{2,53} = 4.84$, $p = 0.032$, $\eta_p^2 = 0.09$). The ASD group in response to targets showed more negative amplitude bilaterally (-3.44 ± 3.45 µV vs. -1.46 ± 2.47 µV, F = 5.22, $p = 0.027$). There was significant *Stimulus* (target, novel) X *Group* (ASD, TD) interaction ($F_{1,54} = 4.82$, $p = 0.033$, $\eta_p^2 = 0.08$), that can be described as comparable N200 amplitude to targets and novels in the ASD group, while in the TD group amplitude was larger for novel stimuli. Latency of N200 component was significantly longer in the ASD group across all 3 categories of stimulation without any hemispheric differences (targets, $F_{1,54} = 9.33$, $p = 0.004$; standards, $F_{1,54} = 6.84$, $p = 0.012$; novels, $F_{1,54} = 6.96$, $p = 0.011$).

P3a (Novelty P3). Rare *Stimulus* (target, novel) type had moderate main effect on P3a amplitude across both hemispheres ($F_{2,53} = 4.22$, $p = 0.041$, $\eta_p^2 = 0.08$). Group differences were found only for novel distracters, in particular, the ASD group had bilaterally higher amplitude as compared to the TD group (5.03 ± 3.33 µV vs. 2.88 ± 3.96 µV, $F_{1,54} = 4.44$, $p = 0.04$). Children with ASD as compared to the TD children had as well higher P3a amplitude to standards ($F_{1,54} = 7.56$, $p = 0.008$), but amplitude of P3a did not show any group differences in response to targets. Group differences for P3a latency were found only in the left hemisphere for all three categories of stimuli, and all of them featured a more prolonged latency in the ASD group (left frontal ROI- targets, $F_{1,54} = 4.88$, $p = 0.031$; standards, $F_{1,54} = 5.07$, $p = 0.028$; novels, $F_{1,54} = 4.73$, $p = 0.034$, see Figures 4 and 5). *Hemisphere* (left, right) X emphGroup (ASD, TD) interaction was significant, and can be described as more prolonged latency of the P3a component at the left hemisphere in the ASD group ($F_{1,54} = 6.73$, $p = 0.012$, $\eta_p^2 = 0.11$).

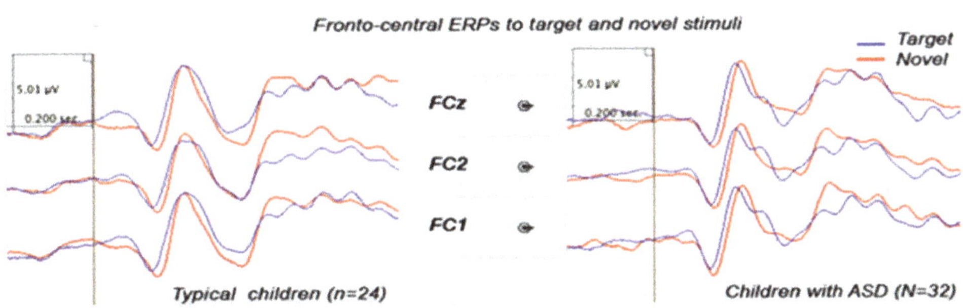

Figure 4. Screenshot of fronto-central ERPs to target and novel stimuli in ASD and TD children. The ASD children showed more negative N1, prolonger N2a and augmented P3a in response to unattended novel distracters.

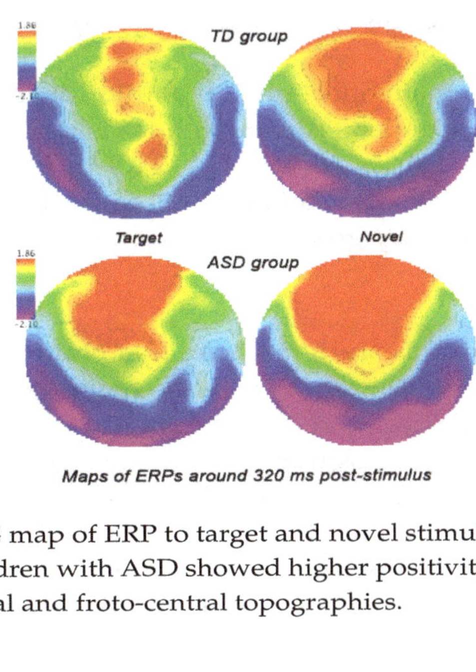

Figure 5. Grandaverage qEEG map of ERP to target and novel stimuli around 320 ms post-stimulus in ASD and TD children. Children with ASD showed higher positivity (P3a ERP component) to both targets and novels at the frontal and froto-central topographies.

3.3.2. Parietal and Parieto-Occipital ERPs

P1. *Stimulus* type (target, standard, novel) had marginal bilateral main effect on amplitude of the posterior P100 component ($F_{2,53} = 3.20$, $p = 0.049$, $\eta_p^2 = 0.05$). Group differences were expressed in a higher amplitude in the ASD group to standards (3.57 ± 2.08 μV vs. 2.33 ± 2.41 μV, $F_{1,54} = 4.15$, $p = 0.046$) and to novels (4.24 ± 2.36 vs. 2.55 ± 2.26, $F_{1,54} = 7.34$, $p = 0.009$, see Figure 6). Comparison of P1 amplitude to target and novel stimuli showed moderate *Stimulus* X *Group* interaction ($F_{1,54} = 4.36$, $p = 0.042$, $\eta_p^2 = 0.08$) where the ASD group showed higher response to novels as compared to the TD group. There were found no latency group differences for this component.

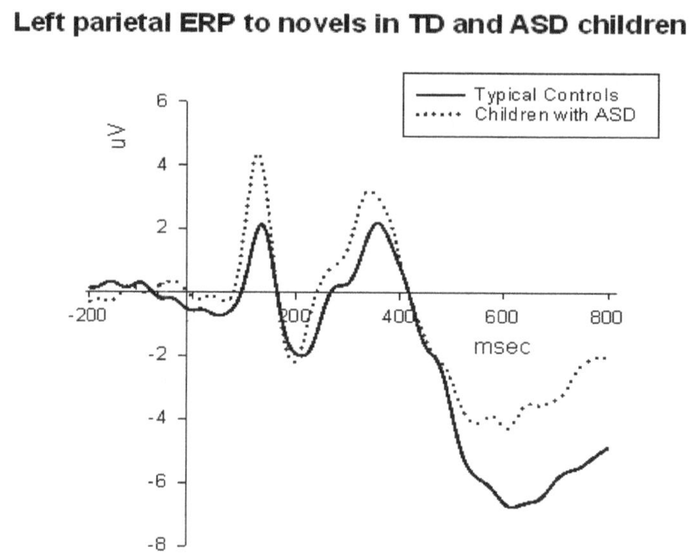

Figure 6. Left parietal ERPs to novels in ASD and TD children. The ASD group showed higher amplitude of P1 and P3b ERP components in response to novel distracters.

N2b. Amplitude of the parietal N2b component did not show any group differences. On the other hand, latency of N2b was globally delayed in the ASD group to all stimuli, and this effect was more pronounced on the left ROI (targets, 257.1 ± 34.1 ms in ASD vs. 222.5 ± 41.0 ms in TD, $F_{1,54} = 10.78$, $p = 0.002$; standards, 253.7 ± 40.2 ms vs. 211.1 ± 59.9 ms, $F_{1,54} = 9.38$, $p = 0.004$; novels, 248.1 ± 35.6 ms vs. 216.5 ± 53.5 ms, $F_{1,54} = 6.45$, $p = 0.014$). *Stimulus* (target, novel) X *Group* interaction was significant ($F_{1,54} = 6.08$, $p = 0.017$, $\eta_p^2 = 0.11$) and this effect was featured by a prolonged latency to targets in the ASD group.

P3b. *Stimulus* type had large main effect on P3b amplitude in both hemispheres ($F_{2,53} = 43.75$, $p < 0.001$, $\eta_p^2 = 0.62$). Analysis of the parietal P3b amplitude yielded group differences only in response to novel stimulus (7.24 ± 3.02 μV in ASD vs. 4.93 ± 4.32 μV in TD, $F_{1,54} = 5.63$, $p = 0.021$). Stimulus factor also had strong main effect on the latency of P3b peak ($F_{2,53} = 8.76$, $p < 0.001$; $\eta_p^2 = 0.24$). However, we didn't find any P3b latency group differences or any significant interactions.

4. Discussion

The reaction time findings in this study indicate that children with ASD had a less accurate behavioral performance. Committed motor response errors were not followed by a normative post-error slowing of reaction time. Error-related negativity was less pronounced and prolonged in the ASD group, though error-relative positivity only tended to be delayed. Both early (P1, N1) and late (P3a, P3b) ERP components in response to novel distracters were enhanced and showed larger amplitude in the ASD group when compared to the TD group. The N2 component showed delayed latency to all categories of stimuli at the frontal and parietal regions of interest. Results partially replicate our earlier ERP findings in autism. Our prior studies showed similar group differences in reaction time tasks using two different types of visual three-stimulus oddball tests, including one with illusory Kanizsa figures as the stimuli [3–6,8,9].

In numerous research studies and reviews autistic children have been found to differ from typical children mainly with respect to the P3 in regular oddball tasks (reviewed in Cui et al. [36]). Kemner et al. [37–39] reported abnormally small occipital and reduced central P3 in response to visual stimuli. At the same time, these authors also reported that the parietal N2 and P3b was larger in autistic children and interpreted their results in terms of differences in attentional resource allocation, as the parietal P3b is more sensitive to such task manipulations as stimulus relevance and probability [40] and less dependent on modality as compared to the occipital P3 [39]. In general, studies using a simple visual target detection, as compared to cross-modal (e.g., audio-visual integration) tasks have found no significant differences in the P3b to targets in children with autism compared to typical controls, while abnormalities were present in dissociations of frontal (delayed) and posterior (relatively intact) P3 in visual attention tasks [41]. It should be noted, that in most ERP studies using oddball tasks, the focus was on ERP responses to target stimuli, and less attention was paid to atypically large ERP magnitude to non-target stimuli (i.e., standards and/or novel distracters). Our results in this study, as well as in our prior research studies [3–9] emphasize the need to perform more detailed analysis of the specifics of excessive reactivity to task-irrelevant items in oddball tests in children with ASD.

The finding of increased amplitude of the frontal P3a to novels in children with autism is of special interest as this ERP measure is directly related to orienting to novelty. The frontal novelty P3a is less explored in autism and results are not consistent [41–43]. It was reported that the frontal P300 which reflects attention orienting was delayed or missing in subjects with autism and this finding was interpreted by the authors as a disruption of both parieto-frontal and cerebello-frontal networks critical for efficient cross-modal integration. Kemner et al. [37] reported that the visual N200 to novel distracters is larger when a person with autism is performing a task even when these novel stimuli are not relevant to the task in question. Abnormalities in central sensory processing both in auditory and visual modalities have been described by different authors in autism [37,39,43–45]. However, most of these studies analyzed and reported findings relating P3b to targets [42,46,47] and only a few P3a to standards or novels [41,43]. Despite the large number of studies published on ERPs in autism, there are not many reports about ERP components similar to those analyzed in this study. Most of the studies outline hyperactivation as well as an abnormal pattern of primary perceptual processes (e.g., low selectivity), abnormal top-down attentional control (e.g., orienting to novelty) and irregular information integration processes [48,49]. In control subjects the frontal P3a occurs earlier and commonly precedes parietal P3b, but in autistic subjects the P3a and P3b components were found to peak almost at the same time over the frontal and parietal sites in a spatial visual attention task [41]. In our study, novel stimuli elicited a delayed P3a component in the autism group. The latency of this component usually is associated with speed of attentional orienting to stimulus and reflects prefrontal working memory processes. Even less explored are early ERPs potentials in oddball tasks in ASD. The role of exogenous components and contribution to abnormalities of behavior in autism deserves further investigation.

In our prior ERP studies [3,5] on novelty processing in ASD, we reported that children with ASD showed significantly higher amplitudes and longer latencies of early frontal ERPs and delayed latency of P3a to novel distractor stimuli. The current study replicates those results mostly in terms of larger amplitudes of early potentials (P1, N1) and augmented magnitude of late potentials (P3a, P3b) to novel distracters. Our results suggest low selectivity in modality specific pre-processing of stimulus. Higher amplitude of the early frontal negativity and parietal positivity in the autism group with minimal differentiation of response magnitude to either target or non-target stimuli is an interesting finding that replicates our previous reports [6–9] where different types of visual oddball tasks were used. The visual N1 is considered to be an index of stimulus discrimination [50]. The visual N1 generally is augmented during pre-attentional stimulus processing [51], and is larger towards task-relevant target stimuli rather than unattended stimuli [52]. The ASD group shows clearly augmented and delayed frontal P3a that might result in an impaired early differentiation of target and non-target items (e.g., on N1 stage) and more effortful compensatory strategies involved for successful target identification, and following correct motor response selection. In general, the autistic group showed prolonged latencies to standard and rare non-target cues in visual oddball task. These results suggest that individuals with autism probably over-process information needed for the successful differentiation of target and distractor stimuli.

Cortical activity during different stages of visual information processing can be detected with ERPs, as they represent stimulus-driven corticoelectric field potentials. The early ERP components are a series of potentials that are recorded at the scalp following sensory stimulation that usually occur between 40 and 200 ms post-stimulation. These components are also characterized by being exogenous in nature (i.e., they are predictably generated by delivering sensory stimulation without a need for the subject to perform any mental operations). This characteristic differentiates the early latency ERPs from endogenous ERPs (e.g., P3b), which require the performance of a cognitive task such as a novelty task used in our study. Dysfunctional selective filtering of the stimuli may occur at the levels of P1 and N1 response related to the sensory gating stage. Sensory gating is based on selective attention concepts as attention towards one stimulus requires automatic concurrent inhibition of attention towards another one. Habituation to irrelevant sensory input is an important function for the information processing by the brain, because the failure might be associated with mental disturbances. The relationship between sensory gating and oversensitivity of individuals with autism to sensory stimulation other than auditory stimulation remains understudied and the clinical correlates of visual P100 and N100 ERP components in autism are yet to be examined in-depth.

A number of potentially interesting correlations were found between P1 and N1 sensory gating measures and P3 variables in schizophrenia [53]. Among these correlations, the positive interdependence between the N1 and P3 (P3b) latency is of interest as it is relevant to the findings of our previous [3,5,8] and current study. The study of Boutros et al. [53] suggests that decreased gating at the N1 phase of information processing negatively impacts the speed of information processing as measured by P3b latency. The further observation that this correlation was stronger in schizophrenia patients [53] emphasizes the possible deleterious effects of abnormal P1 and N1 level gating on information processing. This finding raises the possibility that the early sensory gating deficit may also impact the resource allocation capacity of the cortex as measured by P3b amplitude.

Belmonte and Yurgelin-Todd [48,49] suggested that perceptual filtering of incoming stimulation in autism can be considered as occurring in an all-or-none manner with low specificity for the task relevance of the stimulus. This notion assumes that filtering of perceptual items may primarily be driven by the control of general arousal level rather than the activation of only modality-specific cortical areas. According to the latter authors the attention of individuals with autism seems to be founded more on the coarse control of general arousal than on selective activation of specific perceptual systems. It is reasonable to suggest that an active inhibition of irrelevant distracters is not properly functioning and allows both task-relevant and task-irrelevant stimuli to pass through earlier filtering processes creating the overload on the later stages of stimuli processing in the context of task. It is unsurprising in this context that an increased ratio of excitation/inhibition in key neural systems and high "cortical noise" has been considered as a core abnormality of autism [54,55].

In this study, and similar to our studies on error monitoring in autism [7,8], we found that the ERN component of the response-locked ERP was substantially decreased in children with autism. In particular, the amplitude of ERN was less negative and the latency of ERN was prolonged in the ASD group as compared to the TD children. The ERN is an electroencephalographic measure associated with the commission of errors, thought to be independent of conscious perception [33], while the Pe is thought to reflect the motivational or emotional significance of the error or, in other words, the conscious evaluation of the error [56]. It cannot be ruled out that ERN impairments are influenced by deficits in earlier perceptual processes, or attentional and working memory processes in children with autism, that might be reflected in altered stimulus-locked early and late ERPs.

It has been suggested [57,58] that both the response-locked ERN and the stimulus-locked frontal N2 might reflect similar processes (i.e., response conflict detection and monitoring) and have similar neural correlates (i.e., dipole in the ACC, see also van Veen and Carter [59]). On the behavioral level, we found no group differences in RT, and only group differences between the percentages of commission (and not omission) error in the visual novelty oddball. After an error, ASD patients did not show accuracy improvement through post-error RT slowing as typical controls did. This finding replicates our previous reports [5–8]. Normally, performance on these trials is improved as a result of a change in speed–accuracy strategy which reflects executive control functioning [60]. The atypical post-error performance of ASD children (i.e., speeding instead of normative slowing) suggests the presence of an executive control deficiency. The impairment of adaptive error-correction behavior may have important consequences in daily life as optimal error-correction is necessary for adequate behavioral responses.

As demonstrated in previous studies [61], the posterior medial frontal cortex, and more specifically the rostral ACC division, is the main brain area responsible for error processing, suggesting that ASD patients have reduced posterior medial frontal cortex functioning. This area is involved when there is a need for adjustments to achieve goals [61]. The findings pointing that children with ASD have an impaired ability to improve their response accuracy by slowing down the response speed on post-error trials agrees with this notion. However, it is necessary to take into account that observed significant group differences between ASD and typical controls are manifested not only in the behavioral performance measures on reaction time tasks and associated response monitoring indices such as ERN and Pe. Group differences were also noted in terms of amplitude and latency characteristics of early ERP components preceding motor response selection (frontal and parietal P1, N1, N2) and those reflecting context update and closure (e.g., P3b) in visual oddball task [5] and various auditory tasks [44]. The sum of the group differences across these behavioral and stimulus- and response-averaged ERP indices of the ASD patients' performance is that it reflects global deficits in attentional processes, more specifically deficits in effective differentiation of target and novel distracter stimuli. This latter interpretation is supported by the significant differences between the ASD patients and typically developing controls in terms of both the stimulus-locked and response-locked ERP amplitudes and latencies.

Post-error adaptive correction of responses might be explained by some recent neurobiological findings. There are reports about an excessive preservation of short-distance connections (i.e., local over-connectivity) and relatively poor long-distance connections (i.e., distant under-connectivity) in the neocortex of individuals with autism [62–65]. These cortical connectivity abnormalities may explain why persons with autism tend to focus on details rather than perceiving the whole Gestalt. This over-focusing on details may imply an excessively laborious and ineffective way of handling each trial in the cognitive test, and lower availability of resources after an error when effort is needed to react appropriately. This may result in insufficient activation of the ACC [66], and thus error detection and post-error reaction may be hampered [67,68]. Structural and functional deficiencies of the ACC may contribute to the atypical development of joint attention and social cognition in autism [69]. Such interpretation of the results of the ERN/Pe deficits found in several studies [6,7,66,70] is consistent with many aspects of theory and research suggesting that ACC-mediated response monitoring may contribute to social-emotional and social-cognitive development in autism [69]. However, while emphasizing the possible role of ACC-related self-monitoring deficits in autism, Mundy [69] also noted that according to Devinsky and Luciano [71] this ACC impairment related behavioral deficits emerge only when they are combined with disturbances in other related functional neural networks, e.g., dorsolateral prefrontal cortex (DLPFC). Another factor that might affect variability of ERN is related to developmental changes, as performance monitoring in children and adolescents endures changes due to maturation processes [72], while our sample included both young children (9–12 years old range) and adolescents (i.e., teenagers in 13–18 years old range) and the wide range of participants in our study should be considered as a certain limitation.

Abnormalities of early exogenous ERPs such as N1 and P1 components can negatively affect endogenous potentials (e.g., N2 and P3) as well as response-locked potentials (ERN and Pe). The deficits in identification of distinct categories of stimuli at the early sensory stage result in a need to delegate task of differentiation of target stimulus from irrelevant one to the later, higher level of information processing stage. It is possible to suggest that individuals with ASD may engage some compensatory strategies necessary for successful target detection.

5. Conclusions

The results of the study indicate an atypical manner of processing distracters and orienting attention to novelty in children with autism. The findings are in-keeping with our prior studies using different tasks with visual and auditory stimuli. Augmented early potentials and a delayed frontal P3a and parietal P3b to novel stimuli suggest low selectivity in pre-processing of distracters resulting in excessive information processing at later stages. This may indicate a reduction in the discriminative ability of the ASD group. These results may reflect a locally over-connected network where sensory inputs evoke abnormally large ERPs for unattended stimuli with signs of a reduction in selectivity. This may incur a high load at the later stages of perceptual and cognitive processing and response selection when novel distracter stimuli are differentiated from targets.

Acknowledgments: Funding for this study was provided by the NIH grant R01 MH086784 to Manuel F. Casanova.

Author Contributions: All authors contributed substantially to the work reported in this paper. Manuel Casanova and Estate Sokhadze conceived and designed the experiment and data analysis strategy, participated in oddball test data collection, statistical analysis and interpretation of results. Estate Sokhadze administered visual oddball test to patients and collected raw data. Eva Lamina and Emily Casanova participated in ERP data collection, preprocessing and statistical analysis and also contributed in preparation of figures; Irma Khachidze participated in reaction time and accuracy data processing and statistical analysis; Ioan Opris analyzed reaction time data and assisted in preparation of methodological part related to behavioral data handling, analysis and interpretation; Manuel Casanova and Desmond Kelly participated in patients clinical records analysis and in interpretation of data and discussion, they also reviewed the manuscript and edited the final version.

References

1. *Diagnostic and Statistical Manual of Mental Disorders (DSM-V)*, 5th ed.; American Psychiatric Publishing, Inc.: Washington, DC, USA, 2013; ISBN 089042554X.
2. Gomes, E.; Pedroso, F.S.; Wagner, M.B. Auditory hypersensitivity in the autistic spectrum disorder. *Pro Fono* **2008**, *20*, 279–284. [CrossRef] [PubMed]
3. Baruth, J.M.; Casanova, M.F.; Sears, L.; Sokhadze, E. Early-stage visual processing abnormalities in autism spectrum disorder (ASD). *Transl. Neurosci.* **2010**, *1*, 177–187. [CrossRef] [PubMed]
4. Casanova, M.F.; Baruth, J.M.; El-Baz, A.; Tasman, A.; Sears, L.; Sokhadze, E. Repetitive transcranial magnetic stimulation (rTMS) modulates event-related potential (ERP) indices of attention in autism. *Transl. Neurosci.* **2012**, *3*, 170–180. [CrossRef] [PubMed]
5. Sokhadze, E.; Baruth, J.; Tasman, A.; Sears, L.; Mathai, G.; El-Baz, A.; Casanova, M.F. Event-related potential study of novelty processing abnormalities in autism. *Appl. Psychophysiol. Biofeedback* **2009**, *34*, 37–51. [CrossRef] [PubMed]
6. Sokhadze, E.; Baruth, J.; Tasman, A.; Mansoor, M.; Ramaswamy, R.; Sears, L.; Mathai, G.; El-Baz, A.; Casanova, M.F. Low-frequency repetitive transcranial magnetic stimulation (rTMS) affects event-related potential measures of novelty processing in autism. *Appl. Psychophysiol. Biofeedback* **2010**, *35*, 147–161. [CrossRef] [PubMed]
7. Sokhadze, E.; Baruth, J.; El-Baz, A.; Horrell, T.; Sokhadze, G.; Carroll, T.; Tasman, A.; Sears, L.; Casanova, M. Impaired error monitoring and correction function in autism. *J. Neurother.* **2010**, *14*, 79–95. [CrossRef] [PubMed]

8. Sokhadze, E.M.; Baruth, J.M.; Sears, L.; Sokhadze, G.E.; El-Baz, A.S.; Williams, E.; Klapheke, R.; Casanova, M.F. Event related potentials study of attention regulation during illusory figure categorization task in ADHD, autism spectrum disorders, and typical children. *J. Neurother.* **2012**, *16*, 12–31. [CrossRef] [PubMed]
9. Sokhadze, E.M.; Baruth, J.; Tasman, A.; Casanova, M.F. Event-related potential studies of cognitive processing abnormalities in autism. In *Imaging the Brain in Autism*; Casanova, M.F., El-Baz, A.S., Suri, J.S., Eds.; Springer: New York, NY, USA, 2013; pp. 61–86, ISBN 978-1-4614-6843-1.
10. Casanova, M.F.; Sokhadze, E.; Opris, I.; Wang, Y.; Li, X. Autism spectrum disorders: Linking neuropathological findings to treatment with transcranial magnetic stimulation. *Acta Pediatr.* **2015**, *104*, 346–355. [CrossRef] [PubMed]
11. Sokhadze, E.M.; Casanova, M.F.; Casanova, E.; Kelly, D.P.; Khachidze, I.; Wang, Y.; Li, X. Applications of ERPs in autism research and as functional outcomes of neuromodulation treatment. In *Event-Related Potential (ERP): Methods, Outcomes and Research Insights*; Harris, S.R., Ed.; NOVA Science Publishers: Hauppauge, NY, USA, 2017; pp. 27–88, ISBN 1536108057.
12. Duncan, C.C.; Barry, R.J.; Connolly, J.F.; Fischer, C.; Michie, P.T.; Näätänen, R.; Polich, J.; Reinvang, I.; van Petten, C. Event-related potentials in clinical research: Guidelines for eliciting, recording, and quantifying mismatch negativity, P300, and N400. *Clin. Neurophysiol.* **2009**, *120*, 1883–1908. [CrossRef] [PubMed]
13. Picton, T.W. The P300 wave of the human event-related potential. *J. Clin. Neurophysiol.* **1992**, *9*, 456–479. [CrossRef] [PubMed]
14. Polich, J. Updating P300: An integrative theory of P3a and P3b. *Clin. Neurophysiol.* **2007**, *118*, 2128–2148. [CrossRef] [PubMed]
15. Pritchard, W. Psychophysiology of P300. *Psychol. Bull.* **1981**, *89*, 506–540. [CrossRef] [PubMed]
16. Coles, M.G.H.; Rugg, M.D. Event-related brain potentials: An introduction. In *Electrophysiology of Mind. Event-Related Brain Potentials and Cognition*; Rugg, M.D., Coles, M.G.H., Eds.; Oxford University Press: Oxford, UK, 1995; pp. 1–26, ISBN 0198524161.
17. Herrmann, C.S.; Knight, R.T. Mechanisms of human attention: Event related potentials and oscillations. *Neurosci. Biobehav. Rev.* **2001**, *25*, 465–476. [CrossRef]
18. Patel, S.H.; Azzam, P.N. Characterization of N200 and P300: Selected studies of the event-related potential. *Int. J. Med. Sci.* **2005**, *2*, 147–154. [CrossRef] [PubMed]
19. Hoffman, J.E. Event-related potentials and controlled processes. In *Event-Related Brain Potentials: Basic Issues and Applications*; Rohrbaugh, J.W., Parasuraman, R., Johnson, R., Jr., Eds.; Oxford University Press: New York, NY, USA, 1990; pp. 145–157, ISBN 0195048911.
20. Katayama, J.; Polich, J. Stimulus context determines P3a and P3b. *Psychophysiol.* **1998**, *35*, 23–33. [CrossRef]
21. Polich, J. Theoretical overview of P3a and P3b. In *Detection of Change: Event-related Potential and fMRI Findings*; Polich, J., Ed.; Kluwer Academic Press: Boston, MA, USA, 2003; pp. 83–98, ISBN 978-1-4613-5008-8.
22. American Psychiatric Association. *Diagnostic and Statistical Manual of Mental Disorders (DSM-IV-TR)*, 4th ed.; Text Revised; American Psychiatric Publishing, Inc.: Washington, DC, USA, 2000; ISBN 0890420629.
23. Le Couteur, A.; Lord, C.; Rutter, M. *The Autism Diagnostic Interview—Revised (ADI-R)*; Western Psychological Services: Los Angeles, CA, USA, 2003.
24. Wechsler, D. *Wechsler Intelligence Scale for Children—Fourth Edition (WISC-IV)*; Harcourt Assessment, Inc.: San Antonio, TX, USA, 2003.
25. Roid, G.H. *Stanford-Binet Intelligence Scales Technical Manual*, 5th ed.; Riverside Publishing: Itasca, IL, USA, 2003.
26. Wechsler, D. *Wechsler Abbreviated Scale for Intelligence*; Psychological Corporation: San Antonio, TX, USA, 1999.
27. First, M.B.; Spitzer, R.L.; Gibbon, M.; Williams, J.B.W. *Structured Clinical Interview for DSM-IV-TR Axis I Disorders—Non-Patient Edition (SCID-NP)*; New York State Psychiatric Institute: New York, NY, USA, 2002.
28. *Net Station Acquisition Technical Manual*; Electrical Geodesics, Inc.: Eugene, OR, USA, 2003.
29. Fletcher, E.M.; Kussmaul, C.L.; Mangun, G.R. Estimation of interpolation errors in scalp topographic mapping. *Electroctoencephalogr. Clin. Neurophysiol.* **1996**, *98*, 422–434. [CrossRef]
30. Luu, P.; Tucker, D.M.; Englander, R.; Lockfeld, A.; Lutsep, H.; Oken, B. Localizing acute stroke-related EEC changes: assessing the effects of spatial undersampling. *J. Clin. Neurophysiol.* **2001**, *18*, 302–317. [CrossRef] [PubMed]

31. Perrin, E.; Pernier, J.; Bertrand, O.; Giard, M.; Echallier, J.F. Mapping of scalp potentials by surface spline interpolation. *Electroencephalogr. Clin. Neurophysiol.* **1987**, *66*, 75–81. [CrossRef]
32. Srinivasan, R.; Tucker, D.M.; Murias, M. Estimating the spatial Nyquist of the human EEG. *Behav. Res. Methods* **1998**, *30*, 8–19. [CrossRef]
33. Franken, H.A.; van Strien, J.W.; Franzek, E.J.; van de Wetering, B.J. Error-processing deficits in patients with cocaine dependence. *Biol. Psychol.* **2007**, *75*, 45–51. [CrossRef] [PubMed]
34. Opris, I.; Lebedev, M.A.; Nelson, R.J. Neostriatal neuronal activity correlates better with movement kinematics under certain reward. *Front. Neurosci.* **2016**, *10*, 336. [CrossRef] [PubMed]
35. Levine, T.R.; Hullett, C.R. Eta squared, partial eta squared, and misreporting of effect size in communication research. *Hum. Commun. Res.* **2002**, *28*, 612–625. [CrossRef]
36. Cui, T.; Wang, P.P.; Liu, S.; Zhang, X. P300 amplitude and latency in autism spectrum disorder: A meta-analysis. *Eur. Child Adolesc. Psychiatry* **2017**, *26*, 177–190. [CrossRef] [PubMed]
37. Kemner, C.; Verbaten, M.N.; Cuperus, J.M.; Camfferman, G.; Van Engeland, H. Visual and somatosensory event-related brain potentials in autistic children and three different control groups. *Electroencephalogr. Clin. Neurophysiol.* **1994**, *92*, 225–237. [CrossRef]
38. Kemner, C.; Verbaten, M.N.; Cuperus, J.M.; Camfferman, G.; Van Engeland, H. Auditory event- related potentials in autistic children and three different control groups. *Biol. Psychiatry* **1995**, *38*, 150–165. [CrossRef]
39. Kemner, C.; van der Gaag, R.J.; Verbaten, M.; van Engeland, H. ERP differences among subtypes of pervasive developmental disorders. *Biol. Psychiatry* **1999**, *46*, 781–789. [CrossRef]
40. Donchin, E.; Coles, M.G. Is the p300 component a manifestation of context updating? *Behav. Brain Sci.* **1988**, *11*, 357–374. [CrossRef]
41. Townsend, J.; Westerfield, M.; Leaver, E.; Makeig, S.; Jung, T.; Pierce, K.; Courchesne, E. Event-related brain response abnormalities in autism: Evidence for impaired cerebello-frontal spatial attention networks. *Brain Res. Cogn. Brain Res.* **2001**, *11*, 127–145. [CrossRef]
42. Ciesielski, K.T.; Courchesne, E.; Elmasian, R. Effects of focused attention tasks on event-related potentials in autistic and normal individuals. *Electroencephalogr. Clin. Neurophysiol.* **1990**, *75*, 207–220. [CrossRef]
43. Ferri, R.; Elia, M.; Agarwal, N.; Lanuzza, B.; Musumeci, S.A.; Pennisi, G. The mismatch negativity and the P3a components of the auditory event-related potentials in autistic low-functioning subjects. *Clin. Neurophysiol.* **2003**, *114*, 1671–1680. [CrossRef]
44. Bomba, M.D.; Pang, E.W. Cortical auditory evoked potentials in autism: A review. *Int. J. Psychophysiol.* **2004**, *53*, 161–169. [CrossRef] [PubMed]
45. Verbaten, M.N.; Roelofs, J.W.; van Engeland, H.; Kenemans, J.K.; Slangen, J.L. Abnormal visual event-related potentials of autistic children. *J. Autism Dev. Disord.* **1991**, *21*, 449–470. [CrossRef] [PubMed]
46. Courchesne, E.; Lincoln, A.J.; Yeung-Courchesne, R.; Elmasian, R.; Grillon, C. Pathophysiologic findings in nonretarded autism and receptive developmental disorder. *J. Autism Dev. Disord.* **1989**, *19*, 1–17. [CrossRef] [PubMed]
47. Lincoln, A.J.; Courchesne, E.; Harms, L.; Allen, M. Contextual probability evaluation in autistic, receptive developmental disorder and control children: Event-related potential evidence. *J. Autism Dev. Disord.* **1993**, *23*, 37–58. [CrossRef] [PubMed]
48. Belmonte, M.K.; Yurgelun-Todd, D.A. Functional anatomy of impaired selective attention and compensatory processing in autism. *Brain Res. Cogn. Brain Res.* **2003**, *17*, 651–664. [CrossRef]
49. Belmonte, M.K.; Yurgelun-Todd, D.A. Anatomic dissociation of selective and suppressive processes in visual attention. *Neuroimage* **2003**, *19*, 180–189. [CrossRef]
50. Hopf, J.M.; Vogel, E.; Woodman, G.; Heinze, H.J.; Luck, S.J. Localizing visual discrimination processes in time and space. *J. Neurophysiol.* **2002**, *88*, 2088–2095. [CrossRef] [PubMed]
51. Hillyard, S.A.; Anllo-Vento, L. Event-related brain potentials in the study of visual selective attention. *Proc. Natl. Acad. Sci. USA* **1998**, *95*, 781–787. [CrossRef] [PubMed]
52. Luck, S.J.; Heinze, H.; Mangun, G.R.; Hillyard, S.A. Visual event-related potentials index focused attention within bilateral stimulus arrays. II. Functional dissociation of P1 and N1 components. *Electroencephalogr. Clin. Neurophysiol.* **1990**, *75*, 528–542. [CrossRef]
53. Boutros, N.N.; Korzyukov, O.; Jansen, B.; Feingold, A.; Bell, M. Sensory gating deficits during the mid-latency phase of information processing in medicated schizophrenia patients. *Psychiatry Res.* **2004**, *126*, 203–215. [CrossRef] [PubMed]

54. Casanova, M.F.; Buxhoeveden, D.; Gomez, J. Disruption in the inhibitory architecture of the cell minicolumn: Implications for autism. *Neuroscientist* **2003**, *9*, 496–507. [CrossRef] [PubMed]
55. Rubenstein, J.L.; Merzenich, M.M. Model of autism: Increased ratio of excitation/inhibition in key neural systems. *Genes Brain Behav.* **2003**, *2*, 255–267. [CrossRef] [PubMed]
56. Overbeek, T.J.M.; Nieuwenhuis, S.; Ridderinkhof, K.R. Dissociable components of error processing. *J. Psychophysiol.* **2005**, *19*, 319–329. [CrossRef]
57. Yeung, N.; Botvinick, M.M.; Cohen, J.D. The neural basis of error detection: Conflict monitoring and the error-related negativity. *Psychol. Rev.* **2004**, *111*, 931–959. [CrossRef] [PubMed]
58. Yeung, N.; Cohen, J.D. The impact of cognitive deficits on conflict monitoring. Predictable dissociations between the error-related negativity and N2. *Psychol. Sci.* **2006**, *17*, 164–171. [CrossRef] [PubMed]
59. Van Veen, V.; Carter, C.S. The timing of action-monitoring process in the anterior cingulate cortex. *J. Cogn. Neurosci.* **2002**, *14*, 593–602. [CrossRef] [PubMed]
60. Burle, B.; Vidal, F.; Tandonnet, C.; Hasbroucq, T. Physiological evidence for response inhibition in choice reaction time tasks. *Brain Cogn.* **2004**, *56*, 153–164. [CrossRef] [PubMed]
61. Ridderinkhof, K.R.; Ullsperger, M.; Crone, E.A.; Nieuwenhuis, S. The role of the medial frontal cortex in cognitive control. *Science* **2004**, *306*, 443–447. [CrossRef] [PubMed]
62. Casanova, M.F. Minicolumnar pathology in autism. In *Recent Developments in Autism Research*; Casanova, M.F., Ed.; Nova Biomedical Books: New York, NY, USA, 2005; pp. 133–143, ISBN 1-59454-497-2.
63. Casanova, M.F. Neuropathological and genetic findings in autism: The significance of a putative minicolumnopathy. *Neuroscientist* **2006**, *12*, 435–441. [CrossRef] [PubMed]
64. Just, M.A.; Cherkassky, V.; Keller, T.A.; Minshew, N.J. Cortical activation and synchronization during sequence comprehension in high-functioning autism: Evidence of underconnectivity. *Brain* **2004**, *127*, 1811–1821. [CrossRef] [PubMed]
65. Williams, E.L.; Casanova, M.F. Autism and dyslexia: A spectrum of cognitive styles as defined by minicolumnar morphometry. *Med. Hypotheses* **2009**, *74*, 59–62. [CrossRef] [PubMed]
66. Bogte, H.; Flamma, B.; van der Meere, J.; van Engeland, H. Post-error adaptation in adults with high functioning autism. *Neuropsychologia* **2007**, *45*, 1707–1714. [CrossRef] [PubMed]
67. Bauman, M.L.; Kemper, T.L. Structural brain anatomy in autism: What is the evidence? In *The Neurobiology of Autism*, 2nd ed.; Bauman, M.L., Kemper, T.L., Eds.; John Hopkins University Press: Baltimore, MD, USA, 2005; pp. 121–135, ISBN 0801880475.
68. Minshew, N.J.; Sweeney, J.A.; Bauman, M.L.; Webb, S.J. Neurological aspects of autism. In *Handbook of Autism and Pervasive Developmental Disorders, Diagnosis, Development, Neurobiology, and Behavior*, 3rd ed.; Volkmar, F.R., Paul, R., Klin, A., Cohen, D., Eds.; Wiley: New York, NY, USA, 2005; Volume 1, pp. 473–514, ISBN 0471716960.
69. Mundy, P. Annotation: The neural basis of social impairments in autism: The role of the dorsal medial-frontal cortex and anterior cingulate system. *J. Child Psychol. Psychiatry* **2003**, *44*, 793–809. [CrossRef] [PubMed]
70. Henderson, H.; Schwartz, C.; Mundy, P.; Burnette, C.; Sutton, S.; Zahka, N.; Pradella, A. Response monitoring, the error-related negativity, and differences in social behavior in autism. *Brain Cogn.* **2006**, *61*, 96–109. [CrossRef] [PubMed]
71. Devinsky, O.; Luciano, D. The contributions of cingulate cortex to human behavior. I. In *Neurobiology of Cingulate Cortex and Limbic Thalamus: A Comprehensive Handbook*; Gabriel, M., Vogt, B.A., Eds.; Birkhauser: Boston, MA, USA, 1993; pp. 527–556, ISBN 978-1-4899-6706-0.
72. Tamnes, C.K.; Walhovd, K.B.; Torstveit, M.; Sells, V.T.; Fjell, A.M. Performance monitoring in children and adolescents: A review of developmental changes in the error-related negativity and brain maturation. *Dev. Cogn. Neurosci.* **2013**, *6*, 1–13. [CrossRef] [PubMed]

9

NLRP12 Inflammasome Expression in the Rat Brain in Response to LPS during Morphine Tolerance

Sulie L. Chang [1,2,*], Wenfei Huang [1], Xin Mao [1] and Sabroni Sarkar [1]

1 Institute of NeuroImmune Pharmacology, Seton Hall University, 400 South Orange Avenue, South Orange, NJ 07079, USA; wenfei.huang@shu.edu (W.H.); ninnamao@yahoo.com.cn (X.M.); Sabroni.Sarkar@gmail.com (S.S.)
2 Department of Biological Sciences, Seton Hall University, 400 South Orange Avenue, South Orange, NJ 07079, USA
* Correspondence: sulie.chang@shu.edu

Academic Editor: Donna Gruol

Abstract: Morphine, an effective but addictive analgesic, can profoundly affect the inflammatory response to pathogens, and long-term use can result in morphine tolerance. Inflammasomes are protein complexes involved in the inflammatory response. The nucleotide-binding oligomerization domain-like receptor (NLR) Family Pyrin Domain Containing (NLRP) 12 (NLRP12) inflammasome has been reported to have anti-inflammatory activity. In this study, we examined the expression of NLRP12 inflammasome related genes in the adult F344 rat brain in response to the bacterial endotoxin lipopolysaccharide (LPS) in the presence and absence of morphine tolerance. Morphine tolerance was elicited using the 2 + 4 morphine-pelleting protocol. On Day 1, the rats were pelleted subcutaneously with 2 pellets of morphine (75 mg/pellet) or a placebo; on Days 2 and 4 pellets were given. On Day 5, the animals were randomly assigned to receive either 250 μg/kg LPS or saline (i.p.). The expression of 84 inflammasome related genes in the rat brain was examined using a Ploymerase Chain Reaction (PCR) array. In response to LPS, there was a significant increase in the expression of the pro-inflammatory cytokine/chemokine genes interleukin-1 beta (Il-1β), interleukin-6 (Il-6), C-C motif chemokine ligand 2 (Ccl2), C-C motif chemokine ligand 7 (Ccl7), C-X-C motif chemokine ligand 1 (Cxcl1), and C-X-C motif chemokine ligand 3 (Cxcl3) and a significant decrease in the anti-inflammatory NLRP12 gene in both morphine-tolerant and placebo-control rats compared to saline-treated rats, although the changes were greater in the placebo-control animals. The Library of Integrated Network-Based Cellular Signatures' (LINCS) connectivity map was used to analyze the list of affected genes to identify potential targets associated with the interactions of LPS and morphine tolerance. Our data indicate that, in the morphine tolerant state, the expression of NLRP12 and its related genes is altered in response to LPS and that the Vacuolar protein-sorting-associated protein 28 (VPS28), which is involved in the transport and sorting of proteins into sub-cellular vesicles, may be the key regulator of these alterations.

Keywords: morphine tolerance; NLRP12 inflammasome; LPS

---

1. Introduction

Morphine is a potent analgesic that is widely used clinically for pain management. However, long-term use of morphine can lead to morphine tolerance and addiction [1]. In addition, morphine can profoundly and detrimentally affect the body's immune system, at both the cellular and molecular levels. Morphine suppresses lymphocyte trafficking; decreases natural killer cell activity; inhibits the production of pro-inflammatory cytokines, such as tumor necrosis factor-alpha (TNF-α) and interleukin-1 beta (IL-1β) [2–4]; and induces atrophy of immune organs, such as the spleen and thymus [5–9].

Morphine-induced immunosuppression significantly increases the risk of bacterial infection [10]. Although the immunosuppressive effects of morphine have been widely studied, the mechanisms involved in the body's inflammatory response to pathogens during morphine tolerance have not been fully investigated.

Inflammasomes are multi-protein complexes assembled from nucleotide oligomerization domain receptor proteins known as nucleotide-binding oligomerization domain (NOD)-like receptors (NLR) [11]. They function as important mediators of innate immunity. Inflammasomes play a key role in the regulation of inflammation and immune responses by participating in the production of pro-inflammatory cytokines, including IL-1β and interleukin-18 (IL-18) [11–13]. Both IL-1β and IL-18 produce a wide variety of biological effects associated with infection, inflammation, and autoimmune processes.

There have been about 20 NLR inflammasomes identified in humans. The most commonly studied ones include NLR Family Pyrin Domain Containing 1 (NLPR1), NLR family apoptosis inhibitory protein 6 (NAIP2), NLR Family Pyrin Domain Containing 3 (NLRP3), NLR Family Pyrin Domain Containing 5 (NLRP5), NLR Family Pyrin Domain Containing 6 (NLRP6), NLR Family Pyrin Domain Containing 12 (NLRP12), NLR family member X1 (NLRPX1), and NLR Family CARD Domain Containing 4 (NLRC4) [14]. Inflammasomes have been sub-divided into two groups; pro-inflammatory inflammasomes and anti-inflammatory inflammasomes. The pro-inflammatory inflammasomes include NLRP3 and NLRC4, and their functions have been widely studied. The anti-inflammatory inflammasomes include NLRP12, NLRX1, NLRC3, and NLRC5. They appear to function by limiting or suppressing a pro-inflammatory response; however, this group has not been well studied to date.

There have been a few recent reports characterizing the anti-inflammatory properties of NLRP12 [15,16]. NLRP12 can inhibit NF-κB signaling through both the canonical and non-canonical pathways, which are important in the control and regulation of innate immune responses [15,16]. NLRP12 inhibits IL-1 receptor-associated kinase 1 (IRAK1), a downstream component of the pathogen activated Toll-like receptor (TLR) pathway, which, in turn, decreases the signaling of the canonical NF-κB pathway [17]. In the non-canonical NF-κB pathway, NLRP12 interacts with and rapidly degrades NF-κB-inducing kinase (NIK), thereby suppressing NF-κB signaling [18].

The Library of Integrated Network-Based Cellular Signatures (LINCS) [19] is a database which implements a biological network-based strategy to make assessments regarding the impact of drugs, genetics, and related biological perturbations (alterations induced by external or internal mechanisms) on cellular states. The library database is based on the philosophy that typical human pathology, biology, and pharmacology are most aptly understood using a systems-level approach. It was constructed to generate a robust approach for perturbing a diversity of cell types, measuring cellular responses, integrating and analyzing data, and visualizing and interrogating the database for a variety of biomedical research applications [19]. This library allows researchers to access a wide variety of data by using a matrix consisting of cell type by experimental treatment by phenotypic assay. Using LINCS, researchers are able to inquire about information regarding mechanism-based relationships among the effects of different drug responses and their targets (perturbents) as well as associations among responding cellular components, in the format of network interactions and structure-function relationships [20].

In this study, we used an inflammasome PCR array containing 84 inflammasome-related genes to investigate the expression of inflammasomes during an inflammatory response to the bacterial endotoxin, lipopolysaccharide (LPS), in the rat brain during morphine tolerance. LINCS was then used to project possible candidate targets from the mRNA gene expression profiles generated from the PCR array analysis.

2. Materials and Methods

2.1. Animals

Fisher/NHsd 344 (F344) rats were purchased from Harlan Laboratories (Indianapolis, IN, USA). The animals were housed in groups of 3–5 animals in a temperature controlled (21 °C–22 °C) animal holding room, under a 12-h light/12-h dark illumination cycle (lights on at 7:00 a.m.). Food and tap water were provided ad libitum. The Institutional Animal Care and Use Committee (IACUC) at Seton Hall University, South Orange, NJ, USA approved the experimental protocol.

2.2. Morphine and LPS Administration

A 2 + 4 regimen was used to produce morphine tolerance in 7–8 mo old (250–350 g) male F344 rats [5,21–24]. The rats ($n = 16$) were randomly assigned into two groups. The morphine-tolerant group received two 75 mg morphine sulfate pellets (NIDA, Rockville, MD, USA) on Day 1 via subcutaneous (s.c.) implantation and four pellets on Day 2, whereas the control group received placebo pellets on both days. On Day 5, the two groups were randomly assigned to receive either LPS (250 μg/kg, Sigma, St. Louis, MO, USA) or saline (vehicle) [5,21–24]. Thus, the four experimental groups were placebo-control + saline, placebo-control + LPS, morphine-tolerant + saline, and morphine-tolerant + LPS. Two hours after the treatment with LPS or saline, the animals were euthanized and the brains were harvested.

2.3. RNA Isolation and Preparation of cDNA

Total RNA was extracted from the brain tissue using TRIZOL (Invitrogen, Carlsbad, CA, USA), following the manufacturer's protocol. To remove contaminating DNA, the total RNA samples were treated with RNase-free DNase (Qiagen, Valencia, CA, USA), followed by further purification using an RNeasy Mini Kit (Qiagen, Valencia, CA, USA). The RNA quality and quantity were assessed using a nanodrop spectrophotometer (Thermo Scientific, Waltham, MA, USA). An equal amount of RNA (400 ng) from each sample was then converted into first-strand cDNA using a RT^2 First Strand Kit (SABiosciences, Frederick, MD, USA) for a PCR array.

2.4. Real-Time PCR Array

The expression of 84 key genes involved in the function of inflammasomes, general NLR signaling, and cytokine and chemokine genes was quantified using a custom PCR array and RT^2 SYBR Green Fluorescein qPCR Master Mix (SABiosciences, Frederick, MD, USA), according to the manufacturer's protocol. Using an ABI Prism 7900HT Fast Detection System (Applied Biosystems, Foster, CA, USA), real-time PCR was performed by first denaturing the PCR mix at 95 °C for 10 min, followed by 40 cycles at 95 °C for 15 s and at 60 °C for 1 min.

2.5. PCR Array Data Analysis

The expression of each gene was normalized to housekeeping genes and calculated using the $\Delta\Delta$Ct method. The threshold and baseline values were set manually, and the resulting threshold cycle values (Ct) were analyzed using the PCR array data analysis template supplied on the manufacturer's website [25]. The mean fold change in mRNA expression from 3 to 5 biological replicates was considered significant at $p < 0.05$. The gene profile signatures were created for every two groups compared.

2.6. LINCS Analysis

The differentially expressed genes were input into the Query App (apps.lincscloud.org/query), as described previously [26,27]. Based on the LINCS database, LincsCloud utilized gene profile signatures generated from the PCR array to generate a report, including probability outcomes in terms of gene knockdown effects and drug mimics. The scores given in the report evaluated how much a particular set of gene regulation features (named pertubagens) was likely to be connected with the genes listed in the LINCS report. Positive readings in the Consensus Knockdown Connections in the report indicate that knockdown of the genes listed in the LINCS report would match the gene changes input into the Query App, and thus the genes with high scores represent potential target genes for the experimental treatment.

3. Results

3.1. Expression Profile of Inflammasome-Related Genes Following an LPS Challenge, with and without Morphine Tolerance

Alterations in gene expression were measured in rats challenged with LPS, with and without morphine tolerance, using a PCR array containing 84 genes related to inflammasome activation and function. NLRP12 expression was significantly decreased in response to LPS in both the morphine-tolerant (morphine-tolerant + LPS) and control (placebo-control + LPS) rats, compared to the rats given saline (morphine-tolerant + saline and placebo-control + saline) (Figure 1, Table 1). However, the decrease was greater in the placebo-control rats (−7.3 fold; $p < 0.01$) than in the morphine-tolerant rats (−4.5 fold; $p < 0.05$).

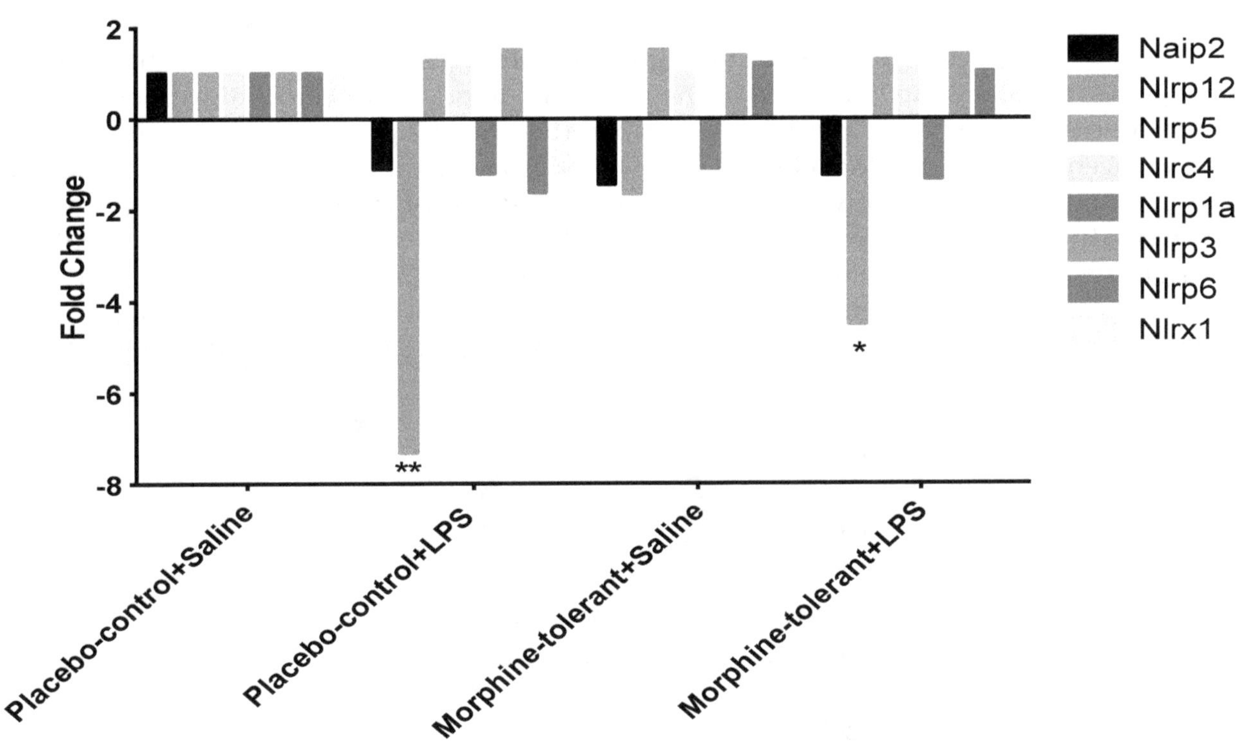

Figure 1. Inflammasome-related gene expression in the rat brain in response to lipopolysaccharide (LPS), with and without morphine tolerance. The expression of the inflammasome-related NOD-like receptor (NLR) genes (Naip2, Nlrp12, Nlrp5, Nlrc4, Nlrp1a, Nlrp3, Nlrp6, And Nlrx1) in the brains of rats given an i.p. injection of either 250 µg/kg LPS or saline, with and without morphine tolerance (n = 3–5 rats per group), was determined using a PCR array. Data were calculated using the ΔΔCT method, relative to the control group (placebo-control +saline), and are represented as a fold change. * $p < 0.05$, ** $p < 0.01$. Naip2: NLR family, apoptosis inhibitory protein 6; Nlrp12: NLR Family Pyrin Domain Containing 12; Nlrp5: NLR Family Pyrin Domain Containing 5; Nlrc4: NLR Family CARD Domain Containing 4; Nlrp1a: NLR family, pyrin domain containing 1A; Nlrp3: NLR Family Pyrin Domain Containing 3; Nlrp6: NLR Family Pyrin Domain Containing 6; Nlrpx1: NLR family member X1.

Table 1. Expression profile of inflammasomes and NLR genes in the rat brain in response to lipopolysaccharides (LPS), with and without morphine tolerance.

	morphine-tolerant + saline/placebo control + saline		placebo control + LPS/placebo control + saline		morphine-tolerant + LPS/morphine-tolerant + saline	
Gene	**Fold Change**	***p*-value ***	**Fold Change ****	***p*-value ***	**Fold Change ****	***p*-value ***
Card6	−1.2347	0.078926	−1.5292	0.004159	−1.714	0.017499
Casp1	1.1505	0.299299	1.2132	0.276593	1.2764	0.02969
Casp12	1.0972	0.462347	1.5422	0.003614	1.4249	0.092085
Casp8	−1.0402	0.612597	−1.1363	0.391056	−1.2652	0.139999
Naip2	−1.4483	0.067329	−1.1031	0.619799	−1.2316	0.25758
Nlrp12	−1.6504	0.674422	−7.31	0.002731	−4.5124	0.025372
Nlrp5	1.494	0.054876	1.274	0.20786	1.2819	0.027352
Nlrc4	1.0028	0.915792	1.1349	0.159712	1.1003	0.445719
Nlrp1a	−1.0898	0.470844	−1.2027	0.001147	−1.3308	0.1379
Nlrp3	1.3773	0.134647	1.5114	0.054565	1.3956	0.02407
Nlrp6	1.205	0.420019	−1.6225	0.358997	1.0293	0.784547
Nlrx1	−1.1574	0.24832	−1.1494	0.191026	1.039	0.679959
Nod2	−1.6257	0.650152	1.0901	0.811946	1.2826	0.50395
Pycard	−1.0575	0.610143	−1.0285	0.797363	−1.2363	0.030115

* For *p*-value, letters in red mean $p < 0.05$. ** For Fold Change, letters in red mean fold change >2 and letters in blue mean the fold change <−2. For the color lines, : 6–10 fold decrease; : 2–5 fold decrease; : <2 fold; : 2–5 fold increase; : 6–10 fold increase; : 11–30 fold increase; : 31–50 fold increase.

3.2. Expression Profile of Inflammasome-Related Downstream Signaling Genes Following an LPS Challenge, With and Without Morphine Tolerance

With a few exceptions, there were no significant changes in expression of the downstream signaling genes in response to LPS in either the morphine-tolerant rats (morphine-tolerant + LPS) or the control animals (placebo-control + LPS), compared to the rats given saline (morphine-tolerant + saline and placebo-control + saline) (Table 1). However, Baculoviral IAP Repeat-Containing 3 (Birc3), an important regulator gene involved in the downstream effects of inflammasomes, was significantly increased in response to LPS in both the morphine-tolerant (21.5 fold; $p < 0.05$) and control (21 fold; $p < 0.01$) groups, compared to the rats given saline (Figure 2, Table 2). In addition, NF-Kappa-B Inhibitor Alpha (Nfkbia), an inhibitor protein of NF-κB, was increased in both groups given LPS (morphine-tolerant + LPS, 3.4 fold, $p < 0.01$; placebo-control + LPS, 3.9 fold, $p < 0.01$) (Figure 2, Table 2).

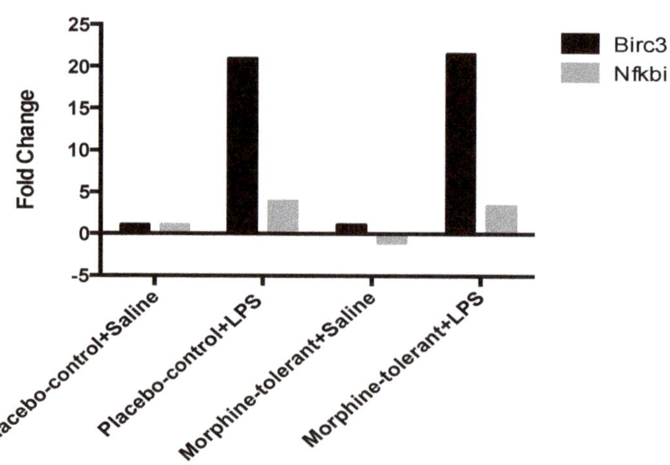

Figure 2. Inflammasome-related downstream gene expression in the rat brain in response to Lipopolysaccharides (LPS), with and without morphine tolerance. The expression of the inflammasome-related downstream signaling genes Baculoviral IAP Repeat-Containing 3 (Birc3) and NF-Kappa-B Inhibitor Alpha (Nfkbia) in the brains of rats given an i.p. injection of either 250 μg/kg LPS or saline, with and without morphine tolerance (n = 3–5 rats per group), was determined using a Polymerase Chain Reaction (PCR) array. The data were calculated using the ΔΔCT method relative to the control group (placebo-control + saline) and are represented as fold change.

Table 2. Expression profile of inflammasome-related downstream signaling genes in the rat brain in response to lipopolysaccharides (LPS), with and without morphine tolerance. Full name of the genes were provided in Table A1.

	morphine-tolerant + saline/placebo control + saline		placebo control + LPS/placebo control + saline		morphine-tolerant + LPS/morphine-tolerant + saline	
Gene	Fold Change	*p*-value *	Fold Change **	*p*-value *	Fold Change **	*p*-value *
Bcl2	1.0469	0.863233	1.0586	0.845254	1.2398	0.339246
Bcl2l1	−1.1256	0.01111	1.0572	0.476643	−1.0291	0.671184
Birc2	1.0509	0.586337	−1.0281	0.622487	1.0699	0.531417
Birc3	1.0648	0.587513	20.9356	0.011065	21.5025	0.001873
Cflar	1.0226	0.697346	1.3021	0.004748	1.2155	0.140978
Chuk	1.1867	0.119108	−1.0233	0.754891	1.1593	0.073058
Ciita	−1.0617	0.750879	1.0619	0.873363	1.4678	0.39646
Ctsb	−1.0009	0.978499	−1.0656	0.617885	−1.1046	0.493204
Fadd	−1.1261	0.258884	1.1235	0.252486	1.0306	0.71174
Hsp90aa1	1.2774	0.114349	1.0391	0.743375	1.189	0.149024
Hsp90ab1	1.0752	0.376876	−1.0968	0.305427	1.1579	0.18515
Ikbkb	1.0718	0.550623	−1.0011	0.962992	1.1799	0.201955
Ikbkg	1.0924	0.324904	−1.0402	0.492725	1.1419	0.079202
Irak1	1.1549	0.062648	1.0287	0.755395	1.2213	0.242955
Map3k7	−1.2495	0.002404	−1.1008	0.434596	−1.2497	0.114056
Map3k7ip1	−1.0335	0.664499	−1.1151	0.369226	1.02	0.864431
Map3k7ip2	−1.2869	0.000867	−1.1169	0.456355	−1.3427	0.007785
Mapk1	−1.0527	0.468581	−1.0887	0.159097	1.0316	0.724595
Mapk11	−1.0673	0.530192	−1.0706	0.578016	−1.0633	0.571223
Mapk12	1.1424	0.420684	1.1889	0.372287	−1.0255	0.780819
Mapk13	−1.1629	0.924422	−1.5423	0.355826	1.0504	0.651078
Mapk14	1.0018	0.940725	−1.0318	0.81795	1.0335	0.709962
Mapk3	−1.1294	0.224192	−1.121	0.372958	−1.0495	0.76638
Mapk8	1.0383	0.883566	−1.0215	0.798267	1.0037	0.911563
Mapk9	−1.1252	0.03886	−1.0075	0.87718	−1.0805	0.288977
Mefv	1.2572	0.278807	1.2582	0.463496	1.9192	0.028283
Myd88	1.0211	0.791137	1.0103	0.917416	1.2185	0.03802
Nfkb1	1.1098	0.279116	1.2919	0.089881	1.3323	0.033357
Nfkbia	−1.0294	0.835021	3.885	0.001215	3.3744	0.001348
Nfkbib	−1.1473	0.330475	−1.0153	0.762037	−1.1167	0.643504
P2rx7	−1.1586	0.428492	1.0742	0.625549	1.0578	0.661519
Panx1	−1.076	0.275575	1.1455	0.406863	1.1101	0.334734
Pea15a	−1.0943	0.291531	−1.043	0.625202	−1.0802	0.492135
Pstpip1	−1.1041	0.527175	−1.1018	0.680263	−1.0232	0.87342
Ptgs2	−1.08	0.499364	1.5126	0.000571	1.1762	0.323717
Rage	1.0729	0.478448	−1.1273	0.17423	1.1854	0.16574
Rela	1.0171	0.804744	1.1801	0.417806	1.2504	0.106174
Ripk2	−1.1057	0.237762	1.2913	0.028006	1.1199	0.389288
Sugt1	1.0063	0.918273	−1.1023	0.519396	−1.1264	0.106262
Tirap	−1.3098	0.094434	−1.0971	0.535721	1.0809	0.374146
Hsp90b1	1.0475	0.680071	−1.0334	0.69801	−1.0877	0.314466
Traf6	−1.0344	0.915204	−1.0171	0.943304	1.0988	0.437323
Txnip	−1.0761	0.70951	−1.0718	0.699702	−1.0187	0.789181
Xiap	1.0572	0.503462	−1.0558	0.471524	1.0089	0.93573

* For *p*-value, letters in red mean $p < 0.05$. ** For Fold Change, letters in red mean fold change >2 and letters in blue mean the fold change <−2. For the color line, : 6–10 fold decrease; : 2–5 fold decrease; : <2 fold; : 2–5 fold increase; : 6–10 fold increase; : 11–30 fold increase; : 31–50 fold increase.

3.3. *Expression Profile of Inflammasome-Related Chemokine and Cytokine Genes after an LPS Challenge, with and without Morphine Tolerance*

Cytokine and chemokine gene expression in response to LPS was greater in the control rats (placebo-control + LPS) compared to the morphine-tolerant animals (morphine-tolerant + LPS) (Table 3). The cytokines IL-1β and IL-6 were significantly increased 7- and 12-fold, respectively ($p < 0.01$–0.001), in the control rats given LPS (placebo-control + LPS), whereas in the morphine-tolerant group (morphine-tolerant + LPS) the fold changes were not statistically significant (3- and 7-fold, respectively) compared to the rats given saline (Figure 3, Table 3).

Table 3. Expression profile of the cytokine and chemokine genes in the rat brain in response to LPS, with and without morphine tolerance.

	morphine-tolerant + saline/placebo control + saline		placebo control + LPS/placebo control + saline		morphine-tolerant + LPS/morphine-tolerant + saline	
Gene	**Fold Change ****	***p*-value ***	**Fold Change ****	***p*-value ***	**Fold Change ****	***p*-value ***
Ccl11	−2.4662	0.023104	−2.8639	0.16576	−2.7346	0.249229
Ccl12	−1.4362	0.646529	2.0214	0.219015	2.1108	0.399119
Ccl2	1.1756	0.521412	23.7845	0.001354	9.1497	0.106064
Ccl5	−1.105	0.472434	1.2909	0.290174	−1.0949	0.766893
Ccl7	−1.0841	0.688167	10.7188	0.000259	6.9528	0.163034
Cxcl1	1.0131	0.944854	36.8609	0	14.4718	0.130008
Cxcl3	1.6208	0.019673	8.1909	0.000076	3.6477	0.170486
Cd40lg	−2.2796	0.215753	1.1119	0.704126	−2.4054	0.273798
Ifnb1	1.2519	0.936419	1.6899	0.391302	1.5695	0.513801
Ifng	1.5355	0.290413	1.1698	0.767882	2.2615	0.088346
Il12a	1.05	0.57557	1.1178	0.33855	1.0837	0.456191
Il12b	2.5587	0.26828	8.1055	0.102341	2.077	0.198782
Il18	1.068	0.60015	1.0484	0.707002	−1.1151	0.48359
Il1b	−1.2476	0.284501	6.7366	0.001383	3.3136	0.089312
Il33	1.2342	0.054615	1.0407	0.583823	1.1978	0.072613
Il6	2.023	0.45937	12.0303	0.008058	7.0943	0.083969
Irf1	1.1299	0.521156	3.4575	0.000386	3.4104	0.01276
Irf2	−1.1481	0.050782	1.0027	0.916481	1.0556	0.593809
Irf3	−1.2824	0.024657	−1.3225	0.225481	−1.2478	0.088625
Irf4	−1.1491	0.43182	−1.0557	0.846866	1.0263	0.858979
Irf5	−1.1024	0.38296	−1.1468	0.376953	1.0391	0.841777
Irf6	1.1055	0.413463	1.012	0.792025	1.118	0.272222
Tnfsf11	−1.6077	0.800779	−1.362	0.519436	−1.3266	0.965379
Tnfsf14	−1.396	0.243156	−1.8445	0.126355	−1.4278	0.629476
Tnfsf4	−1.0175	0.997398	−1.0887	0.790199	−1.3422	0.420711

* For *p*-value, letters in red mean $p < 0.05$. ** For Fold Change, letters in red mean fold change >2 and letters in blue mean the fold change <−2. For the color lines, : 6–10 fold decrease; : 2–5 fold decrease; : <2 fold; : 2–5 fold increase; : 6–10 fold increase; : 11–30 fold increase; : 31–50 fold increase.

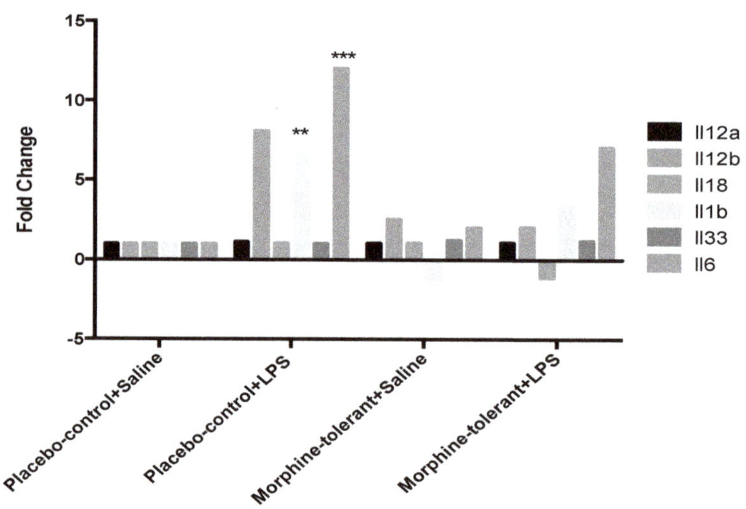

Figure 3. Cytokine gene expression in the rat brain in response to lipopolysaccharides (LPS), with and without morphine tolerance. Gene expression of interleukins Interleukin (Il)-1β, Il-6, Il-12a, Il-12b, Il-18, and Il-33 in the brains of rats, with and without morphine tolerance, following an i.p. injection of either 250 μg/kg LPS or saline ($n = 3$–5 rats per group) was determined using a Polymerase Chain Reaction (PCR) array. Data were calculated using the ΔΔCT method relative to the control group (placebo-control + saline) and are represented as a fold change. * $p < 0.05$, ** $p < 0.01$, *** $p < 0.001$

Similarly, Ccl2, Ccl7, Cxcl1, and Cxcl3 chemokine expression was significantly increased 24-, 11-, 37-, and 8-fold, respectively ($p < 0.01$–0.001), in response to LPS in the control rats (placebo-control +

LPS), whereas in the morphine-tolerant (morphine-tolerant + LPS) group the fold changes (9-, 7-, 14-, and 3-fold, respectively) were not statistically significant (Figure 4, Table 3).

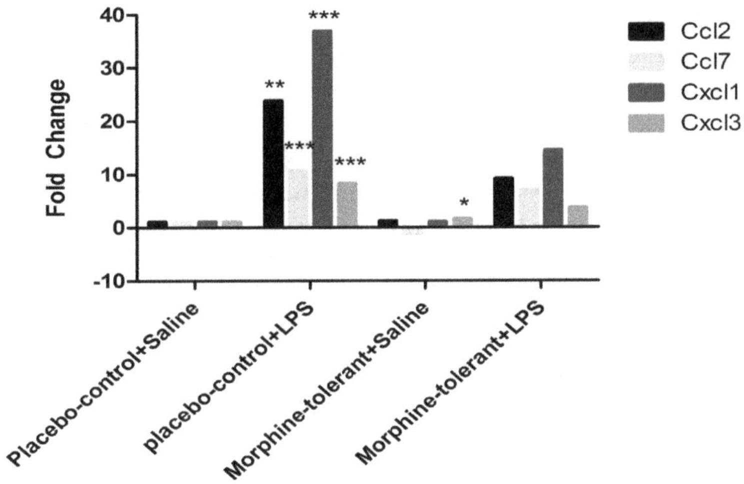

Figure 4. Chemokine gene expression in the rat brain in response to Lipopolysaccharides (LPS), with and without morphine tolerance. Gene expression of the chemokines C-C motif chemokine ligand (Ccl)2, Ccl5, Ccl7, Ccl11, Ccl12, C-X-C motif chemokine ligand (Cxcl)1, and Cxcl3 in the brains of rats with and without morphine tolerance, following an i.p. injection of either 250 μg/kg LPS or saline (n = 3–5 rats per group), was determined using a Polymerase Chain Reaction (PCR) array. Data were calculated using the ΔΔCT method relative to the control group (placebo-control + saline) and are represented as a fold change. * $p < 0.05$, ** $p < 0.01$, *** $p < 0.001$

3.4. LINCS Analysis of the Differentially Expressed Genes

Differentially expressed genes in the morphine-tolerant + saline versus morphine-tolerant + LPS rats and in the placebo-control + saline versus placebo-control + LPS rats as well as gene changes in rats the placebo-control + saline versus morphine-tolerant + saline rats were input into the Query App (apps.lincscloud.org/query). One report was generated by LINCS for each set of genes input. The genes with a high positive score in Consensus Knockdown Connections were considered to be potential gene targets (Table 4). In the placebo-control + saline versus placebo-control + LPS report, VPS28, protein C receptor (PROCR), and charged multivesicular body protein 2A (CHMP2A) were the top three with the highest scores. VPS28 is an ESCRT-I complex subunit that functions in the transport and sorting of proteins into sub-cellular vesicles. PROCR is endothelial protein C receptor involved in the blood coagulation pathway. CHMP2A is a component of the endosomal sorting complex required for transport III, which is involved in the degradation of surface receptor proteins and the formation of endocytic multivesicular bodies.

In the placebo-control + saline versus morphine-tolerant + saline report, SWI/SNF related, matrix associated, actin dependent regulator of chromatin, subfamily e, member 1 (SMARCE1), aryl-hydrocarbon receptor repressor (AHRR), and glutathione peroxidase 7 (GPX7) were the most likely targets predicted by LINCS. SMARCE1 is required for the transcriptional activation of genes normally repressed by chromatin. AHRR mediates dioxin toxicity and is involved in the regulation of cell growth and differentiation. GPX7 is involved with cellular senescence and insulin secretion.

In the morphine-tolerant + saline versus morphine-tolerant + LPS group, AHR (aryl hydrocarbon receptor), UBE2L6 (ubiquitin-conjugating enzyme E2L 6), and PAFAH1B3 (platelet-activating factor acetylhydrolase 1b, Catalytic Subunit 3) were the top three candidates. AHR is involved in the regulation of biological responses to planar aromatic hydrocarbons; UBE2L6 targets abnormal or short-lived proteins for degradation; and PAFAH1B3 functions in brain development and is associated with mental retardation, ataxia, and atrophy of the brain.

The predicted potential targets in each group were different from those in other groups, both in targets and their possibility rankings. VPS28 was the only one that appeared in both the Top 100 lists of placebo-control + saline versus placebo-control + LPS (No. 1 in Table 4) and morphine-tolerant + saline versus morphine-tolerant + LPS (No. 4 in Table 4).

Table 4 shows the top three potential target genes from each set of gene comparisons. There was no similarity in the gene rankings in the three sets of gene comparisons.

Table 4. LINCS Consensus Knockdown Connections from differentially expressed genes in the rat brain in response to lipopolysaccharides (LPS), with and without morphine tolerance. (A) Top 10 Consensus Knockdown Connections in the three sets of gene comparisons; (B) Rankings of the top three Consensus Knockdown Connections in the three sets of gene comparisons. Full name of the genes were provided in Table A2.

	Rank	placebo-Saline vs. Placebo-LPS	Placebo-Saline vs. Morphine-Tolerant-Saline	Morphine-Tolerant-Saline vs. Morphine-Tolerant-LPS
(A)	1	VPS28	SMARCE1	AHR
	2	PROCR	AHRR	UBE2L6
	3	CHMP2A	GPX7	PAFAH1B3
	4	MB	ATP5F1	VPS28
	5	ZNF768	CALR	JUNB
	6	RBPJ	GPR110	RYK
	7	WARS2	CHMP2A	ARG1
	8	TBX2	ELF4	PROC
	9	MRPS2	FGFR1	ZNF324
	10	MAP3K14	F7	ATP5D
	Gene Rank	**Placebo-Saline vs. Placebo-LPS**	**Placebo-Saline vs. Morphine-Tolerant-Saline**	**Morphine-Tolerant-Saline vs. Morphine-Tolerant-LPS**
(B)	VPS28	1	42	4
	PROCR	2	491	681
	CHMP2A	3	7	177
	SMARCE1-1	675	1	504
	AHRR	2383	2	460
	GPX7	488	3	2137
	AHR	46	769	1
	UBE2L6	89	545	2
	PAFAH1B3	95	622	3

4. Discussion

Inflammasomes recognize a variety of pathogen-associated molecular patterns (PAMPs), including endotoxins such as LPS. Depending on the NLR proteins that constitute inflammasomes, an inflamasome can be pro-inflammatory or anti-inflammatory in nature [28]. For pro-inflammatory inflammasomes such as NLRP3, in vitro studies have shown that the activation and release of pro-inflammatory cytokines requires two signals. The first signal, triggered by PAMPs, leads to the activation of inflammasomes, which then provide the second signal. The activated inflammasomes, through caspase 1 activation, promote the production of the pro-inflammatory cytokines, IL-1β and IL-18. However, the signaling pathways during infection or inflammation in vivo are not yet completely defined [29], and the characteristics of anti-inflammatory inflammasomes such as NLRP12 have not yet been extensively investigated. To our knowledge, our study is one of the first to report the modulation of NLRP12 expression in response to LPS and morphine in vivo.

Recently, NLRP12 was designated as an anti-inflammatory NLR inflammasome protein. It is believed to be a negative regulator of the NF-κB signaling pathway by inhibiting downstream signaling of TLRs, particularly IRAK-1 [28,30]. Our results showed that NLRP12 expression decreased in the brains of both the control (placebo-control + LPS) and morphine-tolerant (morphine-tolerant + LPS) rats in response to an LPS challenge, indicating that one of the mechanisms by which LPS induces an inflammatory response is by inhibiting the expression of the anti-inflammatory NLRP12 inflammasome.

Although NLRP12 expression was decreased in both groups given LPS, the decrease was significantly greater in the control rats than in the morphine-tolerant rats, which suggests that the LPS-induced NLRP12 decrease is countered during morphine tolerance. Hence morphine may also modulate NLRP12 activity, directly or indirectly, thereby exerting its immunosuppressive effects and opposing the LPS-induced decrease in NLRP12 in the presence of morphine tolerance.

Birc3, a downstream regulator of inflammasome signaling, is essential for controlling the synthesis of cytokines and chemokines in the inflammatory Mapk and NF-κB pathways. It is also required for inflammasome activation, subsequent caspase 1 activity, and IL-1β formation [31]. In our study, Birc3 expression was significantly increased in both the placebo-control and morphine-tolerant rats in response to LPS, indicating that LPS is able to induce an inflammatory response through Birc3 activity, following inhibition of the anti-inflammatory NLRP12. However, in response to LPS, Birc3 expression in the morphine-tolerant rats did not change in comparison to the placebo-control rats. This indicates that morphine may not be able to modulate Birc3 expression, and therefore there is no change, increase or decrease, in its expression in the morphine tolerant state.

NF-κB is important in the activation of inflammatory mediators such as cytokines and chemokines [16]. Previous studies have reported that NLRP12 inhibits both canonical and non-canonical NF-κB activation [16,28] and that Nfkbia, a downstream regulator of inflammasomes, inhibits the activity of dimeric NF-κB/Rel complexes [32]. In our study, Nfkbia was significantly increased in response to LPS in both the placebo-control and morphine-tolerant rats. During an inflammatory response, one would expect the expression and activity of a positive regulator of inflammation to be increased, whereas that of a negative regulator would be decreased. However, from a physiological standpoint, there is a constant effort to balance pro- and anti-inflammatory activity [33,34]. This quest to balance the pro- and anti-inflammatory responses could be one of the reasons for an increase in Nfkbia, which is known to inhibit the activity of the pro-inflammatory dimeric NF-κB/REL, thus reducing the production of pro-inflammatory mediators.

As expected, we found that the expression of pro-inflammatory cytokines (IL-1β and IL-6) and chemokines (Ccl2, Ccl7, Cxcl1, and Cxcl3) was increased in response to LPS in the placebo-control rats [35–37]. In the morphine-tolerant rats, however, the LPS-induced cytokine and chemokine expression levels were lower, suggesting that NLRP12 inhibition in response to LPS may be opposed or subdued in the morphine tolerant state.

In a previous study, we observed that, in peripheral immune organs such as the spleen, NLRP3 expression, but not NLRP12 expression, is altered in response to LPS, with and without morphine tolerance [38], suggesting that the mechanism(s) of inflammasome activation in response to pathogens may be different in peripheral immune organs, compared to the central nervous system. During morphine tolerance, the LPS-induced expression of NLRP3, as well as that of cytokines and chemokines, is reduced in comparison to the placebo-control rats given LPS [38]. These observations are consistent with previous studies showing that immune activation, including an inflammatory response, is diminished during morphine tolerance [39]. Therefore, the data from the present study, as well as from our previous report [38], collectively indicate that morphine may exert its effects through both pro- and anti-inflammatory inflammasomes.

LINCS analysis is able to predict potential target genes based on a certain treatment and the gene profile signatures in its database. In our study, LINCS was able to generate a report of potential targets with a p value of <0.05 from the list of genes with altered expression in response to LPS in control rats (placebo-control + saline versus placebo-control + LPS) but not from the other two comparisons (placebo-control + saline versus morphine-tolerant + saline, morphine-tolerant + saline versus morphine-tolerant + LPS), because there were not enough significant gene features in those two groups. When enlarging the set of gene features for the comparison of placebo-control + saline versus placebo-control + LPS to a p-value of <0.1, LINCS generated a report with similar potential targets. Thus, the gene features were then studied with a p-value of <0.1 on all three sets of comparisons. VPS28, PROCR, and CHMP2A were the top three with the highest scores in LINCS report generated based on placebo-control + saline versus placebo-control + LPS gene alternations, suggesting that Vps28, Procr and Chmp2a were potential targets of LPS. In the report for placebo-control + saline versus morphine-tolerant + saline, SMARCE1, AHRR, and GPX7 were the most likely targets altered in morphine tolerance predicted by LINCS. In the morphine-tolerant + saline versus morphine-tolerant + LPS report, AHR, UBE2L6, and PAFAH1B3 were the top three candidates that potentially responsible for the LPS-induced immune responses during morphine tolerance in rats. In the LINCS reports, the listed potential targets had different rankings using the different sets of gene features. This confirms that the response to LPS by those inflammosome-related genes could be affected by morphine tolerance.

Moreover, among the targets listed above, while VPS28 was No. 1 in the control rats in response to LPS, it was No. 4 in morphine-tolerant rats (Table 4). The VPS28 protein functions in transporting and sorting proteins into sub-cellular vesicles. In our study, LINCS analysis suggests that the actions of VPS28 in response to LPS could be dampened during morphine tolerance.

5. Conclusions

The results from our study indicate that, in the rat brain, LPS-induced inflammation involves both the inhibition of the NLRP12 anti-inflammatory inflammasome and the stimulation of downstream regulators such as Birc3, thereby increasing the expression of pro-inflammatory chemokines and cytokines. However, in the morphine tolerant state, the response to LPS is dampened, as indicated by the reduced expression of inflammasome-related genes. LINCS analysis confirmed that the response to LPS is altered during morphine tolerance and indicated that VPS28 may be one of the genes responsible for the alterations associated with morphine tolerance.

Acknowledgments: The authors thank Louaine L. Spriggs for her excellent editorial assistance. Funding for this study was provided, in part, by National Institutes of Health (NIH)/National Institute on Drug Abuse (NIDA) grants R01 DA007058 and K02 DA016149 to Sulie L. Chang.

Author Contributions: Sulie L. Chang designed the studies, participated in data collection, data analysis, and manuscript preparation, and approved the manuscript submission. Wenfei Wang conducted the LINCS analysis and participated in manuscript preparation. Sabroni Sarkar participated in the PCR array data analysis and in manuscript preparation. Xin Ma conducted the animal treatments, tissue collection, and PCR array analysis.

Appendix A

Table A1. Genes analyzed in PCR Array.

Gene Symbol	Full Name	mRNA Entry
Card6	caspase recruitment domain family, member 6	NM_001106413.1
Casp1	caspase 1	NM_012762.2
Casp12	caspase 12	NM_130422.1
Casp8	caspase 8	NM_022277.1
Naip2	NLR family, apoptosis inhibitory protein 6	XM_008760697.2
Nlrp12	NLR family, pyrin domain containing 12	NM_001169142.1
Nlrp5	NLR family, pyrin domain containing 5	NM_001107474.1
Nlrc4	NLR family, CARD domain containing 4	NM_001309432.1
Nlrp1a	NLR family, pyrin domain containing 1A	NM_001145755.2
Nlrp3	NLR family, pyrin domain containing 3	NM_001191642.1
Nlrp6	NLR family, pyrin domain containing 6	NM_134375.3
Nlrx1	NLR family member X1	NM_001025010.1
Nod2	nucleotide-binding oligomerization domain containing 2	NM_001106172.1
Pycard	PYD and CARD domain containing	NM_172322.1
Bcl2	BCL2, apoptosis regulator	NM_016993.1
Bcl2l1	BCL2 like 1	NM_001033670.1
Birc2	baculoviral IAP repeat-containing 2	NM_021752.2
Birc3	baculoviral IAP repeat-containing 3	NM_023987.3
Cflar	CASP8 and FADD-like apoptosis regulator	NM_001033864.2
Chuk	conserved helix-loop-helix ubiquitous kinase	NM_001107588.1
Ciita	class II, major histocompatibility complex, transactivator	NM_001270803.1
Ctsb	cathepsin B	NM_022597.2
Fadd	Fas associated via death domain	NM_152937.2
Hsp90aa1	heat shock protein 90, alpha (cytosolic), class A member 1	NM_175761.2
Hsp90ab1	heat shock protein 90 alpha family class B member 1	NM_001004082.3
Ikbkb	inhibitor of kappa light polypeptide gene enhancer in B-cells, kinase beta	NM_053355.2
Ikbkg	inhibitor of kappa light polypeptide gene enhancer in B-cells, kinase gamma	NM_199103.1
Irak1	interleukin-1 receptor-associated kinase 1	NM_001127555.1
Map3k7	mitogen activated protein kinase kinase kinase 7	NM_001107920.2
Map3k7ip1	TGF-beta activated kinase 1/MAP3K7 binding protein 1	NM_001109976.2
Map3k7ip2	TGF-beta activated kinase 1/MAP3K7 binding protein 2	NM_001012062.1
Mapk1	mitogen activated protein kinase 1	NM_053842.2
Mapk11	mitogen-activated protein kinase 11	NM_001109532.2

Table A1. *Cont.*

Gene Symbol	Full Name	mRNA Entry
Mapk12	mitogen-activated protein kinase 12	NM_021746.1
Mapk13	mitogen activated protein kinase 13	NM_019231.2
Mapk14	mitogen activated protein kinase 14	NM_031020.2
Mapk3	mitogen activated protein kinase 3	NM_017347.2
Mapk8	mitogen-activated protein kinase 8	NM_053829.2
Mapk9	mitogen-activated protein kinase 9	NM_001270544.1
Mefv	Mediterranean fever	NM_031634.1
Myd88	myeloid differentiation primary response 88	NM_198130.1
Nfkb1	nuclear factor kappa B subunit 1	NM_001276711.1
Nfkbia	NFKB inhibitor alpha	NM_001105720.2
Nfkbib	NFKB inhibitor beta	NM_030867.2
P2rx7	purinergic receptor P2X 7	NM_019256.1
Panx1	Pannexin 1	NM_001270548.1
Pea15a	phosphoprotein enriched in astrocytes 15	NM_001013231.1
Pstpip1	proline-serine-threonine phosphatase-interacting protein 1	NM_001106824.2
Ptgs2	prostaglandin-endoperoxide synthase 2	NM_017232.3
Rage	MOK protein kinase	NM_001010965.1
Rela	RELA proto-oncogene, NF-kB subunit	NM_199267.2
Ripk2	receptor-interacting serine-threonine kinase 2	NM_001191865.1
Sugt1	SGT1 homolog, MIS12 kinetochore complex assembly cochaperone	NM_001013051.1
Tirap	TIR domain containing adaptor protein	XM_017596001.1
Hsp90b1	heat shock protein 90 beta family member 1	NM_001012197.2
Traf6	TNF receptor associated factor 6	NM_001107754.2
Txnip	thioredoxin interacting protein	NM_001008767.1
Xiap	E3 ubiquitin-protein ligase XIAP	NM_022231.2
Ccl11	C-C motif chemokine ligand 11	NM_019205.1
Ccl12	chemokine (C-C motif) ligand 12	NM_001105822.1
Ccl2	C-C motif chemokine ligand 2	NM_031530.1
Ccl5	C-C motif chemokine ligand 5	NM_031116.3
Ccl7	C-C motif chemokine ligand 7	NM_001007612.1
Cxcl1	C-X-C motif chemokine ligand 1	NM_030845.1
Cxcl3	C-X-C motif chemokine ligand 3	NM_138522.1
Cd40lg	CD40 ligand	NM_053353.1
Ifnb1	interferon beta 1	NM_019127.1
Ifng	interferon gamma	NM_138880.2
Il12a	interleukin 12A	NM_053390.1
Il12b	interleukin 12B	NM_022611.1
Il18	interleukin 18	NM_019165.1
Il1b	interleukin 1 beta	NM_031512.2
Il33	interleukin 33	NM_001014166.1
Il6	interleukin 6	NM_012589.2
Irf1	interferon regulatory factor 1	NM_012591.1
Irf2	interferon regulatory factor 2	NM_001047086.1
Irf3	interferon regulatory factor 3	NM_001006969.1
Irf4	interferon regulatory factor 4	NM_001106108.1
Irf5	interferon regulatory factor 5	NM_001106586.1
Irf6	interferon regulatory factor 6	NM_001108859.1
Tnfsf11	tumor necrosis factor superfamily member 11	NM_057149.1
Tnfsf14	tumor necrosis factor superfamily member 14	NM_001191803.1
Tnfsf4	tumor necrosis factor superfamily member 4	NM_053552.1

Table A2. Top 10 scored Genes in LINCS report.

Gene Symbol	Full name
VPS28	VPS28, ESCRT-I subunit
PROCR	protein C receptor
CHMP2A	charged multivesicular body protein 2A
MB	myoglobin
ZNF768	zinc finger protein 768
RBPJ	recombination signal binding protein for immunoglobulin kappa J region
WARS2	tryptophanyl tRNA synthetase 2 (mitochondrial)
TBX2	T-box 2
MRPS2	mitochondrial ribosomal protein S2
MAP3K14	mitogen-activated protein kinase kinase kinase 14
SMARCE1	SWI/SNF related, matrix associated, actin dependent regulator of chromatin, subfamily e, member 1
AHRR	aryl-hydrocarbon receptor repressor
GPX7	glutathione peroxidase 7
ATP5F1	ATP synthase, H+ transporting, mitochondrial Fo complex subunit B1
CALR	calreticulin
GPR110	G protein-coupled receptor 110
ELF4	E74 like ETS transcription factor 4
FGFR1	fibroblast growth factor receptor 1
F7	coagulation factor VII
AHR	aryl hydrocarbon receptor
UBE2L6	ubiquitin-conjugating enzyme E2L 6
PAFAH1B3	platelet-activating factor acetylhydrolase 1b, catalytic subunit 3
JUNB	JunB proto-oncogene, AP-1 transcription factor subunit
RYK	receptor-like tyrosine kinase
ARG1	arginase 1
ZNF324	zinc finger protein 324
ATP5D	ATP synthase, H+ transporting, mitochondrial F1 complex, delta subunit

References

1. Ossipov, M.H.; Lai, J.; King, T.; Vanderah, T.W.; Malan, T.P., Jr.; Hruby, V.J.; Porreca, F. Antinociceptive and nociceptive actions of opioids. *J. Neurobiol.* **2004**, *61*, 126–148. [CrossRef] [PubMed]
2. Bonnet, M.P.; Beloeil, H.; Benhamou, D.; Mazoit, J.X.; Asehnoune, K. The μ opioid receptor mediates morphine-induced tumor necrosis factor and interleukin-6 inhibition in toll-like receptor 2-stimulated monocytes. *Anesth. Analg.* **2008**, *106*, 1142–1149. [CrossRef] [PubMed]
3. Hutchinson, M.R.; Coats, B.D.; Lewis, S.S.; Zhang, Y.; Sprunger, D.B.; Rezvani, N.; Baker, E.M.; Jekich, B.M.; Wieseler, J.L.; Somogyi, A.A.; et al. Proinflammatory cytokines oppose opioid-induced acute and chronic analgesia. *Brain Behav. Immun.* **2008**, *22*, 1178–1189. [CrossRef] [PubMed]
4. Mohan, S.; Davis, R.L.; DeSilva, U.; Stevens, C.W. Dual regulation of *mu* opioid receptors in SK-N-SH neuroblastoma cells by morphine and interleukin-1beta: Evidence for opioid-immune crosstalk. *J. Neuroimmunol.* **2010**, *227*, 26–34. [CrossRef] [PubMed]
5. Ocasio, F.M.; Jiang, Y.; House, S.D.; Chang, S.L. Chronic morphine accelerates the progression of lipopolysaccharide-induced sepsis to septic shock. *J. Neuroimmunol.* **2004**, *149*, 90–100. [CrossRef] [PubMed]
6. Flores, L.R.; Wahl, S.M.; Bayer, B.M. Mechanisms of morphine-induced immunosuppression: Effect of acute morphine administration on lymphocyte trafficking. *J. Pharmacol. Exp. Ther.* **1995**, *272*, 1246–1251. [PubMed]
7. Gomez-Flores, R.; Weber, R.J. Inhibition of interleukin-2 production and downregulation of IL-2 and transferrin receptors on rat splenic lymphocytes following pag morphine administration: A role in natural killer and T cell suppression. *J. Interferon Cytokine Res.* **1999**, *19*, 625–630. [CrossRef] [PubMed]
8. Patel, N.A.; Romero, A.A.; Zadina, J.E.; Chang, S.L. Chronic exposure to morphine attenuates expression of interleukin-1 beta in the rat hippocampus. *Brain Res.* **1996**, *712*, 340–344. [CrossRef]
9. Roy, S.; Charboneau, R.G.; Barke, R.A. Morphine synergizes with lipopolysaccharide in a chronic endotoxemia model. *J. Neuroimmunol.* **1999**, *95*, 107–114. [CrossRef]
10. Hilburger, M.E.; Adler, M.W.; Truant, A.L.; Meissler, J.J., Jr.; Satishchandran, V.; Rogers, T.J.; Eisenstein, T.K. Morphine induces sepsis in mice. *J. Infect. Dis.* **1997**, *176*, 183–188. [CrossRef] [PubMed]
11. Martinon, F.; Burns, K.; Tschopp, J. The inflammasome: A molecular platform triggering activation of inflammatory caspases and processing of proil-beta. *Mol. Cell* **2002**, *10*, 417–426. [CrossRef]
12. Guarda, G.; Zenger, M.; Yazdi, A.S.; Schroder, K.; Ferrero, I.; Menu, P.; Tardivel, A.; Mattmann, C.; Tschopp, J. Differential expression of NLRP3 among hematopoietic cells. *J. Immunol.* **2011**, *186*, 2529–2534. [CrossRef] [PubMed]
13. Martinon, F.; Mayor, A.; Tschopp, J. The inflammasomes: Guardians of the body. *Annu. Rev. Immunol.* **2009**, *27*, 229–265. [CrossRef] [PubMed]
14. Strowig, T.; Henao-Mejia, J.; Elinav, E.; Flavell, R. Inflammasomes in health and disease. *Nature* **2012**, *481*, 278–286. [CrossRef] [PubMed]
15. Allan, S.M.; Tyrrell, P.J.; Rothwell, N.J. Interleukin-1 and neuronal injury. *Nat. Rev. Immunol.* **2005**, *5*, 629–640. [CrossRef] [PubMed]
16. Allen, I.C.; Wilson, J.E.; Schneider, M.; Lich, J.D.; Roberts, R.A.; Arthur, J.C.; Woodford, R.M.; Davis, B.K.; Uronis, J.M.; Herfarth, H.H.; et al. NLRP12 suppresses colon inflammation and tumorigenesis through the negative regulation of noncanonical NF-kappab signaling. *Immunity* **2012**, *36*, 742–754. [CrossRef] [PubMed]
17. Williams, K.L.; Lich, J.D.; Duncan, J.A.; Reed, W.; Rallabhandi, P.; Moore, C.; Kurtz, S.; Coffield, V.M.; Accavitti-Loper, M.A.; Su, L.; et al. The caterpiller protein monarch-1 is an antagonist of toll-like receptor-, tumor necrosis factor alpha-, and mycobacterium tuberculosis-induced pro-inflammatory signals. *J. Biol. Chem.* **2005**, *280*, 39914–39924. [CrossRef] [PubMed]
18. Lich, J.D.; Williams, K.L.; Moore, C.B.; Arthur, J.C.; Davis, B.K.; Taxman, D.J.; Ting, J.P. Monarch-1 suppresses non-canonical NF-kappab activation and P52-dependent chemokine expression in monocytes. *J. Immunol.* **2007**, *178*, 1256–1260. [CrossRef] [PubMed]
19. National Institute of Health (NIH) Library of Network-Based Cellular Signatures (LINCS) Program. Available online: http://www.lincsproject.org/ (accessed on 11 June 2016).
20. Lamb, J.; Crawford, E.D.; Peck, D.; Modell, J.W.; Blat, I.C.; Wrobel, M.J.; Lerner, J.; Brunet, J.P.; Subramanian, A.; Ross, K.N.; et al. The connectivity map: Using gene-expression signatures to connect small molecules, genes, and disease. *Science* **2006**, *313*, 1929–1935. [CrossRef] [PubMed]

21. Chang, S.L.; Moldow, R.L.; House, S.D.; Zadina, J.E. Morphine affects the brain-immune axis by modulating an interleukin-1 beta dependent pathway. *Adv. Exp. Med. Biol.* **1996**, *402*, 35–42. [PubMed]
22. Graf, J.A.; Patel, J.A.; Chang, S.L. Chronic exposure to morphine, but not ethanol, attenuates the expression of interleukin-1 beta converting enzyme in rat spleen. *Immunol. Lett.* **1997**, *58*, 153–157. [CrossRef]
23. Zadina, J.E.; Kastin, A.J.; Harrison, L.M.; Ge, L.J.; Chang, S.L. Opiate receptor changes after chronic exposure to agonists and antagonists. *Ann. N. Y. Acad. Sci.* **1995**, *757*, 353–361. [CrossRef] [PubMed]
24. House, S.D.; Mao, X.; Wu, G.; Espinelli, D.; Li, W.X.; Chang, S.L. Chronic morphine potentiates the inflammatory response by disrupting interleukin-1beta modulation of the hypothalamic-pituitary-adrenal axis. *J. Neuroimmunol.* **2001**, *118*, 277–285. [CrossRef]
25. RT2 Profiler PCR Array Date Analysis version 3.5. Available online: http://pcrdataanalysis.sabiosciences.com/pcr/arrayanalysis.php (accessed 22 January 2017).
26. Ma, J.; Malladi, S.; Beck, A.H. Systematic analysis of sex-linked molecular alterations and therapies in cancer. *Sci. Rep.* **2016**, *6*, 19119. [CrossRef] [PubMed]
27. Siavelis, J.C.; Bourdakou, M.M.; Athanasiadis, E.I.; Spyrou, G.M.; Nikita, K.S. Bioinformatics methods in drug repurposing for Alzheimer's disease. *Brief. Bioinform.* **2016**, *17*, 322–335. [CrossRef] [PubMed]
28. Allen, I.C.; Lich, J.D.; Arthur, J.C.; Jania, C.M.; Roberts, R.A.; Callaway, J.B.; Tilley, S.L.; Ting, J.P. Characterization of NLRP12 during the development of allergic airway disease in mice. *PLoS ONE* **2012**, *7*, e30612. [CrossRef] [PubMed]
29. Dostert, C.; Guarda, G.; Romero, J.F.; Menu, P.; Gross, O.; Tardivel, A.; Suva, M.L.; Stehle, J.C.; Kopf, M.; Stamenkovic, I.; et al. Malarial hemozoin is a NALP3 inflammasome activating danger signal. *PLoS ONE* **2009**, *4*, e6510. [CrossRef] [PubMed]
30. Zaki, M.H.; Vogel, P.; Malireddi, R.K.; Body-Malapel, M.; Anand, P.K.; Bertin, J.; Green, D.R.; Lamkanfi, M.; Kanneganti, T.D. The nod-like receptor NLRP12 attenuates colon inflammation and tumorigenesis. *Cancer Cell* **2011**, *20*, 649–660. [CrossRef] [PubMed]
31. Beug, S.T.; Cheung, H.H.; LaCasse, E.C.; Korneluk, R.G. Modulation of immune signalling by inhibitors of apoptosis. *Trends Immunol.* **2012**, *33*, 535–545. [CrossRef] [PubMed]
32. Scherer, D.C.; Brockman, J.A.; Chen, Z.; Maniatis, T.; Ballard, D.W. Signal-induced degradation of I kappa B alpha requires site-specific ubiquitination. *Proc. Natl. Acad. Sci. USA* **1995**, *92*, 11259–11263. [CrossRef] [PubMed]
33. Homji, N.F.; Mao, X.; Langsdorf, E.F.; Chang, S.L. Endotoxin-induced cytokine and chemokine expression in the HIV-1 transgenic rat. *J. Neuroinflamm.* **2012**, *9*, 3. [CrossRef] [PubMed]
34. Del Fresno, C.; Garcia-Rio, F.; Gomez-Pina, V.; Soares-Schanoski, A.; Fernandez-Ruiz, I.; Jurado, T.; Kajiji, T.; Shu, C.; Marin, E.; Gutierrez del Arroyo, A.; et al. Potent phagocytic activity with impaired antigen presentation identifying lipopolysaccharide-tolerant human monocytes: Demonstration in isolated monocytes from cystic fibrosis patients. *J. Immunol.* **2009**, *182*, 6494–6507. [CrossRef] [PubMed]
35. Fang, H.; Pengal, R.A.; Cao, X.; Ganesan, L.P.; Wewers, M.D.; Marsh, C.B.; Tridandapani, S. Lipopolysaccharide-induced macrophage inflammatory response is regulated by ship. *J. Immunol.* **2004**, *173*, 360–366. [CrossRef] [PubMed]
36. Martich, G.D.; Boujoukos, A.J.; Suffredini, A.F. Response of man to endotoxin. *Immunobiology* **1993**, *187*, 403–416. [CrossRef]
37. Porter, K.J.; Gonipeta, B.; Parvataneni, S.; Appledorn, D.M.; Patial, S.; Sharma, D.; Gangur, V.; Amalfitano, A.; Parameswaran, N. Regulation of lipopolysaccharide-induced inflammatory response and endotoxemia by beta-arrestins. *J. Cell Physiol.* **2010**, *225*, 406–416. [CrossRef] [PubMed]
38. Mao, X.; Sarkar, S.; Chang, S.L. Involvement of the NLRP3 inflammasome in the modulation of an LPS-induced inflammatory response during morphine tolerance drug and alcohol dependence. *Drug Alcohol Depend.* **2013**, *132*, 38–46. [CrossRef] [PubMed]
39. Limiroli, E.; Gaspani, L.; Panerai, A.E.; Sacerdote, P. Differential morphine tolerance development in the modulation of macrophage cytokine production in mice. *J. Leukoc. Biol.* **2002**, *72*, 43–48. [PubMed]

10

Rotating and Neurochemical Activity of Rats Lesioned with Quinolinic Acid and Transplanted with Bone Marrow Mononuclear Cells

Teresa Serrano Sánchez [1,*], María Elena González Fraguela [1], Lisette Blanco Lezcano [2], Esteban Alberti Amador [3], Beatriz Caballero Fernández [4], María de los Ángeles Robinson Agramonte [1], Lourdes Lorigados Pedre [1] and Jorge A Bergado Rosado [2]

1 Immunochemical Department, International Center for Neurological Restoration, 25th Ave, Playa, 15805, Havana PC 11300, Cuba; marie@neuro.ciren.cu (M.E.G.F.); robin@neuro.ciren.cu (M.d.l.Á.R.A.); lourdesl@neuro.ciren.cu (L.L.P.)

2 Experimental Neurophysiology Department, International Center of Neurological Restoration (CIREN) Ave. 25 No. 15805 e/158 and 160, Playa, Havana 11300, Cuba; lblanco@neuro.ciren.cu (L.B.L.); jorgebergado@yahoo.com (J.A.B.R.)

3 Molecular biology Department, International Center of Neurological Restoration (CIREN) Ave. 25 No. 15805 e/158 and 160, Playa, Havana 11300, Cuba; alberti@neuro.ciren.cu

4 Policlínico 26 de Julio, Calle 72 #1313. A. Almendares, Playa, Havana 11300, Cuba; bettycfdez@infomed.sld.cu

* Correspondence author: teresa@neuro.ciren.cu

Abstract: Huntington's disease (HD) is an inherited, neurodegenerative disorder that results from the degeneration of striatal neurons, mainly GABAergic neurons. The study of neurochemical activity has provided reliable markers to explain motor disorders. To treat neurodegenerative diseases, stem cell transplants with bone marrow (BM) have been performed for several decades. In this work we determine the effect of mononuclear bone marrow cell (mBMC) transplantation on the rotational behavior and neurochemical activity in a model of Huntington's disease in rats. Four experimental groups were organized: Group I: Control animals (n = 5); Group II: Lesion with quinolinic acid (QA) in the striatum (n = 5); Group III: Lesion with QA and transplant with mBMC (n = 5); Group IV: Lesion with QA and transplant with culture medium (Dulbecco's modified Eagle's medium (DMEM) injection) (n = 5). The rotational activity induced by D-amphetamine was evaluated and the concentration of the neurotransmitter amino acids (glutamate and GABA) was studied. The striatal cell transplantation decreases the rotations induced by D-amphetamine ($p < 0.04$, Wilcoxon matched pairs test) and improves the changes produced in the levels of neurotransmitters studied. This work suggests that the loss of GABAergic neurons in the brain of rats lesioned with AQ produces behavioral and neurochemical alterations that can be reversed with the use of bone marrow mononuclear cell transplants.

Keywords: striatum; quinolinic acid; transplantation; mononuclear cell; bone marrow cell; Huntington disease model

---

1. Introduction

Huntington's disease (HD) has been associated with a degeneration of striatal cells, mainly death of medium spiny GABAergic projection neurons within the caudate nucleus and putamen. Although the most pronounced pathology is observed in the basal ganglia, cell death also occurs early in the cerebral cortex [1]. The experimental models play essential roles in the understanding of disease mechanisms, progression, and drug efficacy testing. The injection of quinolinic acid into the striatum is used as a theoretical model of HD [2]. Quinolinic acid (QA) produces loss of GABAergic neurons; in this way there is an imbalance between the healthy and damaged striatum in response to the action of an intact dopaminergic system, which produces an asymmetric motor response to the action of a dopaminergic agonist, D-amphetamine.

The study of the neurochemical activity in the affected brain tissue is a reliable marker to explain the motor disorders that appear in this disease [3]. No therapy has been shown to delay disease onset or slow progression in humans. Unlike other neurodegenerative entities, pharmacological treatment is only a palliative procedure. Thus, there is an urgent need to identify and validate other treatments. Cells isolated from bone marrow are successfully used for transplantation in experimental models of cranial encephalic trauma [4,5] as well as in striatal ischemia to reduce the motor deficit that appears after damage [6]. Recently, autologous bone marrow stem cell transplantation has been used to reverse the cognitive deficit observed in an experimental model of Huntington's disease, which demonstrates that bone marrow cell transplantation is able to reduce the cognitive damage that appears in this model [7]. In general, the repair mechanism consists of the potential to develop into many different types of cells (thus serving as a repair system for the body) and the potential to release trophic factors that repair and regulate other compensatory mechanisms in the damaged area. For this reason, in the last decades, neurorestorative treatment has been tried in experimental models that use stem cells from different sources, such as mononuclear bone marrow cells (mBMC) [8,9].

In the present study, the objective was to determine the effect of mBMC transplantation on the rotational activity induced by systemic administration of D-amphetamine (5 mg/kg intraperitoneal) and the neurochemical activity in two brain areas: the cerebral cortex and striatum. We show evidence that indicates the transplant may be a viable therapeutic option for Huntington's disease.

2. Materials and Methods

2.1. Animals

Adult male Sprague Dawley (SD) rats (total $N = 20$) obtained from the National Center for Laboratory Animals Production (CENPALAB) and weighing 200–250 g (between 9 and 12 weeks of age) were used in this study. Animals were housed in translucent makrolon cages (five animals per cage) under a 12 h light: 12 h darkness cycle with ad libitum access to water and food.

For the behavior and neurotransmission study, four experimental groups were included ($n = 5$ each): Control (C), Group I; QA lesion (QAL), Group II; QA lesion + mononuclear bone marrow cell transplantation (QA+mBMC), Group III; and QA lesion + Dulbecco's modified Eagle's medium (QA+DMEM) injection, Group VI.

2.2. Striatal QA Lesions

Unilateral lesions of the right striatum were produced by the intrastriatal injection of QA. Rats were anesthetized with an intraperitoneal (ip) injection of ketamine (50 mg/mL, ip, IMEFA, Havana, Cuba). QA injections were administered with the help of a stereotaxic apparatus (model 900; David Kopf Instruments, Tujunga, CA, USA). Each rat was injected in the striatum with 1.2 μL of QA (125.5 nmol) (Sigma, Saint Louis, MA, USA) using a 30 G Hamilton syringe at the following coordinates: 1.2 mm anterior and 2.8 mm lateral to the bregma, and 5.5 mm below the dura. The toxin was injected over a period of 1 min, and the cannula was left in place for an additional 10 min before being slowly removed.

2.3. Obtaining Rat Mononuclear Bone Marrow Cells

The mBMC were isolated from the rat femur as described in the work of Woodbury and colleagues [10]. Male SD rats aged between 32 and 48 days old were anesthetized with an intraperitoneal injection of ketamine (50 mg/mL, ip, IMEFA, Havana, Cuba) and a cut on the skin of the hind limbs was performed, separating the tissue parallel to the bone to extract both femurs; then the animals were euthanized with a lethal overdose of chloral hydrate. The extracted bones were placed for 30 min on a Petri dish containing 0.9% physiologic saline, after which the bone marrow was obtained by flushing with sterile phosphate-buffered saline (PBS; NaCl, 8 g/L; KCl, 0.2 g/L; Na_2HPO_4, 1.09 g/L; KH_2PO_4, 0.26 g/L, pH 7.2) through one of the femoral epiphyses. The bone marrow was collected in sterile containers to be later washed by centrifugation.

2.4. Isolation of Mononuclear Bone Marrow Cells

The suspension of bone marrow cells was washed three times with 1× PBS by centrifugation for 10 min at 2000 rpm at 20 °C. An aliquot of 2.5 mL of Ficoll–Hypaque was placed on the bottom of a graduated glass tube, on top of which 5 mL of the cellular suspension in PBS was layered. This was centrifuged for 45 min at 2800 rpm at 20 °C.

The mononuclear cell band was extracted with a pipette and washed immediately, discarding the supernatant into a container with hypochlorite and collecting the cellular pellet, which was suspended in 1× PBS and cell viability was determined by trypam blue exclusion.

2.5. Transplantation

Four weeks after the QA lesion, the animals to be transplanted with mBMCs were deeply anesthetized as previously described. Rats were placed in the stereotactic apparatus and the skin over the skull was reopened. Using a Hamilton syringe, the mBMC suspension (50,000 cells/µL in DMEM) was injected into the lesioned striatum (in two deposits; 1 µL per deposit) at coordinates slightly different from the ones used for the QA lesions: 0.7 mm anterior from the bregma, 2.8 mm lateral from the midline, and 5.5 and 4.6 mm under the dura surface. Cells were injected slowly over a period of 1 min. The needle was left in place for an additional 10 min following injection and then carefully removed. Sham-transplanted animals (DMEM) received an equal volume of tissue culture medium injected in the same way, at the same stereotactic coordinates.

2.6. Behavioral Tests (Rotating Activity Induced by D-Amphetamine)

The rotational activity induced by D-amphetamine (5 mg/kg, ip, Sigma, St. Luis, MO, USA) [11] was studied one week after the QA injury and one month after the mBMC/ DMEM transplant, using an LE 3806 Electronic Multicounter coupled to LE 902 sensors (PanLAB, Barcelona, Spain) that measured the sense of rotation. The measurements were performed for a period of 90 min.

2.7. Obtaining Samples for Neurotransmission Study

After the behavioral test was over, the rats received an overdose of ketamine (100 mg/mL, ip, IMEFA, Havana, Cuba) and were decapitated. Their brains were extracted and washed with cold 0.9% NaCl, after which the striatum (St) and prefrontal cortex was dissected. The obtained tissue was frozen in liquid nitrogen, weighed and stored at −80 °C for further analysis.

2.8. Neurotransmitter Study

The amino acid concentrations in the tissue were determined by high-performance liquid chromatography (HPLC), coupled to a fluorescence detector and using derivatization with o-phthaldialdehyde (OPA). Then, 10 µL of sample was mixed with 10 µL of the OPA derivatizing agent (10 mM OPA dissolved in 0.1 mol/L sodium tetraborate buffer containing 77 mM of 3-mercaptopropionic acid and 10% methanol pH 9.3). The mixture was vortexed for 15 s and the reaction was stopped with 5% acetic acid at 45 s. From this mixture, 20 µL was injected to the chromatograph with a Hamilton syringe. The derivatized amino acids were passed through a reverse phase column (HR-80, 8 cm long with a4.6-mm internal diameter, ESA), with a similar stationary phase precolumn, by means of an isocratic chromatographic pump (Philips PU, Amsterdam, The Netherlands) 4100) and were detected by a fluorescence detector with excitation λ = 340 nm and emission λ = 460 nm (Philips PU 4027).

The chromatograms were recorded using the program CHROMATEPC version 4.24 (Philips). A mobile phase composed of 0.1 mol/L NaH_2PO_4 and 20% methanol was used to separate the amino acids.

2.9. Ethical Considerations

Experiments were carried out in accordance with the Cuban Regulations for the Use of Laboratory Animals (CENPALAB 1997) and the Canadian Council on Animal Care (CCAC) [12] This work was approved by the Ethical Committee of the International Center for Neurological Restoration. Efforts were made to minimize the pain and discomfort of the animals, as well as the number of animal used for experiments.

2.10. Statistical Processing

Statistical analysis was carried out using Statistical software. The values are expressed as mean ± SEM. The normal distribution and homogeneity of variance of the data were tested by the Kolmogorov–Smirnov and Levene tests, respectively. The comparisons between more than two groups were made by one-way non parametric ANOVA; the Kruskall–Wallis test was applied to aminoacid analysis, and the Wilcoxon test was applied to behavioral evaluations. In all cases, statistically significant differences were considered when $p \leq 0.05$.

3. Results

Our results confirm the hypothesis that the transplantation of bone marrow mononuclear cells in the lesioned striatum of rats reverts the neurochemical alterations that appear in the neurotoxic model of Huntington's disease induced by quinolinic acid. The objective was to evaluate the possible protective effect of transplanted mBMC on the changes induced in motor behavior and neurotransmission in the HD model.

3.1. Rotational Activity

Figure 1 show the ipsilateral to the lesion rotatory activity exhibited by the animals injected with QA in striatum under D-amphetamine effects. The striatal transplant of mBMC diminished the rotation induced by D-amphetamine.

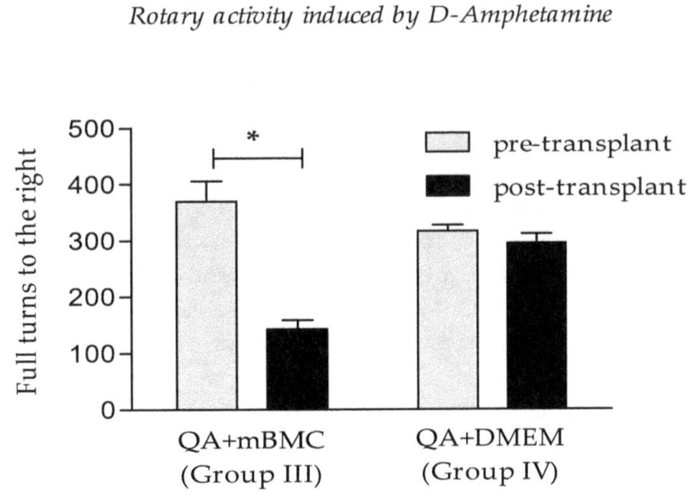

Figure 1. Rotatory activity induced under D-amphetamine. Lesioned group with quinolinic acid + mononuclear bone marrow cell transplant (QA+mBMC, Group III) and lesioned group with QA+Dulbecco's modified Eagle's medium (DMEM) transplant (QA+DMEM, Group IV). Abscissa, number of complete right turns ipsilateral to the lesioned hemisphere. Data are expressed as mean ± standard error of mean (SEM). Ordinates: experimental groups (* equivalent $p \leq 0.04$).

3.2. Neurochemical Activity

3.2.1. Glutamate Concentration

In the Figure 2 the comparison of the glutamate content in the experimental groups for the right striatum (RS) and right cortex (RC) showed significant differences among them (RS $p \leq 0.001$ and RC $p \leq 0.001$). The higher glutamate content was obtained for Group III (QA+mBMC) for both structures.

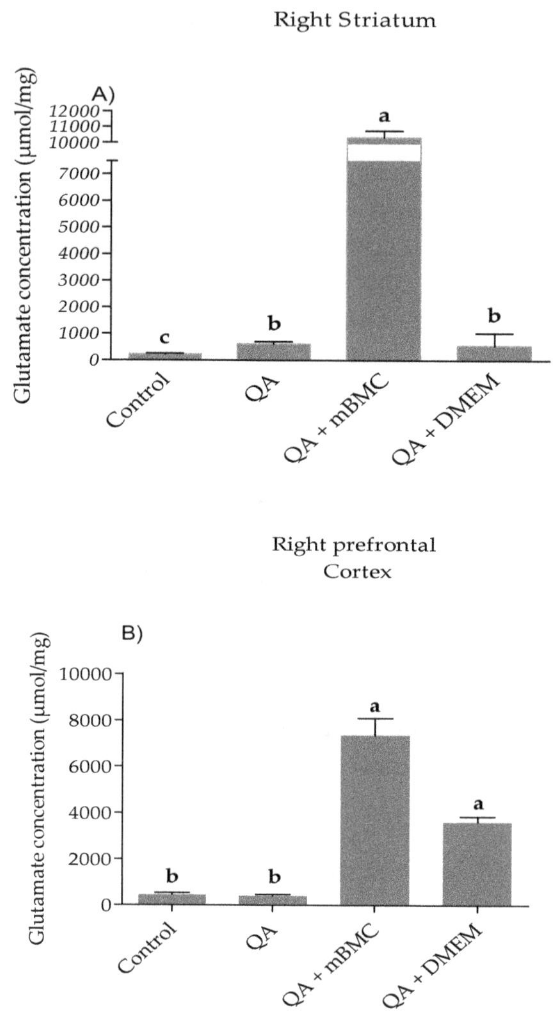

Figure 2. Study of glutamate (GLU) concentration in lesioned rats with transplanted mBMC. (**A**) Comparison of GLU concentration in the right striatum among the experimental groups: H (3, 20) = 16.28, $p < 0.001$. (**B**) GLU concentration in right prefrontal cortex among the experimental groups: H (3, 19) = 15.53, $p < 0.001$. Data are expressed as mean ± SEM. The letters in the top the bar correspond to statistical differences among the experimental groups. The data analysis was carried out through one-way non parametric ANOVA, using the Kruskall–Wallis test (common letters: non-significant differences; different letters; significant differences).QA lesion (Group II); lesioned group with QA + transplant (QA+mBMC, Group III); and lesioned group with QA+DMEM transplant (QA+DMEM, Group IV).

3.2.2. GABA (γ-Aminobutyric Acid) Concentration

Finally, in Figure 3 the comparison of GABA (content in the right striatum (RS) and right cortex (RC) among the experimental groups showed significant differences (RS and RC: ($p \leq 0.001$, the higher GABA content was obtained in both structures for Group III in comparison to the control group.

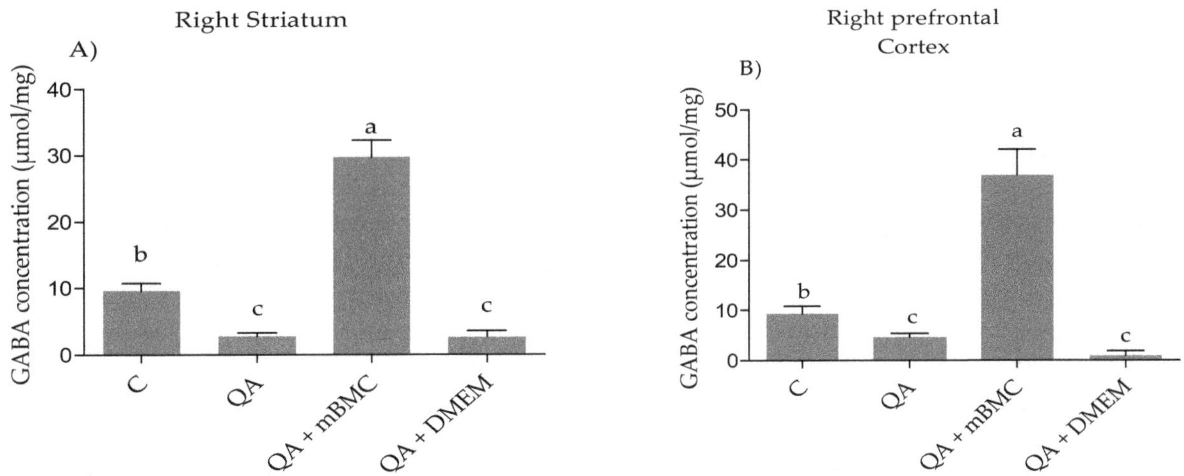

Figure 3. Study of GABA (γ-aminobutyric acid) concentration in lesioned rats + mBMC transplanted. (**A**) Comparison of GABA concentration in the right striatum among experimental groups: H (3, 18) = 12.55, ($p \leq 0.005$). (**B**) GABA concentration in right prefrontal cortex among experimental group: H (3, 15) = 12.72, ($p \leq 0.005$). Data are expressed as mean ± SEM. The letters at the top the bars correspond to statistical differences among experimental groups. The data analysis was carried out through one-way non parametric ANOVA, using the Kruskall–Wallis test (common letters: non-significant differences; different letters; significant differences). QA lesion (Group II); (lesioned group with QA + transplant (QA+mBMC, Group III); and lesioned group with QA+DMEM transplant (QA+DMEM, Group IV).

4. Discussion

It has been suggested that striatum is the most affected structure in Huntington's disease, with major relevance of the spiny neurons of medium size which integrate the nucleus and main receptors of the most important connections with the cerebral cortex [13,14]. The striatum is formed by different types of neural cells, but medium-sized spiny neurons, which use GABA as a neurotransmitter, represent 90–95% of the neurons found and are its main projection cells [15]. The rest of the neuronal types of the striatum are less frequent and include neurons with long dendrites that function as interneurons and use acetylcholine as neurotransmitter. The degeneration of GABAergic cells of medium size of the striatum causes the loss of influence of the neurotransmitter GABA on their targets, affecting by different pathways the "direct" and "indirect" transmission network of the motor circuit [16–18].

In this study, the rotational activity induced by D-amphetamine was evaluated as predictive of the degree of motor deficit present in the rats. This analysis was performed either before or after the mBMC transplant. This dose-dependent motor behavior is usually accompanied by episodes of "rotations" [19,20], which are attributed to an asymmetry of dopamine activity between the lesioned and healthy striatum [21]. The typical stereotyped behavior shown by the healthy group represents a hyperkinetic reaction characteristic of an intact brain before the action of a dopaminergic agonist (data not shown). Hence, the results of this test suggest that the damaged rats developed a rotating activity ipsilateral to the lesioned hemisphere, probably associated with the loss of GABAergic projections, as has already been described by other authors [19].

On the other hand, the rotational activity induced by D-amphetamine decreased significantly in the transplant group, maintaining a certain degree of rotational activity justified by the stereotypic activity caused by D-amphetamine administration. The dopaminergic imbalance observed in the present study does not respond to the decline in the dopamine synthesis process; this dopaminergic imbalance could be related to the neuronal loss of GABAergic striatal neurons which receive the nigrostriatal dopaminergic projections [21]. It is important to emphasize the fact that the rotational behavior induced by D-amphetamine in our study is only an approximate and indirect way of studying neurodegeneration in Huntington's disease. This test only indicates the motor asymmetry that occurs in response to an imbalance in the striatum function product of the ipsilateral lesion by QA.

In this sense, previous data from our group showed that the transplant has a trophic action on the damaged tissue [22], which suggests a mechanism by which the mBMC transplant reduces the dopaminergic asymmetry between the hemispheres. The trophic support could justify the effectiveness of therapy in this area on the recovery of damaged cells, which is in line with authors agreeing on the effectiveness of mBMC transplant for improving behavior in rats lesioned with quinolinic acid [19,23].

The mechanisms by which the transplanted cells produce the recovery of normal neurochemistry in the brain are multifactorial. There is a previous report [22] with the observation that transplant cells express the NeuN protein, suggesting the transformation of them into a GABAergic neural phenotype. In another sense it is possible that the arrival of BDNF (Brain Derived Neurotrophic Factor) from other areas to the lesioned tissue contributes to the positive effect observed after the transplant. It is known that the lesion striatum can stimulate neurogenesis in the subventricular zone and produce trophic factors, including BDNF [24]. However, the possibility that the release of BDNF detected in the study reported by us [22] and that, among other actions, produces an increase in GAD (Glutamate decarboxylase), comes from the cells that are grafted and linked to the microenvironment is not excluded. On the other hand, the transplant offers an appropriate scenario to produce a positive effect in the lesioned area through the activation of other factors such as interleukins and/or growth factors. These agents guarantee the survival of nerve cells, and raise the threshold of resistance to quinolinic acid. Also, these cells are part of the immune system; protective autoimmunity effects are described as a physiological response that occurs after damage [25] that depends directly on the microenvironment where they were implanted.

Although reports of the activity of GABA and glutamate are described in experimental models [26], there is no information available on the changes in the concentration of these amino acids in the experimental model of Huntington's disease induced by quinolinic acid and the effectiveness of mBMC transplantation.

Glutamatergic synapses are the most abundant neurotransmission systems in the central nervous system of mammals [27]. The functional complexity of these synapses is reflected at the presynaptic level by the existence of multiple excitotoxicity mechanisms initiated by the activation of autoreceptors which respond well to glutamate itself or to heterorreceptors that enhance or inhibit the release of the neurotransmitter.

The striatum begins to degenerate before other brain areas, and altered activity at corticostriatal synapses contributes to an imbalance in survival versus death signaling pathways in this brain region. Striatum projection neurons of the indirect pathway are the most vulnerable, and their dysfunction contributes to motor symptoms occurring at early stages of the disease [28]. There is evidence of expression changes in striatal excitatory synaptic activity by decreasing glutamate uptake and increasing signaling at N-methyl-d-aspartate receptors (NMDAR) [29].

In this study, we show the tissue concentration of the neurotransmitters as indicative of synthesis and storage processes. In addition, in the case of the striatum, this study reflects a release process because this structure is the target of cortico-striatal glutamatergic innervation. With this argument, we support the hypothesis that the increase in the glutamate content observed in the transplanted striatum is the result of all the tissue content of the neurotransmitters. Hence, the increase in glutamate in striatum and cortex observed in our results may not be deleterious for these neuronal populations, since the result of the behavior after the transplant was beneficial. More studies must be carried out to clarify this hypothesis. On the other hand, it is observed that the DMEM alone causes an induction of glutamate release. This was an expected result considering that as DMEM contains high levels of amino acids, vitamins, and glucose, it would not be surprising for some benefit to be reported after the local application of it in the lesioned tissue. For example, and in accordance with this result, beneficial effects are reported in the literature with the injection of DMEM on the maintenance and differentiation of epithelial cells [30]. However, none of these effects is as potent as that demonstrated by the mBMC transplant.

The decrease in the concentration of GABA and glutamate in lesioned animals might be related with the injury quinolinic acid and/other eventual loss of GABAergic cells [31–33]. Since several studies show that the administration of the neurotoxin induces cytotoxic effects on various types of neurons, which could be possibly occur though glutamate and GABA recapture systems not being intact or by damage to the blood–brain barrier. In addition, the cell transplantation could produce dendritic growth associated with the appearance of intrinsic GABAergic neuronal circuits. If we take into account the abovementioned information, it is possible that transplantation is an important factor in the establishment of the architecture and the interneuronal communication. Consequently, it modifies the physiology of the synapses of GABAergic type influencing the neurotrasmition system.

GABAergic interneurons play a prominent role in the function of the cerebral cortex since they allow the synchronization of pyramidal neurons and greatly influence their differentiation and maturation during development [34]. A certain retrograde transport of quinolinic acid striatum–cortex with deleterious effects on the interneurons of that region may justify the decrease in GABA found in our study, although future studies must be conducted to corroborate this argument.

In this regard, changes in amino acids are likely to be the product initially of loss of GABAergic cells induced by the lesion at first stage. Previous studies conducted by our group show that transplanted cells survive for a prolonged period of time, producing a trophic action at the implant site [35]. It is also likely that this occurs after the transplant as result of the trophic action of the transplanted cells. In addition, in previous studies, we demonstrated the histopathological changes that occur in the brain lesioned with quinolinic acid and transplanted with mBMCs, through morphological and immunohistochemical studies [36,37]. The observation using cresyl violet allowed a general inspection of the striatal morphology in the different experimental groups, showing the normal cell distribution in this region. QA causes neuronal death and structural alterations, drastically reducing cell density and disrupting the pattern of cell distribution. On the other hand, our group demonstrated through an immunofluorescence study with GFAP and FJC (Fluoro-Jade C) staining that there was intense reactivity for GFAP [31,35] in the striatum of lesioned and DMEM-treated animals, indicating astrocytic gliosis in the tissue. Such a reaction was absent in the striatum of control and transplanted animals. A similar result was seen after marking with FJC, which stains degenerating neurons. Lesioned and DMEM-treated animals showed evidence of intense degeneration, which was not seen in control and transplanted animals. Finally, they were studied through immunofluorescence study by NeuN and FJC staining [36,37] whereby NeuN, a neuronal marker, showed positive reactivity in the control and the transplanted groups. In contrast, these groups were negative for FJC. The merged panel shows positive cellular bodies for NeuN in control and mBMC-transplanted groups, suggesting an integration of transplanted cells and even raising the possibility of neuronal differentiation among the transplanted cells, an aspect that we should consider in future experiments.

5. Conclusions

In the present study, we demonstrated that the loss of GABAergic neurons in the rat striatum as a consequence of AQ injection produces neurochemical and behavioral alterations that can be reversed with a neurorestorative treatment based on the transplantation of mononuclear bone marrow cells. Further studies will be required to understand the mechanisms by which the transplanted cells correct behavioral and neurochemical alterations produced in this model, a novel contribution of this paper.

Author Contributions: T.S.S. Conceived and designed the experiments, performed the review of the literature, and wrote the manuscript. M.E.G.F. participated in the review of the literature and in the study of amino acid determination. L.B.L. participated in the analysis of the data and the writing of the manuscript. E.A.A., B.C.F., M.d.l.Á.R.A., L.L.P and J.A.B.R. participated in the analysis of the data and revision of the manuscript.

Acknowledgments: This study was supported financially by the CIREN Scientific Council.

References

1. Dayalu, P.; Albin, R.L. Huntington disease: Pathogenesis and treatment. *Neurol. Clin.* **2015**, *33*, 101–114. [CrossRef] [PubMed]
2. Davies, S.; Ramsden, D.B. Huntington's disease. *Mol. Pathol.* **2001**, *54*, 409–413. [CrossRef] [PubMed]
3. Araujo, D.M.; Hilt, D.C. Glial cell line-derived neurotrophic factor attenuates the excitotoxin-induced behavioral and neurochemical deficits in a rodent model of Huntington's disease. *Neuroscience* **1997**, *81*, 1099–1110. [CrossRef]
4. Cox, C.S., Jr.; Hetz, R.A.; Liao, G.P.; Aertker, B.M.; Ewing-Cobbs, L.; Juranek, J.; Savitz, S.I.; Jackson, M.L.; Romanowska-Pawliczek, A.M.; Triolo, F.; et al. Treatment of Severe Adult Traumatic Brain Injury Using Bone Marrow Mononuclear Cells. *Stem Cells* **2017**, *35*, 1065–1079. [CrossRef] [PubMed]
5. Hasan, A.; Deeb, G.; Rahal, R.; Atwi, K.; Mondello, S.; Marei, H.E.; Gali, A.; Sleiman, E. Mesenchymal Stem Cells in the Treatment of Traumatic Brain Injury. *Front Neurol.* **2017**, *8*, 28. [CrossRef] [PubMed]
6. Chen, J.; Yang, Y.; Shen, L.; Ding, W.; Chen, X.; Wu, E.; Cai, K.; Wang, G. Hypoxic Preconditioning Augments the Therapeutic Efficacy of Bone Marrow Stromal Cells in a Rat Ischemic Stroke Model. *Cell. Mol. Neurobiol.* **2017**, *37*, 1115–1129. [CrossRef] [PubMed]
7. Lescaudron, L.; Unni, D.; Dunbar, G.L. Autologous adult bone marrow stem cell transplantation in an animal model of huntington's disease: Behavioral and morphological outcomes. *Int. J. Neurosci.* **2003**, *113*, 945–956. [CrossRef] [PubMed]
8. Kerkis, I.; Haddad, M.S.; Valverde, C.W.; Glosman, S. Neural and mesenchymal stem cells in animal models of Huntington's disease: Past experiences and future challenges. *Stem Cell Res. Ther.* **2015**, *6*, 232. [CrossRef] [PubMed]
9. Rossignol, J.; Fink, K.D.; Crane, A.T.; Davis, K.K.; Bombard, M.C.; Clerc, S.; Bavar, A.M.; Lowrance, S.A.; Song, C.; Witte, S.; et al. Reductions in behavioral deficits and neuropathology in the R6/2 mouse model of Huntington's disease following transplantation of bone-marrow-derived mesenchymal stem cells is dependent on passage number. *Stem Cell Res. Ther.* **2015**, *6*, 9. [CrossRef] [PubMed]
10. Woodbury, D.; Schwarz, E.J.; Prockop, D.J.; Black, I.B. Adult rat and human bone marrow stromal cells differentiate into neurons. *J. Neurosci. Res.* **2000**, *61*, 364–370. [CrossRef]
11. Ungerstedt, U.; Arbuthnott, G.W. Quantitative recording of rotational behavior in rats after 6-hydroxy-dopamine lesions of the nigrostriatal dopamine system. *Brain Res.* **1970**, *24*, 485–493. [CrossRef]
12. National Research Council (US). *National Research Council (US) Committee on Guidelines for the Care and Use of Animals in Neuroscience and Behavioral Research*; National Academies Press: Washington, DC, USA, 2003; pp. 1–224.
13. DeLong, M.; Wichmann, T. Changing views of basal ganglia circuits and circuit disorders. *Clin. EEG Neurosci.* **2010**, *41*, 61–67. [CrossRef] [PubMed]
14. DeLong, M.R.; Wichmann, T. Basal Ganglia Circuits as Targets for Neuromodulation in Parkinson Disease. *JAMA Neurol.* **2015**, *72*, 1354–1360. [CrossRef] [PubMed]
15. Ribak, C.E.; Vaughn, J.E.; Roberts, E. The GABA neurons and their axon terminals in rat corpus striatum as demonstrated by GAD immunocytochemistry. *J. Comp. Neurol.* **1979**, *187*, 261–283. [CrossRef] [PubMed]
16. Bergman, H.; Feingold, A.; Nini, A.; Raz, A.; Slovin, H.; Abeles, M.; Vaadia, E. Physiological aspects of information processing in the basal ganglia of normal and parkinsonian primates. *Trends Neurosci.* **1998**, *21*, 32–38. [CrossRef]
17. Kelly, R.M.; Strick, P.L. Macro-architecture of basal ganglia loops with the cerebral cortex: Use of rabies virus to reveal multisynaptic circuits. *Prog. Brain Res.* **2004**, *143*, 449–459. [PubMed]
18. Obeso, J.A.; Rodriguez-Oroz, M.C.; Rodriguez, M.; Lanciego, J.L.; Artieda, J.; Gonzalo, N.; Olanow, C.W. Pathophysiology of the basal ganglia in Parkinson's disease. *Trends Neurosci.* **2000**, *23*, S8–S19. [CrossRef]
19. Hantraye, P.; Riche, D.; Maziere, M.; Isacson, O. A primate model of Huntington's disease: Behavioral and anatomical studies of unilateral excitotoxic lesions of the caudate-putamen in the baboon. *Exp. Neurol.* **1990**, *108*, 91–104. [CrossRef]
20. Schwarcz, R.; Fuxe, K.; Agnati, L.F.; Hokfelt, T.; Coyle, J.T. Rotational behaviour in rats with unilateral striatal kainic acid lesions: A behavioural model for studies on intact dopamine receptors. *Brain Res.* **1979**, *170*, 485–495. [CrossRef]

21. Fuxe, K.; Janson, A.M.; Jansson, A.; Andersson, K.; Eneroth, P.; Agnati, L.F. Chronic nicotine treatment increases dopamine levels and reduces dopamine utilization in substantia nigra and in surviving forebrain dopamine nerve terminal systems after a partial di-mesencephalic hemitransection. *Naunyn Schmiedebergs Arch. Pharmacol.* **1990**, *341*, 171–181. [CrossRef] [PubMed]
22. Serrano, S.T.; Alberti, A.E.; Lorigados, P.L.; Blanco, L.L.; Diaz, A.I.; Bergado, J.A. BDNF in quinolinic acid lesioned rats after bone marrow cells transplant. *Neurosci. Lett.* **2014**, *559*, 147–151. [CrossRef] [PubMed]
23. Rossignol, J.; Fink, K.; Davis, K.; Clerc, S.; Crane, A.; Matchynski, J.; Lowrance, S.; Bombard, M.; Dekorver, N.; Lescaudron, L.; et al. Transplants of adult mesenchymal and neural stem cells provide neuroprotection and behavioral sparing in a transgenic rat model of Huntington's disease. *Stem Cells* **2014**, *32*, 500–509. [CrossRef] [PubMed]
24. Tattersfield, A.S.; Croon, R.J.; Liu, Y.W.; Kells, A.P.; Faull, R.L.; Connor, B. Neurogenesis in the striatum of the quinolinic acid lesion model of Huntington's disease. *Neuroscience* **2004**, *127*, 319–332. [CrossRef] [PubMed]
25. Del Barco, D.G.; Berlanga, J.; Penton, E.; Hardiman, O.; Montero, E. Boosting controlled autoimmunity: A new therapeutic target for CNS disorders. *Expert Rev. Neurother.* **2008**, *8*, 819–825. [CrossRef] [PubMed]
26. Haber, S.N. Neurotransmitters in the human and nonhuman primate basal ganglia. *Hum. Neurobiol.* **1986**, *5*, 159–168. [PubMed]
27. Moberly, A.H.; Czarnecki, L.A.; Pottackal, J.; Rubinstein, T.; Turkel, D.J.; Kass, M.D.; McGann, J.P. Intranasal exposure to manganese disrupts neurotransmitter release from glutamatergic synapses in the central nervous system in vivo. *Neurotoxicology* **2012**, *33*, 996–1004. [CrossRef] [PubMed]
28. Van, D.E.; Reedeker, N.; Giltay, E.J.; Eindhoven, D.; Roos, R.A.; van der Mast, R.C. Course of irritability, depression and apathy in Huntington's disease in relation to motor symptoms during a two-year follow-up period. *Neurodegener. Dis.* **2014**, *13*, 9–16.
29. Lau, A.; Tymianski, M. Glutamate receptors, neurotoxicity and neurodegeneration. *Pflugers Arch.* **2010**, *460*, 525–542. [CrossRef] [PubMed]
30. Ahmado, A.; Carr, A.J.; Vugler, A.A.; Semo, M.; Gias, C.; Lawrence, J.M.; Chen, L.L.; Chen, F.K.; Turowski, P.; da Cruz, L.; Coffey, P.J. Induction of differentiation by pyruvate and DMEM in the human retinal pigment epithelium cell line ARPE-19. *Investig. Ophthalmol. Vis. Sci.* **2011**, *52*, 7148–7159. [CrossRef] [PubMed]
31. Braidy, N.; Grant, R.; Adams, S.; Brew, B.J.; Guillemin, G.J. Mechanism for quinolinic acid cytotoxicity in human astrocytes and neurons. *Neurotox. Res.* **2009**, *16*, 77–86. [CrossRef] [PubMed]
32. Guillemin, G.J. Quinolinic acid, the inescapable neurotoxin. *FEBS J.* **2012**, *279*, 1356–1365. [CrossRef] [PubMed]
33. St'astny, F.; Lisy, V.; Mares, V.; Lisa, V.; Balcar, V.J.; Santamaria, A. Quinolinic acid induces NMDA receptor-mediated lipid peroxidation in rat brain microvessels. *Redox. Rep.* **2004**, *9*, 229–233. [CrossRef] [PubMed]
34. Marin, O. Origin of cortical interneurons: Basic concepts and clinical implications. *Rev. Neurol.* **2002**, *35*, 743–751. [PubMed]
35. Alberti, E.; Los, M.; Garcia, R.; Fraga, J.L.; Serrano, T.; Hernandez, E.; Klonisch, T.; Macias, R.; Martinez, L.; Castillo, L.; de la Cuétara, K. Prolonged survival and expression of neural markers by bone marrow-derived stem cells transplanted into brain lesions. *Med. Sci. Monit.* **2009**, *15*, BR47–BR54. [PubMed]
36. Serrano, T.; Pierozan, P.; Alberti, E.; Blanco, L.; de la Cuétara Bernal, K.; González, M.E.; Pavón, N.; Lorigados, L.; Robinson-Agramonte, M.A.; Bergado, J.A. Transplantation of mononuclear cells from bone marrow in a rat model of Huntington's disease. *Neurorestoratology* **2016**, *4*, 95–105. [CrossRef]
37. Teresa, S.-S. Havana: International Center for Neurological Restoration (CIREN). Ph.D. Thesis, Cuba University, Havana, Cuba, 2017.

11

Astrocytic IL-6 Influences the Clinical Symptoms of EAE in Mice

Maria Erta [1,2], Mercedes Giralt [1,2], Silvia Jiménez [1], Amalia Molinero [1,2], Gemma Comes [1,2] and Juan Hidalgo [1,2,*]

1 Department of Cellular Biology, Physiology and Immunology, Animal Physiology Unit, Faculty of Biosciences, Universitat Autònoma de Barcelona, Bellaterra 08193, Spain; mariaerta@gmail.com (M.E.); merce.giralt@uab.es (M.G.); siljiba@gmail.com (S.J.); amalia.molinero@uab.es (A.M.); gemma.comes@uab.es (G.C.)

2 Institute of Neurosciences, Universitat Autònoma de Barcelona, Bellaterra 08193, Spain

* Correspondence: Juan.Hidalgo@uab.es

Academic Editor: Donna Gruol

Abstract: Interleukin-6 (IL-6) is a multifunctional cytokine that not only plays major roles in the immune system, but also serves as a coordinator between the nervous and endocrine systems. IL-6 is produced in multiple cell types in the CNS, and in turn, many cells respond to it. It is therefore important to ascertain which cell type is the key responder to IL-6 during both physiological and pathological conditions. In order to test the role of astrocytic IL-6 in neuroinflammation, we studied an extensively-used animal model of multiple sclerosis, experimental autoimmune encephalomyelitis (EAE), in mice with an IL-6 deficiency in astrocytes (Ast-IL-6 KO). Results indicate that lack of astrocytic IL-6 did not cause major changes in EAE symptomatology. However, a delay in the onset of clinical signs was observed in Ast-IL-6 KO females, with fewer inflammatory infiltrates and decreased demyelination and some alterations in gliosis and vasogenesis, compared to floxed mice. These results suggest that astrocyte-secreted IL-6 has some roles in EAE pathogenesis, at least in females.

Keywords: interleukin-6; astrocyte; EAE

1. Introduction

Interleukin 6 (IL-6) is a multifunctional four-helix bundle cytokine, originally identified as a B-cell differentiation factor in 1985 [1], which has been linked to numerous biological functions. It is now known to be one of the main cytokines controlling the immune system, and in addition, it acts as a coordinator between the nervous and endocrine systems. IL-6 plays an essential role in the central nervous system (CNS) in many physiological, inflammatory and disease conditions, being able to exert dual actions (for a review, see [2]). Although many cells in the CNS produce IL-6 [3], astrocytes are the main producer [2,4].

Multiple sclerosis (MS) is one of the most common inflammatory disorders of the CNS and a leading cause of disability in young adults. It is estimated that 2–2.5 million people are currently living with this demyelinating disease worldwide [5]. Its pathological hallmarks consist of local demyelination, inflammation and variable axonal destruction. Experimental autoimmune encephalomyelitis (EAE) [6] is a well-known animal model to study this inflammatory condition. Cytokines are key mediators in the pathogenesis of inflammatory lesions in CNS, presenting both helpful and harmful effects [7]. IL-6 plays a crucial role in MS as demonstrated by its presence in acute and chronic active plaques of MS patients [8]. In addition, it has been shown that IL-6-deficient mice are resistant to EAE [9–13] presumably because of a lack of differentiation of naive T cells into MOG-specific T helper cells producing IL-17 (Th17) and the subsequent reduction of their infiltration into the CNS [14], although the exact mechanism is not fully understood.

A thorough understanding of the role of the cellular context in this and other diseases is necessary to clarify the putative roles of IL-6 in the CNS [15,16]. We recently characterized the role of astrocytic IL-6 in normal (basal) conditions by using transgenic mice with astrocyte-specific IL-6 deficiency, showing effects on behavior and body weight in a sex-dependent manner [17,18]. The role of astrocytic IL-6 during pathological situations remained to be assessed, and here, we report the initial studies with EAE.

2. Materials and Methods

2.1. Animals

The generation of astrocyte-IL-6 KO (Ast-IL6 KO) and floxed littermate mice, which served as controls, was as described previously [17]. A number of studies have shown that GFAP is primarily expressed in astrocytes of the CNS, with minimal expression in peripheral regions [19]. All mice were kept under constant temperature with free access to food (Harlan global diet 2918) and water. Ethical approval for the use and experimentation of all mice in this study was obtained from the Animal and Human Experimentation Ethics Committee of the Universitat Autònoma de Barcelona (nº 4017, approved 3 September 2015).

2.2. EAE Induction and Clinical Evaluation

For the induction of EAE, two-month-old male and female mice were used. EAE was induced by active immunization with $MOG_{35–55}$ peptide. On Day 0, all mice, under isoflurane anesthesia, were injected subcutaneously into the hind flanks with an emulsion of 100 μL $MOG_{35–55}$ (3 mg/mL) and 100 μL Complete Freund's Adjuvant (CFA) (Sigma-Aldrich, St. Louis, MO, USA) supplemented with 4 mg/mL *Mycobacterium tuberculosis* H37RA (Difco, Detroit, MI, USA). In addition, animals received an intraperitoneal injection of 500 ng pertussis toxin (Sigma-Aldrich, St. Louis, MO, USA), which was repeated two days later.

After immunization, mice were examined daily, weighed and scored for EAE. The EAE clinical score was assessed for each animal according to the following criteria: 0 = no signs of disease, 0.5 = partial loss of tail tonus, 1 = loss of tail tonus, 2 = moderate hind limb paraparesis, 2.5 = severe hind limb paraparesis, 3 = partial hind limb paralysis, 3.5 = hind limb paralysis, 4 = hind limb paralysis plus partial front leg paralysis, 4.5 = moribund/total paralysis and 5 = death. Finally, for each animal, we determined the time to disease onset (clinical score $\geqslant$1), time to peak disease, peak-score, cumulative score (sum of all scores from disease onset to Day 20) and grade of remission (difference between peak score and outcome).

Three independent EAE experiments were carried out (Table 1). Experiment 1 was carried out for 0–22 days post-immunization (dpi); Experiment 2 was carried out for 0–20 dpi; and Experiment 3 was carried out for 0–46 dpi. For each experiment, littermates were used. Female mice from 20–22 dpi were grouped before comparison to 46 dpi mice. Male Ast-IL-6 KO mice did not differ from male floxed mice at 20–22 dpi and, thus, were not examined at 46 dpi. In all cases, all surviving mice were euthanized at the indicated days post-immunization by decapitation. Spinal cords were immediately removed and fixed for 48 h in 4% paraformaldehyde and embedded in paraffin for immunohistochemistry (IHC) and histochemistry (HC) analyses. Spinal cords from additional healthy female mice were processed in parallel.

Table 1. Number of mice per genotype, sex and experiment.

Genotype	Experiment 1 (0–22 dpi)		Experiment 2 (0–20 dpi)		Experiment 3 (0–46 dpi)
	Males	Females	Males	Females	Females
Floxed	7	3	11	17	8
Ast-IL-6 KO	3	7	8	8	8

dpi, days post-immunization; Ast, astrocyte.

2.3. IHC and HC Analysis

Embedded paraffin tissues were cut into 8 μm-wide sections in a microtome (Leica, Germany) and mounted in Superfrost slides (Thermo Scientific, Waltham, MA, USA).

Microglia were identified by lectin HC (tomato lectin from *Lycopersicon esculentum*, Sigma-Aldrich 1:500 in Tris-buffered saline (TBS) with 0.5% triton X-100 (TBS-t)). Astrocytes were identified by GFAP IHC (rabbit anti-Glial Fibrillary Acidic Protein from DakoCytomation Denmark, 1:1200 in blocking buffer). Lymphocytes were identified by CD3 IHC (rabbit anti-human CD3, Dako A0452, 1:100 in blocking buffer). Spinal cord sections were also stained with hematoxylin-eosin and with Luxol Fast Blue solution (LFB) (0.1%, overnight al 37 °C) and counterstained with Cresyl violet (0.1%, 1 min), to assess the number of cellular infiltrates and demyelination in grey matter, respectively.

Sections for IHC and HC were preincubated for 1 h with the blocking buffer (0.5% BSA in TBS-t) and then incubated with the primary antibodies (GFAP, CD3) or tomato lectin overnight at 4 °C, followed by 1 h at room temperature (RT) (GFAP, CD3) or at 37 °C (lectin). For CD3 IHC, a previous antigen retrieval step was performed with protease type XIV (Sigma P5147). After washing in TBS, sections were incubated with either horseradish peroxidase-coupled streptavidin (Vector Labs, Burlingame, CA, USA, 1:600, 1 h) for HC or biotinylated secondary antibody (Vector Labs, Burlingame, CA, USA, 1:300, 1 h at RT) followed by washes and horseradish peroxidase-coupled streptavidin (Vector Labs, Burlingame, CA, USA, 1:600, 1 h) for IHC. The immunoreactivity was visualized by using 0.033% H_2O_2 in 0.5 mg/mL 3,3-diaminobenzidine-tetrahydrochloride (DAB) in Tris buffer (TB) for 4–30 min at room temperature. Reaction was stopped with TB, washed, dehydrated and mounted in DPX (distyrene-plasticiser-xylene) (Sigma, St Louis, MO, USA). Images at 100× (GFAP) or 200× (lectin, CD3) were taken in a bright field Nikon Eclipse 90i microscope (Nikon Instruments Europe BV, Amsterdam, The Netherlands) and acquired with a Nikon digital camera DXm1200F (Nikon Instruments Europe BV, Amsterdam, The Netherlands) and Nikon Act-1 version 2.70 software (Nikon Instruments Europe BV, Amsterdam, The Netherlands) from different brain areas and spinal cord. Finally, to quantify staining areas, intensity and the number of cells, images were analyzed using ImageJ software (NIH, Bethesda, MD, USA). Histological analyses were performed on at least two sections per mouse. Control sections for non-specific binding analysis (where primary antibody or tomato lectin was not used) were included routinely.

For GFAP IHC, the percentage of stained area (at 100×) was measured in different regions of the spinal cord from EAE-induced mice. Six to twelve images per animal were examined. White and grey matter areas of spinal cords were also analyzed (12 images per animal and area). A threshold was set for each area to better define cells from tissue background. Because tomato lectin HC stains both microglia and vessels, the quantification of staining using ImageJ was supplemented with manual counts of microglial cells showing a basal (ramified), reactive or fully-activated (round) morphology and of the number of vessels; these were assessed in the same regions as for GFAP IHC analysis, at 200×. In addition, total numbers of microglia/macrophage infiltration areas in spinal cord were recorded. For CD3 IHC, the percentage of stained area was measured in the spinal cord (10 images per area and animal). In LFB/Cresyl violet staining, total numbers of cellular infiltrates in grey matter of spinal cord were counted, and afterwards, a color deconvolution plugin from ImageJ software was used in order to separate colors from LFB and Cresyl violet to be able to quantify the demyelination by analyzing the percentage of LFB-stained area in spinal cord. The threshold set gave 100% of area of the spinal cord covered by LFB staining for healthy female mice. To standardize, the same threshold was used for female and male mice. Demyelination and a decrease of the area covered by LFB caused by EAE were readily detected in both male and female mice.

2.4. Statistical Analysis

Values in text and figures are shown as the mean ± standard error of the mean (SEM). Statistical analyses were performed using SPSS statistical software (version 17.0 for Windows, SPSS Inc., Chicago, IL, USA). $p \leqslant 0.05$ was considered significant in all analyses.

For clinical evaluations and body weight changes, we used the general linear model (GzLM) for repeated measures, the generalized estimated equations test (GEE), with genotype (floxed *vs.* Ast-IL-6 KO mice) and sex as the main factors. The *post-hoc* Student *t*-test or the Mann–Whitney *U*-test was used to identify significant differences between Ast-IL-6 KO and floxed animals at specific time periods. For the remaining variables analyzed, two-way ANOVA (with genotype and sex as the main factors) or GzLM was used for each sex separately followed by *post-hoc* tests when appropriate.

3. Results

3.1. Lack of Astrocytic IL-6 Alters the Clinical Course of EAE in Ast-IL-6 KO Mice and Ameliorates EAE Symptomatology in a Sex-Dependent Manner

Both genotypes showed the prototypical ascending paralysis course with body weight loss (Figure 1). The clinical score and the body weight changes observed following MOG_{35-55} immunization up to 20 dpi in the Ast-IL6 KO and floxed mice are shown in Figure 1. Ast-IL6 KO females showed a significantly reduced clinical score and increased body weight with respect to female floxed mice, a genotypic difference that was not observed in the male mice. Average incidence of the disease ranged from 90% to 100%, and there were no significant differences in mortality rate (Table 2).

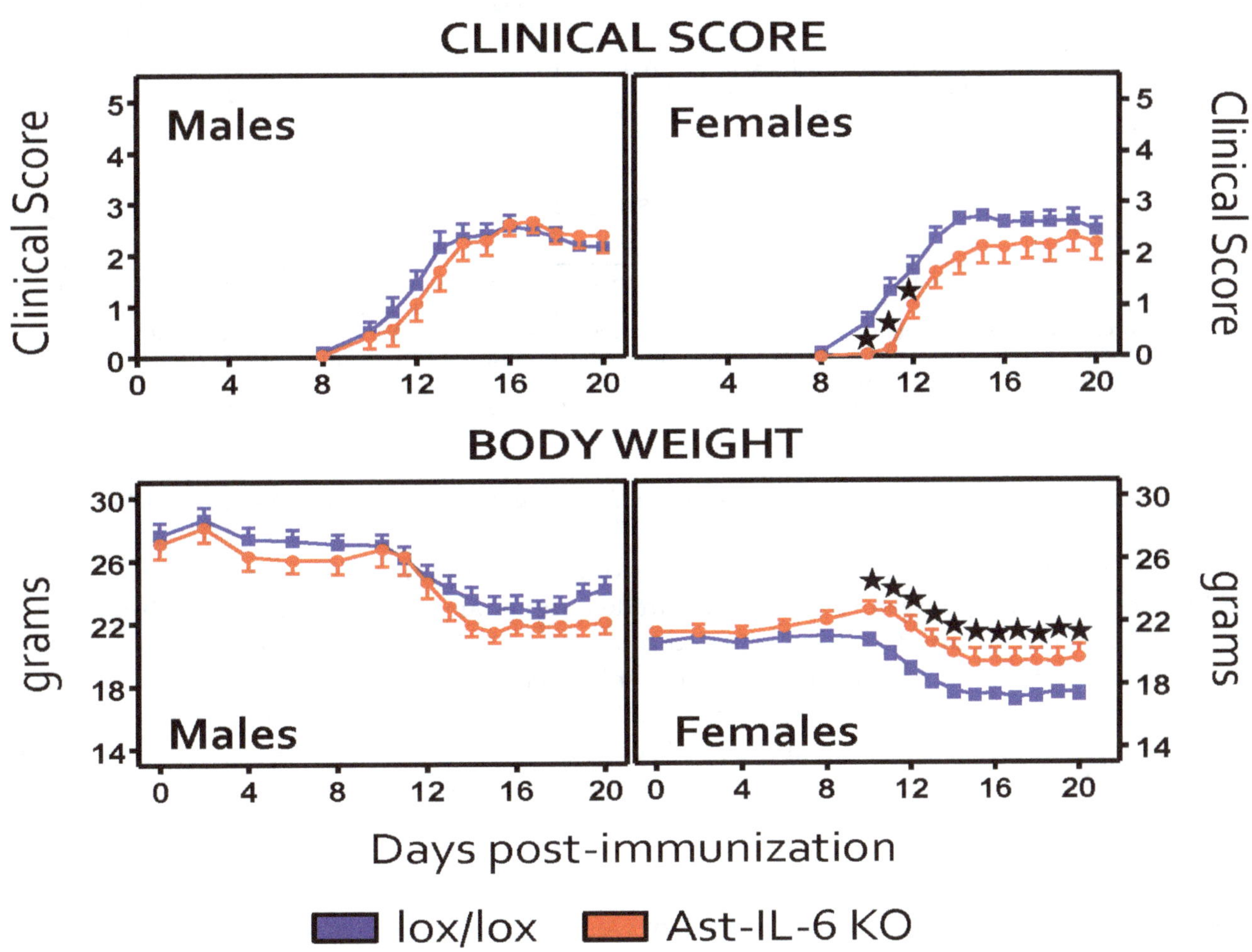

Figure 1. Clinical course of EAE, in both floxed (n = 18 males, 28 females) and Ast-IL-6 KO (n = 11 males, 23 females) mice up to 20 dpi. Results are the mean ± SEM of data pooled from Experiments 1–3 (Days 0–20 dpi; Table 1). ★ p at least <0.05 *versus* floxed mice at specific days following a *post-hoc* analysis.

Table 2. EAE disease.

EAE	Females		Males	
	Ast-IL-6 KO	**Floxed**	**Ast-IL-6 KO**	**Floxed**
Incidence	21/23	28/28	11/11	17/18
Mortality	3/23	0/28	0/11	0/18
Day of onset	13.38 ± 0.59 *	11.57 ± 0.29	12.27 ± 0.52 *	11.65 ± 0.49

Results shown are pooled data from Experiments 1–3 separated by sex and genotype. For each animal, time to disease onset was defined by a clinical score ⩾1. For statistical analysis, a two-way ANOVA for genotype (floxed *vs.* Ast-IL-6 KO mice) and sex as the main factors was performed. * $p < 0.05$ *vs.* floxed mice.

When the day of disease onset was analyzed using sex and genotype as the main factors, a significant genotypic difference was observed for both sexes (Table 2). In contrast, the peak score, cumulative score and grade of remission at 20 dpi were not different between genotypes for either sex (Table 3). These results suggest that while the disease is delayed and the severity is somewhat lower at the early stages in female mice, it is not affected by astrocytic IL-6 deficiency later on.

Table 3. EAE clinical course.

Clinical Course	Females (0–20 dpi)		Females (46 dpi)		Males (0–20 dpi)	
	Ast-IL-6 KO (n = 15)	**Floxed (n = 20)**	**Ast-IL-6 KO (n = 8)**	**Floxed (n = 8)**	**Ast-IL-6 KO (n = 11)**	**Floxed (n = 18)**
Time of peak score	14.30 ± 0.53	14.80 ± 0.49	22.5 ± 2.46 *	15.5 ± 1.92	15.18 ± 0.80	13.76 ± 0.6
Peak score	2.80 ± 0.23	3.45 ± 0.16	3.68 ± 0.50	3.18 ± 0.23	3.18 ± 0.18	3.14 ± 0.12
Cumulative score	19.40 ± 2.55	24.16 ± 1.32	88.87 ± 21.84	72.18 ± 10.35	20.32 ± 1.64	22.61 ± 1.34
Grade of Remission	0.64 ± 0.13	0.91 ± 0.11	1.00 ± 0.34	1.43 ± 0.27	0.82 ± 0.26	20.32 ± 1.64

Results shown are pooled data from Experiments 1–3 separated by sex and genotype. For simplicity, data from 20–22 dpi were grouped and are referred to as 20 dpi. For each animal, we determined time to peak disease, peak-score, cumulative score (sum of all scores from disease onset to Days 20 and 22 combined or 46), and the grade of remission (difference between peak score and outcome). Results are the mean ± SEM. For statistical analysis at 0–20 dpi, a two-way ANOVA for genotype (floxed *vs.* Ast-IL-6 KO mice) and sex as the main factors was performed. For the females at 46 dpi, a one-way ANOVA for genotype (floxed *vs.* Ast-IL-6 KO mice) was performed. * $p < 0.05$ *vs.* floxed mice.

3.2. Reduced Cellular Infiltrates and Demyelination in the Spinal Cord of Ast-IL-6 KO Female Mice

The number of inflammatory infiltrates in the longitudinal lumbar-cervical spinal cord of control and EAE-induced animals was assessed in females and males at 20–22 dpi (for simplicity, data from 20–22 dpi were grouped and are referred to as 20 dpi). Females were also assessed at 46 dpi (Figure 2A,C). The total number of infiltrates in white matter was counted in a Cresyl violet/Luxol Fast Blue staining and in a CD3 IHC counterstained with hematoxylin; a mean value of both stainings was then calculated for each animal and used for statistical analysis. As shown in Figure 2A, there is a significant decrease in the number of infiltrates in Ast-IL6 KO females at both 20–22 and 46 dpi compared to floxed female mice. Ast-IL-6 KO males did not show a significant difference compared to floxed males (Figure 2A).

Demyelination in spinal cord white matter was assessed measuring the percentage of Luxol Fast Blue-stained area (Figure 2B,C). Healthy animals (0 dpi) had 100% area covered by LFB staining. Following EAE, Ast-IL-6 KO females showed a significantly lower Luxol Fast Blue-stained area, indicating greater demyelination, compared to floxed female mice at 20 dpi, but not at 46 dpi (Figure 2B). Ast-IL-6 KO males did not show a significant difference in Luxol Fast Blue-stained area compared to floxed males (Figure 2B).

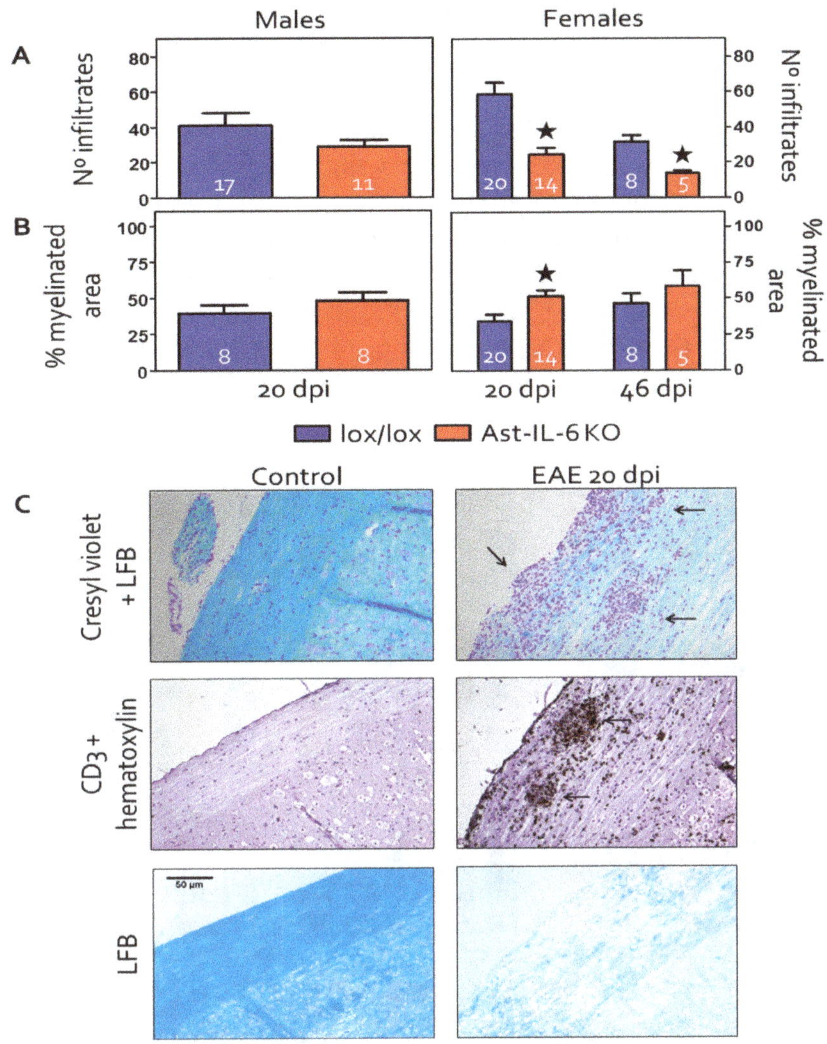

Figure 2. Assessment of the total number of cellular infiltrates (**A**) and demyelination (**B**) in the longitudinal lumbar-cervical spinal cord white matter from EAE-induced animals at 20 dpi (for both females and males Ast-IL6 KO and floxed mice) and 46 dpi (females). Number of mice per group as indicated. ★ $p < 0.05$ between Ast-IL6 KO and floxed mice. (**C**) Representative sections from female mice showing infiltrates (arrows) in spinal cord stained with Cresyl violet (top) and CD3 (middle) in non-immunized (control) and immunized (20 dpi) floxed mice. The bottom panel shows the demyelination of the spinal cord as revealed by Luxol Fast Blue (LFB) staining following color deconvolution. All images at magnification 100×.

3.3. Reduced Gliosis and Vasogenesis in Spinal Cord and Brain of EAE-Induced Ast-IL-6 KO Females

Gliosis was evaluated by GFAP (astrocytes) and lectin (microglia) staining in the spinal cord of the EAE-induced mice (Figure 3A,B,D). The area occupied by GFAP immunostaining was measured in both the grey and white matter (Figure 3A). A significant decrease in GFAP immunostaining in grey matter was observed in Ast-IL-6 KO female mice compared to floxed female mice at 46 dpi, accompanied by a less reactive morphology of astrocytes (Figure 3D, top, left inset). No genotypic difference in GFAP immunostaining was observed for females or males in grey matter at 20 dpi or in the white matter for females and males at the times studied.

Regarding microgliosis in spinal cord (Figure 3D, bottom), quantification of the occupied area did not show significant differences between genotypes (data not shown). As quantification of lectin staining is not able to separate microglia from blood vessels, the number of microglia was counted. No significant genotypic difference in the number of microglia was observed for either females or males in both the grey and white matter of the spinal cord at the days studied (Figure 3B). These results indicated that astrocytic IL-6 deficiency did not impact microgliosis in either the grey or white matter of the spinal cord.

Finally, vasogenesis was analyzed by counting lectin-stained vessels in the spinal cord of EAE-induced mice (Figure 3D, bottom, arrows and insets). In female mice, the number of vessels in the white matter was significantly reduced in Ast-IL-6 KO mice compared to floxed mice at both 20–22 and 46 dpi (Figure 3C). No genotypic difference was observed for the number of vessels in the white matter for males or for the number of vessels in the grey matter for females and males at the times studied.

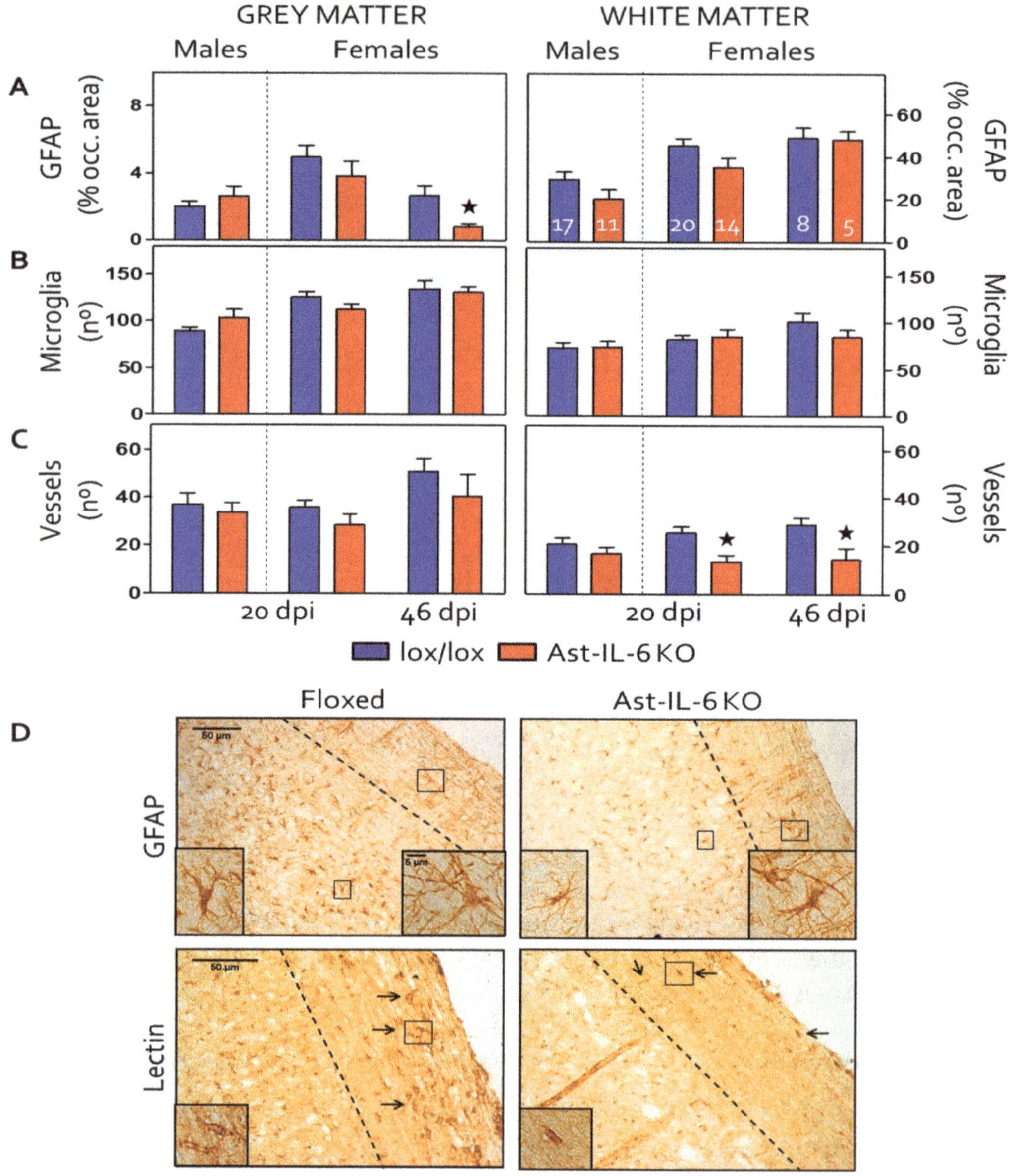

Figure 3. (**A–C**) Results from GFAP and lectin stainings in the spinal cord (grey and white matter) of EAE-induced animals at 20 dpi (for both females and males Ast-IL6 KO and floxed mice) and 46 dpi (females). Number of mice per group as indicated. GFAP overall immunostaining (**A**) and the number of lectin-positive microglia (**B**) and vessels (**C**) are shown. ⋆ $p < 0.05$ *vs.* floxed mice. (**D**) Representative GFAP at 100× (top) and lectin at 150× (bottom) stainings of 46 and 20 dpi females, respectively. Arrows indicate vessels. The discontinuous line separates grey matter (left) from white matter (right). All inserts are at 400×; at the top they, show astrocytic morphology in both grey and white matter, and at the bottom, they show a vessel.

4. Discussion

IL-6 is implicated in the pathogenesis of autoimmune disorders, such as MS in humans [20,21]. A critical role of IL-6 in the animal model of MS, EAE, has been demonstrated by a number of studies: systemic IL-6 KO mice are resistant to EAE [9–13], and neutralization of IL-6 with antibodies leads to a reduced disease [22], by not well-defined mechanisms. Moreover, studies have demonstrated that the transgenic expression of IL-6 in the CNS by viral systems reduces EAE [23] and that the systemic administration of IL-6 also reduces the clinical symptoms in a viral model of EAE [24]. Thus, IL-6 can potentiate, but also inhibit EAE, reflecting the complexity of its actions. Key questions remain, however, including the identity of the key cell types that produce and respond to IL-6 and whether the critical actions of IL-6 are peripheral or central.

Because the production of IL-6 during the course of EAE arises from diverse cellular sources both in the periphery and in the CNS, the specific contribution of each source of IL-6 to the development of the disease needs to be established. We have previously demonstrated a role of CNS IL-6 in regulating EAE, because mice expressing IL-6 only by astrocytes (GFAP-IL6-IL-6 KO mice) were capable of developing the atypical EAE known to occur in GFAP-IL6 mice [13]. Furthermore, in adoptive transfer experiments, EAE is less severe in IL-6KO mice than in wild-type mice, which suggests that IL-6 locally mediates the disease in the CNS [10]. Thus, although EAE has always been considered a disease mostly induced peripherally, it seems that CNS IL-6 may also play an important role. Because astrocytic IL-6 plays a major role in neuroinflammation [25,26] and because astrocytes are the most abundant cell in the CNS, astrocytic IL-6 seemed to be an excellent candidate to examine as the key regulator of EAE in the CNS.

We have previously shown that compared to floxed mice, Ast-IL-6 KO mice exhibit a number of altered behaviors under normal (basal) conditions, including changes in activity, anxiety and learning; a prosurvival role of astrocytic IL-6 is also apparent [17,18]. Here, we present results from studies involving a neuropathological condition, $MOG_{35–55}$-induced EAE. In contrast to results in systemic IL-6 KO mice, astrocytic-specific IL-6 deficiency is unable to prevent typical signs of EAE induction and has no prominent neuropathologic effects. However, astrocyte IL-6 KO mice did show significant delays of the onset of the EAE, at least in female mice, ameliorating the clinical signs in the early stages of EAE.

Autoreactive T-cells can result in inflammatory demyelination of the CNS, and knowing that the frequency of Tregs in MS patients is unchanged from controls [27] (although their function is impaired) could be a clue to the decreased demyelination seen only in Ast-IL-6 KO females, the only group that presented a decrease in T lymphocyte infiltration. Thus, a lower EAE score at early stages could be due to an initial impaired T cell infiltration of the CNS. This possibility is consistent with our results showing that Ast-IL-6 KO female (but not male) mice had a decreased number of infiltrates in the spinal cord and lower scores for clinical signs. However, it is important to note that we only carried out Cresyl violet and CD3 immunostaining for T cells, so we cannot rule out that a change in T cell subpopulations is responsible for the different clinical signs observed in Ast-IL-6 KO female mice. IL-6 has a major role in Th17 cell differentiation from naive $CD4^+$ T-cells (reviewed in [28]), particularly in the EAE model [14,29]. EAE-resistant IL-6 KO mice show a deficiency in Th17 cell infiltrates in the CNS [30]. When responsiveness to IL-6 is experimentally eliminated in T helper cells, mice show resistance to EAE induction, as the IL-21 pathway is intact, but not active in the absence of IL-6 signaling [31]. Th17 cells produce IL-17 (among other cytokines), which enhances IL-6 production by astrocytes, which, in turn, induces the differentiation of Th17 cells in a positive feed-back loop between IL-17 and IL-6 via activation of NF-κB and STAT-3 [32,33]. This loop may be compromised in our Ast-IL-6 KO animals, where astrocyte production of IL-6 has been eliminated. However, since Ast-IL-6 KO mice only show a delay in EAE, but are not resistant to EAE, we can speculate that this astrocytic loop is not necessary for the development of the disease; and/or that neuronal, endothelial and microglial IL-6 could instead allow this positive feedback between IL-17 and IL-6. In order to test these hypotheses, a detailed study of the exact lymphocytic population present in the infiltrates would be important, particularly with further backcrossing to C57/Bl6 mice.

Somewhat surprisingly, considering the importance of astrocytic IL-6 in neuroinflammation [2,4,25,26], we did not observe dramatic effects of astrocytic IL-6 deficiency on either astrocytes or microglia at the times studied. This result makes it unlikely that changes in glial cell reactivity are underlying the differences in clinical signs between Ast-IL-6 KO mice and floxed mice. Nevertheless, overall staining and cell morphologies are limited approaches, and more detailed studies are needed to assess other roles of glial cells (other than IL-6 production by astrocytes) in clinical signs of EAE. Finally, regarding the number of vessels, we observed a decrease in Ast-IL-6 KO mice, which is in agreement with results in mice overexpressing IL-6, which show extensive revascularization, both in basal conditions [25,26] and after an injury [34], indicative of a role of IL-6 in vasogenesis. Other studies also support the idea that IL-6 promotes vasogenesis [35]. Probably, this is secondary to the number and/or type of inflammatory cells present in the spinal cord, since no differences were observed in male mice.

The extent of the reduction of IL-6 in astrocytes of the Ast-IL-6 KO mice *in vivo* has yet to be determined. However, studies of cultured astrocytes from the Ast-IL-6 KO mice demonstrated that the astrocytes are deficient in IL-6 production. In these studies, analysis of culture supernatant after 24 h of stimulation (10 ng/mL of LPS and 10 ng/mL of INF-γ) showed that astrocytes from floxed mice produced approximately 13 ng/mL of IL-6, whereas astrocytes from Ast-IL-6 KO mice only produced 2 ng/mL IL-6 [17,18]. Regardless of the extent of the astrocytic IL-6 deficiency in the Ast-IL-6 KO mice, a delay in onset to clinical symptoms was evident in females, including less demyelination at 20–22 dpi in accordance with the lower clinical scores. However, this was a transient effect, and sometime after 20–22 dpi, the EAE was similar in both genotypes (as indicated by the lack of significant differences in demyelination at 46 dpi), indicating the astrocytic IL-6 no longer played a role.

5. Conclusions

In conclusion, we have shown that lack of astrocytic IL-6 is not sufficient to prevent EAE disease, but it is able to delay the disease and to ameliorate clinical scoring and the inflammatory milieu in female mice. These results support the idea that the local CNS production of IL-6 is important in this disease. Several interesting questions remain to be addressed. For example, due to the delayed onset of clinical signs of disease in Ast-IL-6 KO females, it will be important to analyze in detail the priming and inflammatory infiltrates in the CNS of female and male Ast-IL-6 KO mice and their floxed controls. Furthermore, studies of males at later dpi may reveal genotypic differences at later stages. Moreover, a comparison of the immunized Ast-IL-6 KO and floxed mice with a CFA immunized control group could reveal specific EAE effects in Ast-ILK-6 KO mice. Future studies will address these and other relevant issues relative to the role of astrocytic IL-6 in the EAE.

Acknowledgments: This work was supported by SAF2011-23272 and SFA2014-56546-R to Juan Hidalgo. Maria Erta gratefully acknowledges a PhD fellowship from Universitat Autònoma de Barcelona.

Author Contributions: M.E., M.G., S.J., A.M. and G.C. were involved in several aspects of the experiments carried out. M.E. led most of the experimental work. J.H. conceived of the experiments. M.E. and J.H. wrote the paper.

References

1. Hirano, T.; Taga, T.; Nakano, N.; Yasukawa, K.; Kashiwamura, S.; Shimizu, K.; Nakajima, K.; Pyun, K.H.; Kishimoto, T. Purification to homogeneity and characterization of human B-cell differentiation factor (BCDF or BSFp-2). *Proc. Natl. Acad. Sci. USA* **1985**, *82*, 5490–5494. [CrossRef] [PubMed]
2. Gruol, D.L.; Nelson, T.E. Physiological and pathological roles of interleukin-6 in the central nervous system. *Mol. Neurobiol.* **1997**, *15*, 307–339. [CrossRef] [PubMed]
3. Schöbitz, B.; de Kloet, E.R.; Sutanto, W.; Holsboer, F. Cellular localization of interleukin 6 mRNA and interleukin 6 receptor mrna in rat brain. *Eur. J. Neurosci.* **1993**, *5*, 1426–1435. [CrossRef] [PubMed]

4. Van Wagoner, N.J.; Benveniste, E.N. Interleukin-6 expression and regulation in astrocytes. *J. Neuroimmunol.* **1999**, *100*, 124–139. [CrossRef]
5. Milo, R.; Kahana, E. Multiple sclerosis: Geoepidemiology, genetics and the environment. *Autoimmun. Rev.* **2010**, *9*, A387–A394. [CrossRef] [PubMed]
6. Baxter, A.G. The origin and application of experimental autoimmune encephalomyelitis. *Nat. Rev. Immunol.* **2007**, *7*, 904–912. [CrossRef] [PubMed]
7. Merrill, J.E.; Benveniste, E.N. Cytokines in inflammatory brain lesions: Helpful and harmful. *Trends Neurosci.* **1996**, *19*, 331–338. [CrossRef]
8. Maimone, D.; Guazzi, G.C.; Annunziata, P. IL-6 detection in multiple sclerosis brain. *J. Neurol. Sci.* **1997**, *146*, 59–65. [CrossRef]
9. Eugster, H.-P.; Frei, K.; Kopf, M.; Lassmann, H.; Fontana, A. IL-6 deficient mice resist myelin oligodendrocyte glycoprotein-induced autoimmune encephalomyelitis. *Eur. J. Immunol.* **1998**, *28*, 2178–2187. [CrossRef]
10. Mendel, I.; Katz, A.; Kozak, N.; Ben-Nun, A.; Revel, M. Interleukin-6 functions in autoimmune encephalomyelitis: A study in gene-targeted mice. *Eur. J. Immunol.* **1998**, *28*, 1727–1737. [CrossRef]
11. Okuda, Y.; Sakoda, S.; Bernard, C.C.; Fujimura, H.; Saeki, Y.; Kishimoto, T.; Yanagihara, T. IL-6-deficient mice are resistant to the induction of experimental autoimmune encephalomyelitis provoked by myelin oligodendrocyte glycoprotein. *Int. Immunol.* **1998**, *10*, 703–708. [CrossRef] [PubMed]
12. Samoilova, E.B.; Horton, J.L.; Hilliard, B.; Liu, T.S.; Chen, Y. IL-6-deficient mice are resistant to experimental autoimmune encephalomyelitis: Roles of IL-6 in the activation and differentiation of autoreactive T cells. *J. Immunol.* **1998**, *161*, 6480–6486. [PubMed]
13. Giralt, M.; Ramos, R.; Quintana, A.; Ferrer, B.; Erta, M.; Castro-Freire, M.; Comes, G.; Sanz, E.; Unzeta, M.; Pifarré, P.; *et al.* Induction of atypical EAE mediated by transgenic production of IL-6 in astrocytes in the absence of systemic IL-6. *Glia* **2013**, *61*, 587–600. [CrossRef] [PubMed]
14. Serada, S.; Fujimoto, M.; Mihara, M.; Koike, N.; Ohsugi, Y.; Nomura, S.; Yoshida, H.; Nishikawa, T.; Terabe, F.; Ohkawara, T.; *et al.* IL-6 blockade inhibits the induction of myelin antigen-specific Th17 cells and Th1 cells in experimental autoimmune encephalomyelitis. *Proc. Natl. Acad. Sci. USA* **2008**, *105*, 9041–9046. [CrossRef] [PubMed]
15. Spooren, A.; Kolmus, K.; Laureys, G.; Clinckers, R.; De Keyser, J.; Haegeman, G.; Gerlo, S. Interleukin-6, a mental cytokine. *Brain Res. Rev.* **2011**, *67*, 157–183. [CrossRef] [PubMed]
16. Erta, M.; Quintana, A.; Hidalgo, J. Interleukin-6, a major cytokine in the central nervous system. *Int. J. Biol. Sci.* **2012**, *8*, 1254–1266. [CrossRef] [PubMed]
17. Quintana, A.; Erta, M.; Ferrer, B.; Comes, G.; Giralt, M.; Hidalgo, J. Astrocyte-specific deficiency of interleukin-6 and its receptor reveal specific roles in survival, body weight and behavior. *Brain Behav. Immun.* **2013**, *27*, 162–173. [CrossRef] [PubMed]
18. Erta, M.; Giralt, M.; Esposito, F.L.; Fernandez-Gayol, O.; Hidalgo, J. Astrocytic IL-6 mediates locomotor activity, exploration, anxiety, learning and social behavior. *Horm. Behav.* **2015**, *73*, 64–74. [CrossRef] [PubMed]
19. Su, M.; Hu, H.; Lee, Y.; d'Azzo, A.; Messing, A.; Brenner, M. Expression specificity of GFAP transgenes. *Neurochem. Res.* **2004**, *29*, 2075–2093. [CrossRef] [PubMed]
20. Mycko, M.P.; Papoian, R.; Boschert, U.; Raine, C.S.; Selmaj, K.W. Cdna microarray analysis in multiple sclerosis lesions: Detection of genes associated with disease activity. *Brain* **2003**, *126*, 1048–1057. [CrossRef] [PubMed]
21. Lock, C.; Hermans, G.; Pedotti, R.; Brendolan, A.; Schadt, E.; Garren, H.; Langer-Gould, A.; Strober, S.; Cannella, B.; Allard, J.; *et al.* Gene-microarray analysis of multiple sclerosis lesions yields new targets validated in autoimmune encephalomyelitis. *Nat. Med.* **2002**, *8*, 500–508. [CrossRef] [PubMed]
22. Gijbels, K.; Brocke, S.; Abrams, J.S.; Steinman, L. Administration of neutralizing antibodies to interleukin-6 (IL-6) reduces experimental autoimmune encephalomyelitis and is associated with elevated levels of IL-6 bioactivity in central nervous system and circulation. *Mol. Med.* **1995**, *1*, 795–805. [PubMed]
23. Willenborg, D.O.; Fordham, S.A.; Cowden, W.B.; Ramshaw, I.A. Cytokines and murine autoimmune encephalomyelitis: Inhibition or enhancement of disease with antibodies to select cytokines, or by delivery of exogenous cytokines using a recombinant vaccinia virus system. *Scand. J. Immunol.* **1995**, *41*, 31–41. [CrossRef] [PubMed]
24. Rodriguez, M.; Pavelko, K.D.; McKinne, C.W.; Leibowitz, J.L. Recombinant human IL-6 suppresses demyelination in a viral model of multiple sclerosis. *J. Immunol.* **1994**, *153*, 3811–3821. [PubMed]

25. Campbell, I.L.; Abraham, C.R.; Masliah, E.; Kemper, P.; Inglis, J.D.; Oldstone, M.B.A.; Mucke, L. Neurologic disease in transgenic mice by cerebral overexpression of interleukin 6. *Proc. Natl. Acad. Sci. USA* **1993**, *90*, 10061–10065. [CrossRef] [PubMed]
26. Campbell, I.L.; Erta, M.; Lim, S.L.; Frausto, R.; May, U.; Rose-John, S.; Scheller, J.; Hidalgo, J. Trans-signaling is a dominant mechanism for the pathogenic actions of interleukin-6 in the brain. *J. Neurosci.* **2014**, *34*, 2503–2513. [CrossRef] [PubMed]
27. Costantino, C.M.; Baecher-Allan, C.; Hafler, D.A. Multiple sclerosis and regulatory T cells. *J. Clin. Immunol.* **2008**, *28*, 697–706. [CrossRef] [PubMed]
28. Kimura, A.; Kishimoto, T. Il-6: Regulator of Treg/Th17 balance. *Eur. J. Immunol.* **2010**, *40*, 1830–1835. [CrossRef] [PubMed]
29. Murphy, A.C.; Lalor, S.J.; Lynch, M.A.; Mills, K.H. Infiltration of th1 and Th17 cells and activation of microglia in the CNS during the course of experimental autoimmune encephalomyelitis. *Brain Behav. Immun.* **2010**, *24*, 641–651. [CrossRef] [PubMed]
30. Bettelli, E.; Carrier, Y.; Gao, W.; Korn, T.; Strom, T.B.; Oukka, M.; Weiner, H.L.; Kuchroo, V.K. Reciprocal developmental pathways for the generation of pathogenic effector Th17 and regulatory T cells. *Nature* **2006**, *441*, 235–238. [CrossRef] [PubMed]
31. Korn, T.; Mitsdoerffer, M.; Croxford, A.L.; Awasthi, A.; Dardalhon, V.A.; Galileos, G.; Vollmar, P.; Stritesky, G.L.; Kaplan, M.H.; Waisman, A.; *et al.* IL-6 controls Th17 immunity *in vivo* by inhibiting the conversion of conventional t cells into Foxp3+ regulatory T cells. *Proc. Natl. Acad. Sci. USA* **2008**, *105*, 18460–18465. [CrossRef] [PubMed]
32. Ma, X.; Reynolds, S.L.; Baker, B.J.; Li, X.; Benveniste, E.N.; Qin, H. IL-17 enhancement of the IL-6 signaling cascade in astrocytes. *J. Immunol.* **2010**, *184*, 4898–4906. [CrossRef] [PubMed]
33. Ogura, H.; Murakami, M.; Okuyama, Y.; Tsuruoka, M.; Kitabayashi, C.; Kanamoto, M.; Nishihara, M.; Iwakura, Y.; Hirano, T. Interleukin-17 promotes autoimmunity by triggering a positive-feedback loop via interleukin-6 induction. *Immunity* **2008**, *29*, 628–636. [CrossRef] [PubMed]
34. Swartz, K.R.; Liu, F.; Sewell, D.; Schochet, T.; Campbell, I.; Sandor, M.; Fabry, Z. Interleukin-6 promotes post-traumatic healing in the central nervous system. *Brain Res.* **2001**, *896*, 86–95. [CrossRef]
35. Fee, D.; Grzybicki, D.; Dobbs., M.; Ihyer, S.; Clotfelter, J.; Macvilay, S.; Hart, M.N.; Sandor, M.; Fabry, Z. Interleukin 6 promotes vasculogenesis of murine brain microvessel endothelial cells. *Cytokine* **2000**, *12*, 655–665. [CrossRef] [PubMed]

12

Cellular Redox Imbalance and Neurochemical Effect in Cognitive-Deficient Old Rats

Maria Elena González-Fraguela [1,*], Lisette Blanco-Lezcano [2], Caridad Ivette Fernandez-Verdecia [2], Teresa Serrano Sanchez [1], Maria de los A. Robinson Agramonte [1] and Lidia Leonor Cardellá Rosales [3]

1 Immunochemical Department, International Center for Neurological Restoration, 25th Ave, Playa, 15805, PC 11300 Havana, Cuba; teresa@neuro.ciren.cu (T.S.S.); robin@neuro.ciren.cu (M.d.l.A.R.A.)
2 Experimental Neurophysiology Department, International Center of Neurological Restoration (CIREN) Ave. 25 No. 15805 e/158 and 160, Playa, Havana 11300, Cuba; lblanco@neuro.ciren.cu (L.B.-L.); ivettef@neuro.ciren.cu (C.I.F.-V.)
3 Physiologic Sciences Department, Latin American Medicine School, Carretera Panamericana, Kilómetro 3 1/2 Municipio Playa, Habana 19148, Cuba; lcardella@infomed.sld.cu
* Correspondence: marie@neuro.ciren.cu

Abstract: The purpose of the present study is to access the linkage between dysregulation of glutamatergic neurotransmission, oxidative metabolism, and serine signaling in age-related cognitive decline. In this work, we evaluated the effect of natural aging in rats on the cognitive abilities for hippocampal-dependent tasks. Oxidative metabolism indicators are glutathione (GSH), malondialdehyde (MDA) concentrations, and cytosolic phospholipase A_2 (PLA_2) activity. In addition, neurotransmitter amino acid (*L*-Glutamic acid, γ-aminobutyric acid (GABA), *DL*-Serine and *DL*-Aspartic acid) concentrations were studied in brain areas such as the frontal cortex (FC) and hippocampus (HPC). The spatial long-term memory revealed significant differences among experimental groups: the aged rats showed an increase in escape latency to the platform associated with a reduction of crossings and spent less time on the target quadrant than young rats. Glutathione levels decreased for analyzed brain areas linked with a significant increase in MDA concentrations and PLA_2 activity in cognitive-deficient old rats. We found glutamate levels only increased in the HPC, whereas a reduced level of serine was found in both regions of interest in cognitive-deficient old rats. We demonstrated that age-related changes in redox metabolism contributed with alterations in synaptic signaling and cognitive impairment.

Keywords: aging; learning; memory; neurotransmitter; oxidative stress; phospholipase A_2; serine

---

1. Introduction

The demographic changes that affect a large part of humanity are leading to an increase in life expectancy at birth, which has a high impact on societies and their economies. The increase in health costs are not at the expense of the new generation, in fact they are very reduced, but at the expense of the predominance of pathologies related to aging and other physical and intellectual disabilities associated with advanced age.

Aging is an essential factor for many diseases, specifically in neurodegenerative diseases. Oxidative stress constitutes the most important theory of ageing at the molecular level. The cognitive processes that are mediated by the hippocampus (declarative memory) and the prefrontal cortex (working memory) represent the most vulnerable areas to ageing.

This is due to brain cells that are exposed to rising levels of oxidative stress with the loss of energy homeostasis, and the increase in lipid mediators by phospholipases A_2 (PLA_2) activity, alterations in neurotransmitters, and signal transduction and accumulation of damage in biomolecules [1].

Oxidative stress is characterized by an imbalance in reactive oxygen species production (ROS) or impaired antioxidant protection. Both mechanisms are considered to have an important role in age-related cognitive decline. Glutathione (GSH) is the main mechanism of antioxidant defense against ROS in biological systems [2]. Glutathione concentration decreases with age in several animal models [3–5] and brain areas [6,7]. The reduction in GSH concentration causes an incomplete oxidation of the substrates into the mitochondria inducing the leakage of electrons from the electron transport chain and consequently increasing ROS generation.

A habitual target of ROS are neural membrane lipids, the enhanced phospholipid degradation induces changes in fluidity and permeability in neural membranes with the consequent alteration of ionic channels and modulation in the enzymatic activities coupled to membrane composition [8].

Previous studies have demonstrated the involvement of oxidative signaling pathways in a permanent damage of the neuronal circuitry, especially with glutamatergic neurons. Sustained activation of ionotropic glutamate receptors as the *N*-methyl-D-aspartic acid receptor (NMDAR), could affect intracellular calcium levels leading to activation of proteases, nucleases, and phospholipases [9].

The cytosolic PLA_2 causes the release of arachidonic acid (AA), hydrolyzing the sn-2 fatty acids of membrane phospholipids. This important polyunsaturated fatty acid (PUFA) is the precursor for the synthesis of eicosanoids and prostanoids. Some findings indicate that PLA_2 plays important roles in synaptic functions, long-term potentiation (LTP), learning, and memory [10]. The effect of PLA_2 on cognitive function can be related with the ability of AA to change neuronal metabolism and synaptic activity [11].

Glutamate, an excitatory neurotransmitter in the central nervous system (CNS), plays a recognized role in the regulation of neurogenesis, neuronal survival, synaptic plasticity, and learning and memory processes [12].

Several studies have suggested that the stimulation of PLA_2 is a process mediated by the glutamate receptor in neuronal cultures [10]. Likewise, D-serine is the most effective co-agonist of the glycine site of NMDAR, which is essential for the optimal function of this receptor in physiological and pathological processes [13].

Experimental data has demonstrated that D-serine treatment decreases the extent of neuron death with a neuroprotective effect against apoptosis [14]. At the present time, serine metabolism is the subject of intense investigation to confirm its role in the diagnosis and therapy of neurological disorders, as well as its therapeutic potential in preclinical models [15,16].

The objective of this study was to obtain evidence about the linkage between dysregulation of glutamatergic neurotransmission in oxidative stress conditions and the role of serine signaling in age-related cognitive decline.

2. Materials and Methods

2.1. Animal

Male Sprague–Dawley rats obtained from a national breeder institution (CENPALAB, Artemisa) were housed five per cage in a 12:12-h light-dark cycle with food and water ad libitum, under standard conditions for temperature (25 °C) and relative humidity (60%). All experimental studies were performed during light cycle (7.00–19.00 h). We used two age groups: young, (n = 30; 2 months old) with a body weight 272 $\pm$ 36 g (mean $\pm$ standard deviation, SD); and cognitive-deficient old rats (n = 45; 23 months old, body weight 520 $\pm$ 46 g).

All efforts were made to minimize the number of animals used and their suffering. All procedures concerning animal experimentation were carried out according to the ethical principles for animal research established by the Canadian Council for Animal Care [17] and the Cuban Regulations for the Use of Laboratory Animals (CENPALAB 1997) and were approved by the Ethical Committee of the International Center for Neurological Restoration.

2.2. *Behavioral Test*

Morris Water Maze (MWM)

The MWM tests spatial learning and memory retention in rodents and involves an acquisition phase where the animal learns the location of a "goal or escape platform" target over a period of multiple days [18]. An overhead camera and computer assisted tracking system with videomax software (Spontaneous Motor Activity Recording Tracking SMART 2.0) (PanLab, Barcelona España, Spain) was used to record the position of the rat in the maze (Scheme 1). A cued learning test was used to discriminate motoric or motivational factors. On the first day, animals received four trials in a water maze (no distal cues) with a well visible and distinguished platform located at different quadrants.

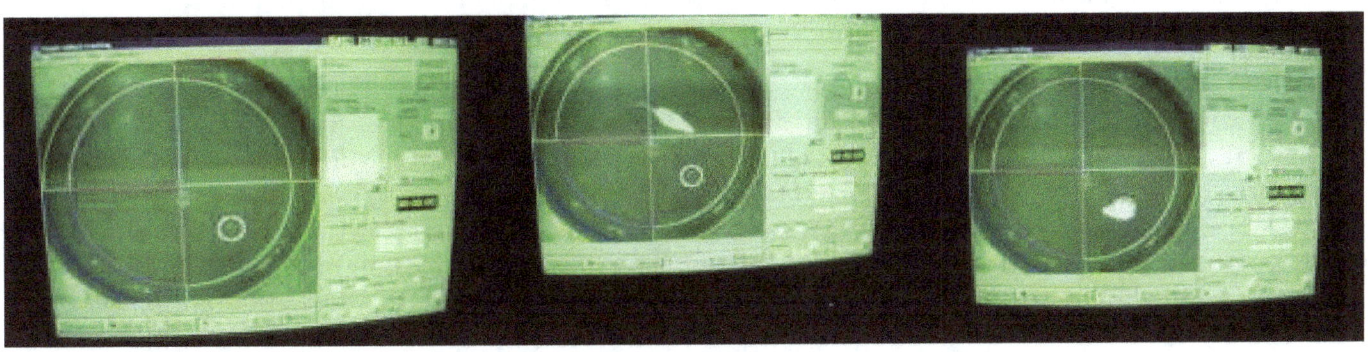

Scheme 1. The software display during data acquisition in the Morris water maze (MWM) task using the Spontaneous Motor Activity Recording Tracking (SMART) system from Panlab S.A.

One day after, a classic spatial acquisition test was introduced. Animals were trained in the MWM with non-visible platform conditions for eight trials per day over four consecutive days. The order of the start position was changed in every trial as well as the sequence of positions along the days. The platform position was kept fixed in the northeast position (NE target quadrant, Q1) throughout the training period (Scheme 2). In each trial, the rat was released from the starting position, facing the wall, and was allowed to search for a hidden escape platform for 60 s. If the animal was unable to find the platform it was gently carried onto it, and allowed a 30 s rest period sitting on the platform. Data from each four trials were grouped into one block (4 days: 32 trials: 8 blocks-B1–B8). On the fifth day (trial 33), the platform was removed and the animal was allowed to search for it for 60 s (probe trial for Q1). This trial evaluated the quality of reference memory. Immediately, the platform was relocated in the same position (Q1) to evaluate four additional trials (34–37, B9) to explore the cognitive flexibility with a previous dissociating stimulus (absence of escape platform). Two days later, the rat's long-term reference memory was evaluated in a single block of four trials (B10) using the above described paradigm (Q1 at NE position).

Aged rats are classified according to the criteria of 2 or 2.5 standard deviations above the average of the young controls latency [19–21].

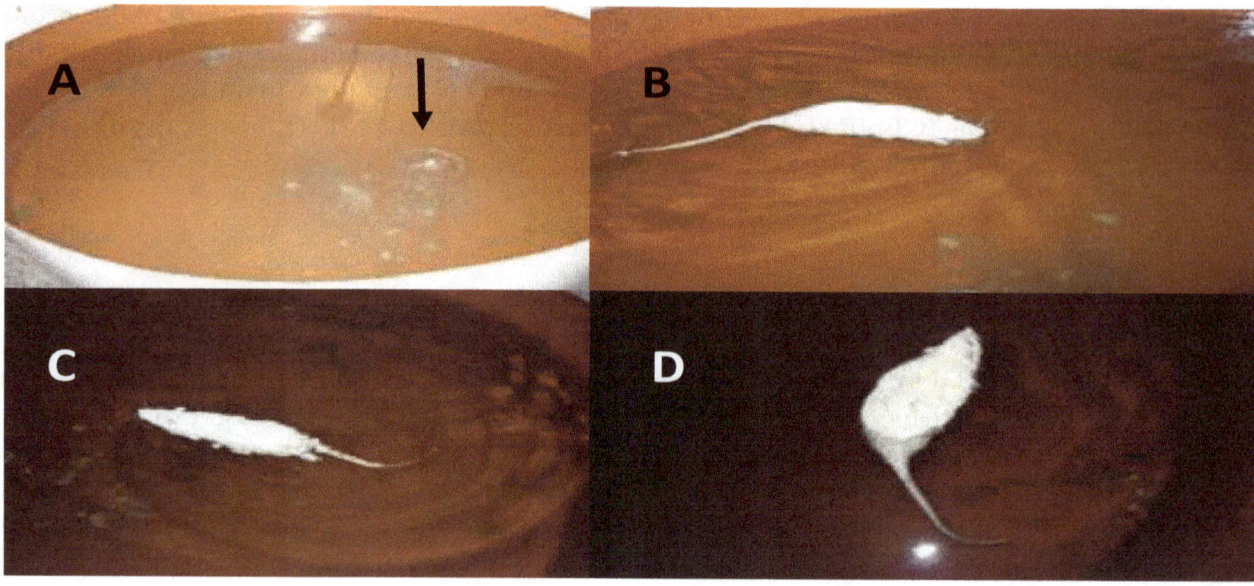

Scheme 2. (**A**) The tank before the task. The arrow shows the location of the platform. (**B–D**) The different moments in which the rat is searching for the platform in the maze and reaching it.

2.3. Sedation and Sample Collection

For the studies that required sedation, an anesthetic mixture of 4 mL of ketalar (ketamine 50 mg/mL, IMEFA, Havana, Cuba), 2 mL of valium (diazepam 5 mg/mL, IMEFA, Havana, Cuba), 1 mL of atropine (atropine, 0.5 mg/mL, IMEFA, Havana, Cuba), and 16 mL of 0.9% sodium chloride solution (0.9% NaCl, IMEFA, Havana, Cuba) was used. The dose regimen was 1 mL of the mixture/100 g of body weight, and immediately the rats were sacrificed by decapitation. Their brains were extracted and rinsed in cold saline; the total frontal cortex (FC) and hippocampus (HPC) were bilaterally dissected. The tissues were frozen in liquid nitrogen, weighed, and stored at −80 °C until the biochemical analysis.

2.4. Biochemical Analysis

2.4.1. Oxidative Stress Markers

Glutathione GSH Quantification

Tissue samples were homogenized in a glass-Teflon potter containing 5% 5-sulfosalicylic acid (1:15, *w*/*v*) and the protein-free supernatant was isolated by centrifugation at 8160× *g* during 10 min. Total GSH was quantified by Tietze's recycling assay as described by Azbill et al. [22]. Aliquots of the supernatants were incubated for 25 min at 37 °C in a medium containing 0.21 mM NADPH, 0.6 mM DTNB (5,5′-ditiobis(2-nitrobenzoico), 6.3 mM EDTA (ethylene diamine tetraacetic acid), and 143 mM sodium phosphate pH 7.5. Following the addition of 0.5 U GRD (glutathione reductasa), the absorbance increase at 412 nm due to the formation of 5-thio-nitrobenzoate was recorded. The concentration values were calculated from a GSH standard curve.

Malondialdehyde (MDA) Quantification

Tissues samples were homogenized in 1 M Tris/0.25 M sucrose buffer (pH 7.4) at a tissue/buffer volume ratio of 1/5. The homogenates were centrifuged at 14,000 rpm for 15 min. Two-hundred microliters of the sample were vortexed with 400 µL of a 0.67% thiobarbituric acid solution in 0.2 M HCl, then incubated for 15 min in a water bath at 100 °C and centrifuged at 2448× *g* for 10 min at room temperature. The resulting supernatant was used for measuring absorbance at 535 nm. The concentration values were calculated from an MDA standard curve [23].

Assay for Calcium-Dependent Cytosolic Phospholipase A2 (PLA2) Activity

PLA_2 enzymatic activity was measured using the protocol recommended by the manufacturer (Cayman Chemical Company, Ann Arbor, MI, USA). Briefly, 10 μL sample were incubated with 1.5 mM arachidonoyl thio-phosphotidylcholine (a PLA_2 substrate) for 1 h at room temperature. Enzyme catalysis was stopped by the addition of beta dystrobrevin/EGTA (Ethylene glycol-bis(2-aminoethylether)-*N,N,N′,N′*-tetraacetic acid), and the optical density of the sample was measured at 405 nm. PLA_2 activity was calculated in accordance to kit instruction and PLA_2 activity was expressed in U/mg [24].

2.4.2. Amino Acid Analysis

Sample Preparation and Derivatization

The brain tissue for amino acid analysis was homogenized in ice-cold 0.2 M perchloric acid including cysteine (4 mL per g of tissue) and sonicated for 5 min. The brain homogenate was centrifuged at 17,000 rpm for 4 min at 4 °C and the supernatant was diluted (1/50), aliquoted, and stored at −20 °C. 20 μL of standard (*L*-Glutamic acid, γ-aminobutyric acid (GABA), *DL*-Serine and *DL*-Aspartate) or sample was added with 20 μL of the derivatization reagent (25 mg OPA (Ophthaldialdehyde) of diluted in 1500 μL of methanol, 100 μL of borate buffer 0.1 M (pH9), and 30 μL of β-mercaptoethanol), the derivatization mixture was vortexed for 1 min at room temperature, After that, 5 μL of 5% acetic acid were added to stop of reaction, then, 20 μL of this final solution was injected into the HPLC system.

Instrumentation and Chromatographic Conditions

For chromatographic analysis, an HPLC system (Agilent 1200 Technologies) (Santa Clara, CA, USA) was used. Chromatographic separation was achieved on a reversed phase column (HR-80, ESA), using an isocratic chromatographic pump (Agilent 1200 series), and detected with a fluorescence detector (Agilent G1321A, 1100 series) set at $\lambda_{excitation}$ 340 nm and $\lambda_{emission}$ 460 nm. The column temperature was maintained at 25 °C and the mobile phase was pumped at a flow rate of 1.0 $mLmin^{-1}$. The chromatographic data were recorded using the Agilent ChemStation B.04.02SP1 software. The mobile phase was composed of 0.1 M NaH_2PO_4/25% methanol.

2.5. Data Processing and Statistical Analysis

The values were expressed as mean ± standard error mean. Normal distribution and homogeneity of variance of the data were tested by the Kolmogorov–Smirnov and Levene tests, respectively. The comparison between experimental groups of the biochemical indicators was performed by a one-way analysis of variance (ANOVA) and the behavioral variables in the MWM were analyzed by analysis of variance for repeated measurements (ANOVA). For post hoc comparisons was used the Tukey honest significant differences test (HSD) and nonparametric comparison with Mann–Whitney U test. Significant differences were considered only if $p < 0.05$.

3. Results

3.1. Behavioural Studies

Morris Water Maze

The post-hoc analysis on spatial long-term memory revealed significant differences between experimental groups for escape latency to platform ($F_{(1, 28)} = 12.39$; $p < 0.001$) related with an increase in aged rats that demonstrated severe spatial memory impairment in this group (Figure 1). Likewise, regarding the number of crossings, the aged rats exhibited a poor performance in the acquisition of the navigation search strategy during the test. The Tukey honest significance differences test, showed a reduction of crossings and time spent on the target quadrant in older animals than younger rats ($F_{(1, 28)} = 8.91$; $p < 0.001$) (Figure 2, Table 1).

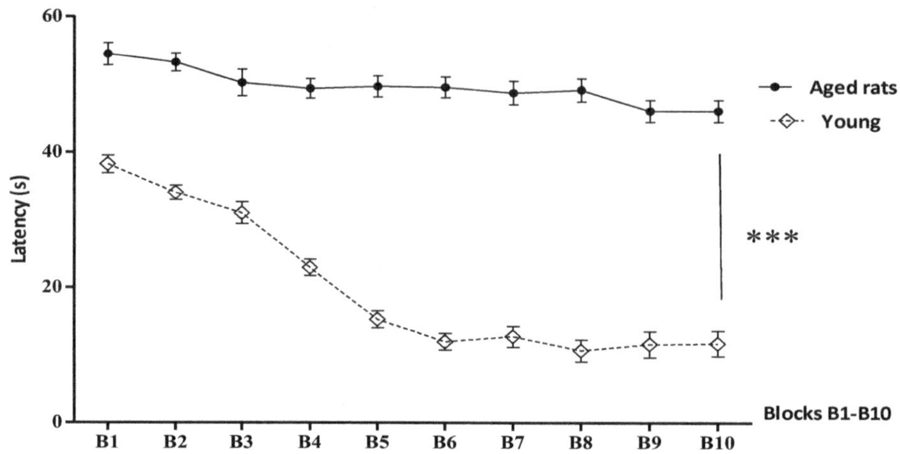

Figure 1. Latency in the MWM (mean ± SD mean are represented) to find the hidden platform during the training sessions grouped into the blocks (B). Classical training (B1–B9) and long-term contextual memory (B10). *** Significant differences between experimental groups: aged rats ($n = 45$) and young ($n = 30$) ($p < 0.001$).

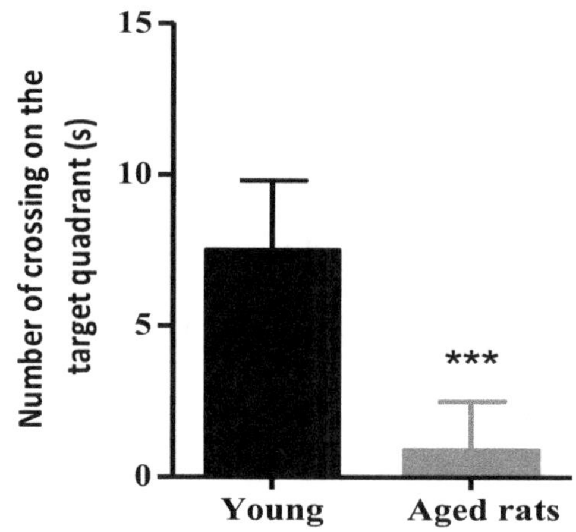

Figure 2. Number of crossings on the target quadrant (mean ± SD mean are represented) *** Significant differences between experimental groups: aged rats ($n = 45$) and young ($n = 30$) ($p < 0.001$).

Table 1. Data (mean ± SD mean) from four trials grouped in blocks (B1–B10) for the *latency* in the MWM and the number of crossings in the target quadrant between experimental groups.

Blocks (B)	Aged Rats (Mean ± SD Mean)	Young (Mean ± SD Mean)
B1	54.5 ± 1.62	38.20 ± 1.32
B2	53.30 ± 1.33	34.02 ± 1.087
B3	50.26 ± 1.97	30.99 ± 1.61
B4	49.41 ± 1.48	22.96 ±1.20
B5	49.7 ± 1.56	15.30 ± 1.27
B6	49..59 ± 1.54	11.96 ± 1.26
B7	48.8 ± 1.70	12.75 ± 1.57
B8	48.2 ± 1.73	10.66 ± 1.59
B9	46.12 ± 1.60	11.58 ± 1.94
B10	46.06 ± 1.7	11.70 ± 1.92
Number of Crossings	0.9 ± 1.6	7.5 ± 2.3

3.2. Biochemical Indicators

The comparison between experimental groups with regard to GSH content showed significant differences in examined brain areas in cognitive-deficient old rats (FC ($Z = 5.41$; $p < 0.001$); HPC ($F_{(1,38)} = 288.6$; $p < 0.001$)). The level of GSH dropped by 82% in FC and 80% in HPC in respect to the control groups. These results are associated with a significant increase in MDA concentrations for aged rats only for hippocampus, a highly sensitive region to oxidative stress. (HPC ($F_{(1,38)} = 837.9$; $p < 0.001$)).

Similarly, a considerable increase was observed in PLA_2 activity for analyzed brain areas. The enzyme activity revealed significant differences among experimental groups (FC ($F_{(1,38)} = 29.15$; $p < 0.001$); HPC ($F_{(1,38)} = 70.96$, $p < 0.001$)) in correspondence with the reduction of GSH content in the studied brain structures GSH: Glutathione, MDA: Malondialdehyde, PLA_2: Phospholipase A_2, GABA: γ-aminobutyric acid. (Figure 3, Table 2).

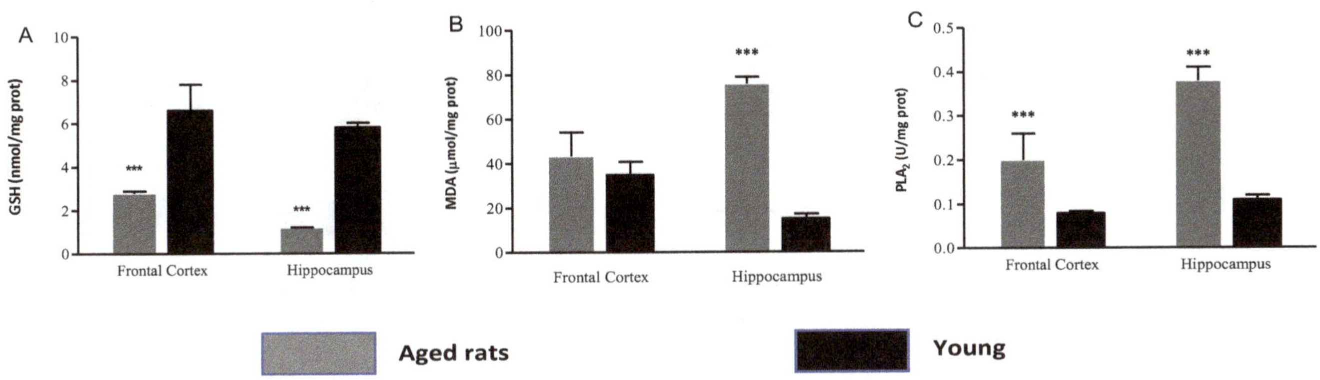

Figure 3. Effect of aging on oxidative metabolism indicators in the examined brain areas. (**A**) Glutathione (GSH), (**B**) Malondialdehyde (MDA), (**C**) Phospholipase A2 (PLA2). *** Corresponds to significant differences between experimental groups ($p < 0.001$).

Table 2. Data (mean ± SD mean) corresponding to biochemical indicators in examined brain areas between experimental groups.

Biochemical Indicators	Frontal Cortex Aged Rats	Frontal Cortex Young Rats	Hippocampus Aged Rats	Hippocampus Young Rats
GSH	1.3 ± 0.1	5.45 ± 1.2	0.76 ± 0.22	5.15 ± 0.2
MDA	43.42 ± 10.6	34.93 ± 5.95	80.31 ± 3.01	15.84 ± 2.02
PLA_2	0.2 ± 0.06	0.08 ± 0.0	0.35 ± 0.03	0.11 ± 0.01
L Glutamate	5.29 ± 0.8	5.17 ± 1.10	10.24 ± 1.2	6.89 ± 1.2
GABA	0.88 ± 0.03	0.94 ± 0.02	1.11 ± 0.03	1.17 ±0.03
DL Serine	4.85 ± 0.8	6.07 ± 0.55	2.13 ± 1.02	5.52 ± 1.2
DL Aspartate	5.35 ± 0.72	5.4 ± 0.55	5.02 ± 1.03	5.16 ± 1.2

Amino Acid Concentrations

The levels of GABA were unchanged compared with controls in brain regions investigated in aged rats (FC ($F_{(1,38)} = 0.17$; $p > 0.05$) and HPC ($F_{(1,38)} = 0.39$; $p > 0.05$)). Furthermore, the aspartate concentrations were not significantly different between groups (FC ($F_{(1,38)} = 0.18$; $p > 0.05$) and HPC ($F_{(1,38)} = 0.70$; $p > 0.05$)). In contrast, the levels of glutamate only increased in HPC in aged rats (HPC ($F_{(1,38)} = 93.32$; $p < 0.001$), whereas a reduced level of serine was found in the regions of interest in cognitive-deficient old rats (FC ($F_{(1,38)} = 58.3$; $p < 0.001$) and HPC ($F_{(1,38)} = 365.1$; $p < 0.001$)) (Figure 4, Table 2).

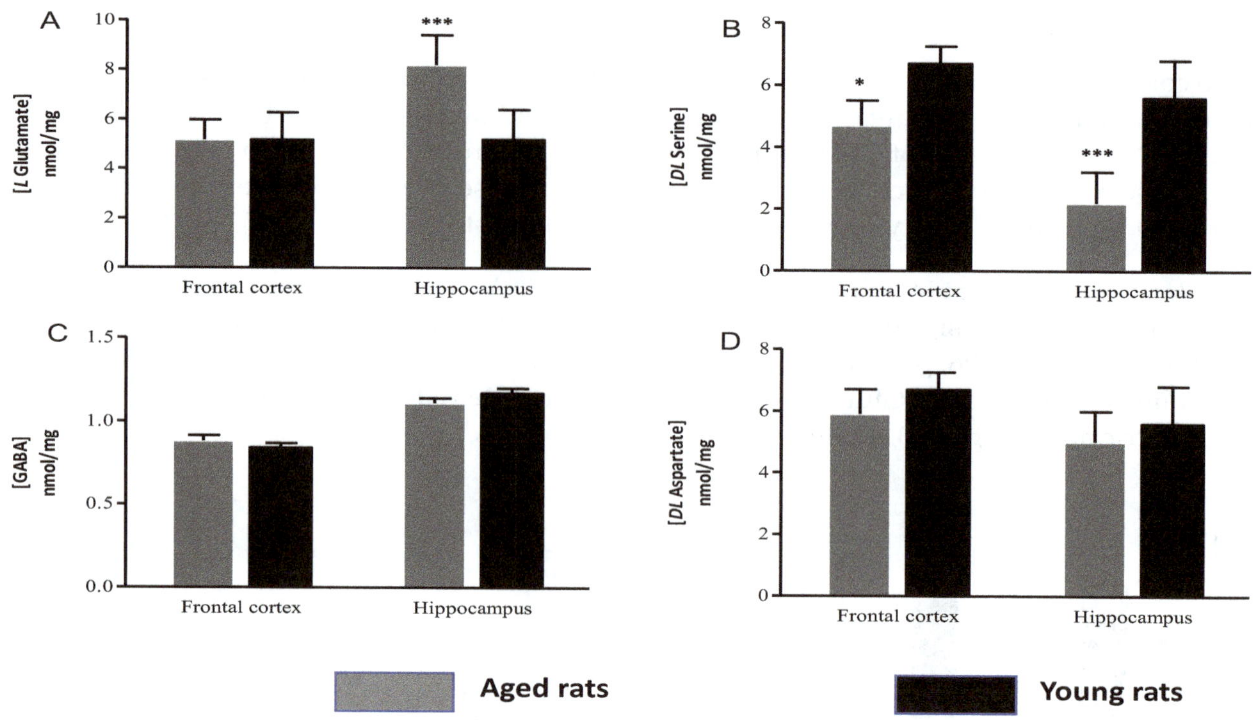

Figure 4. Effect of aging on amino acid concentration in the examined brain areas. (**A**) *L* Glutamate, (**B**) *DL* Serine, (**C**) GABA, (**D**) *DL* Aspartate. *** ($p < 0.001$); * ($p < 0.05$) corresponds to significant differences between experimental groups.

4. Discussion

Some aged animals undergo severe cognitive deficiencies, whereas others preserve their normal cognitive abilities. In particular, spatial memory appears to be significantly affected [25]. The behavioral results allowed us to select aged rats that demonstrated a deficient execution in the acquisition of a successful navigation strategy in the MWM. The metabolic changes originated by GSH depletion in HPC caused increased swim times in the MWM test associated with a reduction of time spent on the target quadrant, confirming a failure in the memory trace formation, and therefore cognitive dysfunction.

We observed a significant GSH depletion in cognitive-deficient old rats, as much in FC as in HPC. Besides its roles in maintenance of oxidant homeostasis within the cell, GSH may serve as a substrate and an allosteric modulator of eicosanoid biosynthesis, in the regulation of NMDAR activity and activation of transcription factors [26]. We found a reduction of more than 70% in the GSH content in cognitive-deficient old rats compared to the young rats. The majority of authors have reported a decreases of tripeptide in brain tissue of around 50% in previous rodent studies [27,28].

The strong GSH decrease observed in our work generates hydrogen peroxide (H_2O_2) and hydroxyl radical (OH) that induce lipid peroxidation in the membrane of neurons and glial cells and damage the (Ca^{2+} and Na^+/K^+) ATPases and glucose transporters [29]. In connection with this result, we observed a significant increase in MDA concentration and PLA_2 activity in aged rats for examined brain areas. The loss of the energy metabolism homeostasis, redox imbalance, and subsequent damage by accumulation of MDA could originate the functional impairment in aged rats.

Due to its numerous functions for maintenance of membrane phospholipid balance and for originating several lipid mediators, PLA_2 activation has been implicated in pathological conditions in the CNS for neurodegenerative diseases among others [8,30–32].

H_2O_2 accumulation induces the redox ambience appropriate for activating the PLA_2 pathway by means of extracellular signal-regulated kinase (ERK) and interleukin 1b [33,34]. In this context,

PLA_2 activity increases the release of AA from the plasma membrane, which directly produce 4-hydroxynonenal and MDA.

Arachidonic acid AA undergoes oxidative modifications and increases the mitochondrial ROS levels in the hippocampus and cerebral cortex [35]. As such, the AA and its metabolites are permeable to the membrane and could affect the function of neighboring neurons with disruption of monolayer integrity and cell death [36].

The results obtained from the cognitive-deficient old rats revealed high PLA_2 enzymatic activity and consequently increased AA generation. It is important to point out that high concentrations of AA cause uncoupling oxidative phosphorylation with a detrimental effect on the ATP-producing capacity of mitochondria, which results in mitochondrial dysfunction and an additional increase in the production of ROS.

These experimental data are in line with clinical studies. Jiang R et al. [37] reported that higher PLA_2 enzymatic activity is associated with increased prevalence of cognitive impairment in the Chinese population. On the other hand, there is evidence that the contribution of PLA_2 activity in regulating neuronal excitatory functions, in cultured primary cortical neurons, trigger NMDAR receptors, which has been demonstrated to activate PLA_2 and AA release [38]. In turn, PLA_2 activity and AA are involved in receptor signaling which is linked with oxidative events which underline important roles in synaptic signaling, LTP, learning and memory [39,40].

In consonance with these studies, the present findings evidence an increase in glutamate concentrations in the HPC of aged rats which is closely associated with the elevation of PLA_2 activity in this region. The LTP dependence of NMDAR activation has been demonstrated in several brain areas, including hippocampal subfields like the dentate gyrus and the CA1 [41].

It is well established now that excessive levels of glutamate can produce toxic effects due to overstimulation of NMDAR, increasing the intracellular Ca^{2+} and activate Ca^{2+}-dependent enzymes including PLA_2. This cascade of events culminates with a Ca^{2+} dysregulation in neurons and astrocytes, which initiates cellular death by a process known as excitotoxicity. This process implicates the activation of proteases, the generation of radical species, and mitochondrial Ca^{2+} overload that affects critical biological molecules including lipids, proteins, and DNA.

However, on the other hand, one of the deleterious consequences of GSH metabolism dysfunction is the NMDAR hypoactivity [42]. The GSH insufficiency in aged rats could induce the formation of disulfide bonds between pairs of cysteine residues on the extracellular portion of the NMDAR generating a selective reduction of NMDAR currents [42], which contrast with the possible excitotoxic effect of NMDAR activation in old rats due to high levels of glutamate.

Previous studies with NMDAR blockade suggested that altered redox states of these extracellular cysteine residues could mediate the decline in NMDAR function during aging [43]. The application of dithiothreitol, a specific reducing agent, increased the NMDAR component and the magnitude of LTP in hippocampal slices from old rodents [43].

The intracellular redox status observed in the aged rats can directly contribute to synaptic inefficiency of NMDAR, caused by changes in neurotransmitter systems in vulnerable brain regions. Liu et al. [44] have reported that H_2O_2 accumulation is associated with the downregulation of the GluN2 subunits of the NMDAR in adult rat hippocampi. Otherwise, recent modeling work has shown that reduced NMDAR signaling into interneurons produced alterations in spatial representations that affected working memory execution [45]. Therefore, the suppression of NMDAR responses could induce changes in memory mechanisms that impaired the cognitive processes in GSH-depleted aged rats.

This previous hypothesis is supported by a reduced level of serine in the brain regions investigated in aged rats. D-serine, an enantiomer of serine, has a crucial characteristic of binding to NMDAR [46]. This amino acid binds to the glycine-site of the GluN1 subunit of NMDAR so that glutamate can link to GluN2 subunits [47].

We found a reduction of around 60% in serine levels in HPC and 30% in FC in cognitive-deficient old rats with regard to younger counterparts. The bond of D-serine is critical to synaptic NMDAR function [48] due to D-serine having three additional hydrogen bonds to the receptor, which may activate the NMDAR more efficiently than glycine [49]. This finding increases the possibility that alterations in serine metabolism could be a contributor to the dysfunctions of memory in the aged rats.

D-serine is converted from L-serine by serine racemase, an enzyme dependent of pyridoxal phosphate, mostly expressed in excitatory neurons in the CNS of rodents [50]. D-serine is especially increased in brain areas involved in cognitive processes, as in the cerebral cortex, hippocampus, and basal ganglia [49].

The pathway responsible for the degradation of D-serine in the CNS is the D-amino acid oxidase (DAAO) [51]. Nevertheless, the reduction in serine concentration could involve an exceptional property of serine racemase which is able to catalyze the degradation of D-serine and L-serine to pyruvate and ammonia [13].

The possibility of serine racemase to enhance pyruvate levels from metabolic availability of serine may represent an important mechanism to obtain energy for mitochondrial oxidative phosphorylation and synthesis of ATP. This alternative of the serine metabolic pathway explains how the increased ROS production secondary to GSH depletion observed in aged rats reduces the synaptic levels of D-serine and exacerbates the NMDAR dysfunction in increased energy demand conditions.

These results are coincidental with reports from others authors who have shown that alterations of LTP expression are associated with a deficiency of NMDAR [52–54] and is recovered in aged rats and senescence-accelerated mice by D-serine treatment [54].

5. Conclusions

These findings suggest that age-related changes in the cellular redox metabolism contributes to memory dysfunctions and cognitive decline. The energy demands of synaptic activity lead to increased ROS production as a by-product of ATP synthesis with elevated utilization of a glutathione-based antioxidant system. Glutathione depletion induces an acute increase in the oxidative stress conditions and may generate NMDAR hypofunction and alterations in synaptic transmission. In the same way, the reduction of serine levels in aged rats, as the most effective co-agonist, could lead to a marked impairment of NMDAR function. The results discussed here support the hypothesis of redox homeostasis as a crucial element that regulates brain function and it will be necessary to further research the molecular mechanism of observed results.

Author Contributions: This work was carried out in collaboration between all authors. M.E.G.-F. was the principal investigator, designed the study, conducted the data analysis and wrote of the paper. L.B.-L. and C.I.F.-V. supervised the statistical analysis and assisted with interpreting the results and revision of the manuscript. T.S.S. and M.d.l.A.R.A. participated in the analysis of the data. L.L.C.R. participated in the analysis of the data and revision of the manuscript. All authors read and approved the final manuscript.

References

1. Zhang, Y.; Li, P.; Feng, J.; Minghu, W. Dysfunction of NMDA receptors in Alzheimer's disease. *Neurol. Sci.* **2016**, *37*, 1039–1047. [CrossRef] [PubMed]
2. Mari, M.; Morales, A.; Colell, A.; Garcia-Ruiz, C.; Fernandez-Checa, J. Mitochondrial Glutathione, a Key Survival Antioxidant. *ARS* **2009**, *11*, 2685–2700. [CrossRef] [PubMed]
3. Bergado, J.A.; Almaguer, W.; Rojas, J.; Capdevila, V.; Frey, J.U. Spatial and emotional memory in aged rats: A behavioral-statistical analysis. *Neuroscience* **2011**, *172*, 256–269. [CrossRef] [PubMed]

4. Krämer, T.; Grob, T.; Menzel, L.; Hirnet, T.; Griemert, E.; Radyushkin, K.; Thal, S.C.; Methner, A.; Schaefer, M.K.E. Dimethyl fumarate treatment after traumatic brain injury prevents depletion of antioxidative brain glutathione and confers neuroprotection. *J. Neurochem.* **2017**, *143* (Suppl. 5), 523–533. [CrossRef] [PubMed]
5. Gemelli, T.; de Andrade, R.B.; Rojas, D.B.; Zanatta, Â.; Schirmbeck, G.H.; Funchal, C.; Wajner, M.; Dutra-Filho, C.S.; Wannmacher, C.M.D. Chronic Exposure to β-Alanine Generates Oxidative Stress and Alters Energy Metabolism in Cerebral Cortex and Cerebellum of Wistar Rats. *Mol. Neurobiol.* **2018**, *55* (Suppl. 6), 5101–5110. [CrossRef] [PubMed]
6. Cruz-Aguado, R.; Almaguer-Melian, W.; Diaz, C.M.; Lorigados, L.; Bergado, J. Behavioral and biochemical effects of glutathione depletion in the rat brain. *Brain Res. Bull.* **2001**, *55* (Suppl. 3), 327–333. [CrossRef]
7. Bonasera, S.; Arikkath, J.; Boska, M.D.; Chaudoin, T.R.; De Korver, N.W.; Goulding, E.H.; Traci, A.; Hoke, T.A.; Mojtahedzedah, V.; Reyelts, C.D.; et al. Age-related changes in cerebellar and hypothalamic function accompany non-microglial immune gene expression, altered synapse organization, and excitatory amino acid neurotransmission deficits. *Aging* **2016**, *8*, 2153–2164. [CrossRef] [PubMed]
8. Chauhan, V.; Chauhan, A. Abnormalities in membrane lipids, membrane-associated proteins, and signal transduction in Autism. In *Austim Oxidative Stress, Inflammation and Immune Abnormalities*; Chauhan, A., Ed.; CRC Press: Boca Raton, FL, USA, 2010; pp. 177–207.
9. Paoletti, P.; Bellone, C.; Zhou, Q. NMDA receptor subunit diversity: Impact on receptor properties, synaptic plasticity and disease. *Nat. Neurosci.* **2013**, *14*, 383–400. [CrossRef] [PubMed]
10. Basselin, M.; Chang, L.; Chen, M.; Bell, J.M.; Rapoport, S. Chronic Administration of Valproic Acid Reduces Brain NMDA Signaling via Arachidonic Acid in Unanesthetized Rats. *Neurochem. Res.* **2008**, *33*, 2229–2240. [CrossRef] [PubMed]
11. Ng, C.Y.; Kannan, S.; Chen, Y.J.; Tan, F.C.; Ong, W.Y.; Go, M.L.; Verma, C.S.; Low, C.M.; Lam, Y. A New Generation of Arachidonic Acid Analogues as Potential Neurological Agent Targeting Cytosolic Phospholipase A2. *Sci. Rep.* **2017**, *7*, 13683. [CrossRef] [PubMed]
12. Wang, R.; Reddy, P.H. Role of glutamate and NMDA receptors in Alzheimer's disease. *J. Alzheimers Dis.* **2017**, *57* (Suppl. 4), 1041–1048. [CrossRef] [PubMed]
13. Billard, J.M. D-serine signalling as a prominent determinant of neuronal-glial dialogue in the healthy and diseased brain. *J. Cell. Mol. Med.* **2008**, *12*, 1872–1884. [CrossRef] [PubMed]
14. Sasabe, J.; Miyoshi, Y.; Suzuki, M.; Mita, M.; Konno, R.; Matsuoka, M.; Hamase, K.; Aiso, S. D-amino acid oxidase controls motoneuron degeneration through D-serine. *Proc. Natl. Acad. Sci. USA* **2012**, *109*, 627–632. [CrossRef] [PubMed]
15. Nuechterlein, K.H.; Subotnik, K.L.; Green, M.F.; Ventura, J.; Asarnow, R.F.; Gitlin, M.J.; Yee, C.M.; Gretchen-Doorly, D.; Mintz, J. Neurocognitive predictors of work outcome in recent-onset schizophrenia. *Schizophr. Bull.* **2011**, *37*, 33–40. [CrossRef] [PubMed]
16. Fujita, Y.; Ishima, T.; Hashimoto, K. Supplementation with D-serine prevents the onset of cognitive deficits in adult offspring after maternal immune activation. *Sci. Rep.* **2016**, *6*, 37261. [CrossRef] [PubMed]
17. Olferd, E.; Cross, B.; McWillian, D.; McWillian, A. *Guidelines for the Use of Animal in Neuroscience Research*; Canadian Council on Care (CCAC), Bradda Printing Services Inc.: Ottawa, ON, Canada, 1997; pp. 163–165.
18. Van Praag, H.; Shubert, T.; Zhao, C.; Gage, F.H. Exercise enhances learning and hippocampal neurogenesis in aged mice. *J. Neurosci.* **2005**, *25* (Suppl. 38), 8680–8685. [CrossRef] [PubMed]
19. Almaguer-Melian, W.; Cruz-Aguado, R.; Riva, C.L.; Kendrick, K.M.; Frey, J.U.; Bergado, J. Effect of LTP-reinforcing paradigms on neurotransmitter release in the dentate gyrus of young and aged rats. *Biochem. Biophys. Res. Commun.* **2005**, *327*, 877–883. [CrossRef] [PubMed]
20. Tombaugh, G.C.; Rowe, W.B.; Chow, A.R.; Michael, T.H.; Rose, G.M. Theta-frequency synaptic potentiation in CA1 in vitro distinguishes cognitively impaired from unimpaired aged Fischer 344 rats. *J. Neurosci.* **2002**, *22*, 9932–9940. [CrossRef] [PubMed]
21. Rowe, W.B.; Spreekmeester, E.; Meaney, M.J.; Quirion, R.; Rochford, J. Reactivity to novelty in cognitively-impaired and cognitively unimpaired aged rats and young rats. *Neuroscience* **1998**, *83*, 669–680. [CrossRef]
22. Tietze, F. Enzymic method for quantitative determination of nanogram amounts of total and oxidized glutathione: Applications to mammalian blood and other tissues. *Anal. Biochem.* **1969**, *27*, 502–522. [CrossRef]
23. Buege, J.A.; Aust, S.D. Microsomal lipid peroxidation. *Methods Enzymol.* **1978**, *52*, 302–310. [PubMed]

24. Lucas, K.K.; Dennis, E.A. Distinguishing phospholipase A2 types in biological samples by employing group-specific assays in the presence of inhibitors. *Prostag. Other Lipid Mediat.* **2005**, *77*, 235–248. [CrossRef] [PubMed]
25. Shukitt-Hale, B.; Casadesus, G.; Cantuti-Castelvetri, I.; Joseph, J.A. Effect of age on object exploration, habituation, and response to spatial and nonspatial change. *Behav. Neurosci.* **2001**, *115*, 1059–1064. [CrossRef] [PubMed]
26. Johnson, W.; Wilson-Delfosse, A.L.; Mieyal, J.J. Dysregulation of Glutathione Homeostasis in Neurodegenerative Diseases. *Nutrients* **2012**, *4*, 1399–1440. [CrossRef] [PubMed]
27. Allam, F.; Dao, T.; Gaurav, C.; Bohar, R.; Farzan, J. Grape Powder supplementation prevents oxidative stress-induced anxiety-like behaviour, memory impairment and high blood pressure in rats. *J. Nutr.* **2013**, *8*, 835–841. [CrossRef] [PubMed]
28. Blanco-Lezcano, L.; Jimenez-Martin, J.; Díaz-Hung, M.L.; Alberti-Amador, E.; Wong-Guerra, M.; González-Fraguela, M.E.; Estupiñán-Díaz, B.; Serrano-Sánchez, T.; Francis-Turner, L.; Delgado-Ocaña, S.; et al. Motor dysfunction and alterations in glutathione concentration, cholinesterase activity, and BDNF expression in substantia nigra pars compacta in rats with pedunculopontine lesion. *Neuroscience* **2017**, *348*, 83–97. [CrossRef] [PubMed]
29. Mattson, M.P. ER calcium and Alzheimer's disease: In a state of flux. *Sci. Signal.* **2010**, *3*, pe10. [CrossRef] [PubMed]
30. Rao, J.S.; Kellom, M.; Reese, E.A.; Rapoport, S.I.; Kim, H.-W. Dysregulated glutamate and dopamine transporters in postmortem frontal cortex from bipolar and schizophrenic patients. *J. Affect. Disord.* **2012**, *136*, 63–71. [CrossRef] [PubMed]
31. Chalimoniuk, M.; Stolecka, A.; Zieminska, E.; Stepien, A.; Langfort, J.; Strosznaider, J.B. Involvement of multiple protein kinases in cPLA2 phosphorylation, arachidonic acid release, and cell death in vivo and in vitro models of 1-methyl-4-phenylpyridinium-induced parkinsonism—The possible key role of PKG. *J. Neurochem.* **2009**, *110*, 307–317. [CrossRef] [PubMed]
32. Last, V.; Williams, A.; Werling, D. Inhibition of cytosolic phospholipase A2 prevents prion peptide-induced neuronal damage and co-localisation with beta iii tubulin. *BMC Neurosci.* **2012**, *13*, 106. [CrossRef] [PubMed]
33. Beckhauser, T.F.; Francis-Oliveira, J.; De Pasquale, R. Reactive Oxygen Species: Physiological and Physiopathological Effects on Synaptic Plasticity. *J. Exp. Neurosci.* **2016**, *10* (Suppl. 1), 23–48. [CrossRef] [PubMed]
34. Serrano, F.; Chang, A.; Hernandez, C.; Pautler, R.G.; Sweatt, J.D.; Klann, E. NADPH oxidase mediates beta-amyloid peptide-induced activation of ERK in hippocampal organotypic cultures. *Mol. Brain* **2009**, *2*, 31. [CrossRef] [PubMed]
35. Adibhatla, R.M.; Hatcher, J.F.; Dempsey, R.J. Phospholipase A2, hydroxyl radicals, and lipid peroxidation in transient cerebral ischemia. *ARS* **2003**, *5* (Suppl. 5), 647–654. [CrossRef] [PubMed]
36. Cocco, T.; Di Paola, M.; Papa, S.; Lorusso, M. Arachidonic acid interaction with the mitochondrial electron transport chain promotes reactive oxygen species generation. *Free Radic. Biol. Med.* **1999**, *27* (Suppl. 1–2), 1–2). [CrossRef]
37. Jiang, R.; Chen, S.; Shen, Y.; Wu, J.; Chen, S.; Wang, A.; Wu, S.; Zhao, X. Higher Levels of Lipoprotein Associated Phospholipase A2 is associated with Increased Prevalence of Cognitive Impairment: The APAC Study. *Sci. Rep.* **2016**, *6*, 33073. [CrossRef] [PubMed]
38. Shelat, P.B.; Chalimoniuk, M.; Wang, J.H.; Strosznajder, J.B.; Lee, J.C.; Sun, A.Y.; Simonyi, A.; Sun, G.Y. Amyloid beta peptide and NMDA induce ROS from NADPH oxidase and AA release from cytosolic phospholipase A2 in cortical neurons. *J. Neurochem.* **2008**, *106* (Suppl. 1), 45–55. [CrossRef] [PubMed]
39. Snyder, E.M.; Nong, Y.; Almeida, C.G.; Paul, S.; Moran, T.; Choi, E.Y.; Nairn, A.C.; Salter, M.W.; Lombroso, P.J.; Gouras, G.K.; et al. Regulation of NMDA receptor trafficking by amyloid-beta. *Nat. Neurosci.* **2005**, *8*, 1051–1058. [CrossRef] [PubMed]
40. Calon, F.; Lim, G.P.; Morihara, T.; Yang, F.; Ubeda, O.; Salem, N., Jr.; Frautschy, S.A.; Cole, G.M. Dietary n-3 polyunsaturated fatty acid depletion activates caspases and decreases NMDA receptors in the brain of a transgenic mouse model of Alzheimer's disease. *Eur. J. Neurosci.* **2005**, *22*, 617–626. [CrossRef] [PubMed]
41. Bergado, A.; Lucas, M.; Richter-Levin, G. Emotional tagging—A simple hypothesis in a complex reality. *Prog. Neurobiol.* **2011**, *94* (Suppl. 1), 64–76. [CrossRef] [PubMed]

42. Baxter, P.S.; Bell, K.F.S.; Hasel, P.; Kaindl, A.M.; Fricker, M.; Thomson, D.; Cregan, S.P.; Gillingwater, T.H.; Hardingham, G.H. Synaptic NMDA receptor activity is coupled to the transcriptional control of the glutathione system. *Nat. Commun.* **2015**, *6*, 6761. [CrossRef] [PubMed]
43. Foster, C.F. Dissecting the age-related decline on spatial learning and memory tasks in rodent models: *N*-methyl-D-aspartate receptors and voltage-dependent Ca^{2+} channels in senescent synaptic plasticity. *Prog. Neurobiol.* **2012**, *96* (Suppl. 3), 283–303. [CrossRef] [PubMed]
44. Liu, C.; Liu, Y.; Yang, Z. Myocardial infarction induces cognitive impairment by increasing the production of hydrogen peroxide in adult rat hippocampus. *Neurosci. Lett.* **2014**, *560*, 112–116. [CrossRef] [PubMed]
45. Murray, J.D.; Antigenic, A.; Gancsos, M.; Ichinose, M.; Corlett, P.R.; Krystal, J.H.; Wang, X.J. Linking microcircuit dysfunction to cognitive impairment: Effects of disinhibition associated with schizophrenia in a cortical working memory model. *Cereb. Cortex* **2014**, *24*, 859–872. [CrossRef] [PubMed]
46. Abe, T.; Suzuki, M.; Sasabe, J.; Takahashi, S.; Unekawa, M.; Mashima, K.; Iizumi, T.; Hamase, K.; Konno, R.; Aiso, S.; et al. Cellular origin and regulation of D- and L serine in in vitro and in vivo models of cerebral ischemia. *J. Cereb. Blood Flow Metab.* **2014**, *34*, 1928–1935. [CrossRef] [PubMed]
47. Balu, D.T.; Coyle, J.T. The NMDA receptor 'glycine modulatory site' in schizophrenia: D-serine, glycine, and beyond. *Curr. Opin. Pharmacol.* **2015**, *20*, 109–115. [CrossRef] [PubMed]
48. Benneyworth, M.A.; Li, Y.; Basu, A.C.; Bolshakov, V.Y.; Coyle, J.T. Cell selective conditional null mutations of serine racemase demonstrate a predominate localization in cortical glutamatergic neurons. *Cell. Mol. Neurobiol.* **2012**, *32*, 613–624. [CrossRef] [PubMed]
49. Suzuki, M.; Imanishi, N.; Mita, M.; Hamase, K.; Aiso, S.; Sasabe, J. Heterogeneity of D-Serine Distribution in the Human Central Nervous System. *ASN Neuro* **2017**, 1–10. [CrossRef] [PubMed]
50. Wolosker, H.; Balu, D.T.; Coyle, J.T. The Rise and Fall of the d-Serine-Mediated Gliotransmission Hypothesis. *Trends Neurosc.* **2016**, *39*, 712–721. [CrossRef] [PubMed]
51. Vanoni, M.A.; Cosma, A.; Mazzeo, D.; Mattevi, A.; Todone, F.; Curti, B. Limited proteolysis and X-ray crystallography reveal the origin of substrate specificity and of the rate-limiting product release during oxidation of D-amino acids catalyzed by mammalian D-amino acid oxidase. *Biochemistry* **1997**, *36*, 5624–5632. [CrossRef] [PubMed]
52. Sasabe, J.; Chiba, T.; Yamada, M.; Okamoto, K.; Nishimoto, I.; Matsuoka, M.; Aiso, S. D-Serine is a key determinant of glutamate toxicity in amyotrophic lateral sclerosis. *EMBO J.* **2007**, *26*, 4149–4159. [CrossRef] [PubMed]
53. Miladinovic, T.; Nashed, M.G.; Singh, G. Overview of Glutamatergic Dysregulation in Central Pathologies. *Biomolecules* **2015**, *5*, 3112–3141. [CrossRef] [PubMed]
54. Yang, S.; Qiao, H.; Wen, L.; Zhou, W.; Zhang, Y. D-serine enhances impaired long-term potentiation in CA1 subfield of hippocampal slices from aged senescence-accelerated mouse prone/8. *Neurosci. Lett.* **2005**, *379*, 7–12. [CrossRef] [PubMed]

13

Stress and Withdrawal from Chronic Ethanol Induce Selective Changes in Neuroimmune mRNAs in Differing Brain Sites

Darin J. Knapp [1,2,†,*], Kathryn M. Harper [1,†], Buddy A. Whitman [1,3,†], Zachary Zimomra [1] and George R. Breese [1,2,3,4,5]

1 Bowles Center for Alcohol Studies, The University of North Carolina at Chapel Hill, CB7178, Chapel Hill, NC 27599-7178, USA; Kathryn_harper@med.unc.edu (K.M.H.); bawhitman@gmail.com (B.A.W.); zzimomra@kent.edu (Z.Z.); george_breese@med.unc.edu (G.R.B.)

2 Department of Psychiatry, The University of North Carolina at Chapel Hill, CB7178, Chapel Hill, NC 27599-7178, USA

3 Curriculum in Neurobiology, The University of North Carolina at Chapel Hill, CB7178, Chapel Hill, NC 27599-7178, USA

4 Department of Pharmacology, The University of North Carolina at Chapel Hill, CB7178, Chapel Hill, NC 27599-7178, USA

5 UNC Neuroscience Center, The University of North Carolina at Chapel Hill, CB7178, Chapel Hill, NC 27599-7178, USA

* Correspondence: Darin_knapp@med.unc.edu

† These authors contributed equally to this work.

Academic Editor: Donna Gruol

Abstract: Stress is a strong risk factor in alcoholic relapse and may exert effects that mimic aspects of chronic alcohol exposure on neurobiological systems. With the neuroimmune system becoming a prominent focus in the study of the neurobiological consequences of stress, as well as chronic alcohol exposure proving to be a valuable focus in this regard, the present study sought to compare the effects of stress and chronic ethanol exposure on induction of components of the neuroimmune system. Rats were exposed to either 1 h exposure to a mild stressor (restraint) or exposure to withdrawal from 15 days of chronic alcohol exposure (i.e., withdrawal from chronic ethanol, WCE) and assessed for neuroimmune mRNAs in brain. Restraint stress alone elevated chemokine (C–C motif) ligand 2 (CCL2), interleukin-1-beta (IL-1β), tumor necrosis factor alpha (TNFα) and toll-like receptor 4 (TLR4) mRNAs in the cerebral cortex within 4 h with a return to a control level by 24 h. These increases were not accompanied by an increase in corresponding proteins. Withdrawal from WCE also elevated cytokines, but did so to varying degrees across different cytokines and brain regions. In the cortex, stress and WCE induced CCL2, TNFα, IL-1β, and TLR4 mRNAs. In the hypothalamus, only WCE induced cytokines (CCL2 and IL-1β) while in the hippocampus, WCE strongly induced CCL2 while stress and WCE induced IL-1β. In the amygdala, only WCE induced CCL2. Finally—based on the previously demonstrated role of corticotropin-releasing factor 1 (CRF1) receptor inhibition in blocking WCE-induced cytokine mRNAs—the CRF1 receptor antagonist CP154,526 was administered to a subgroup of stressed rats and found to be inactive against induction of CCL2, TNFα, or IL-1β mRNAs. These differential results suggest that stress and WCE manifest broad neuroimmune effects in brain depending on the cytokine and brain region, and that CRF inhibition may not be a relevant mechanism in non-alcohol exposed animals. Overall, these effects are complex in terms of their neuroimmune targets and neuroanatomical specificity. Further investigation of the differential distribution of cytokine induction across neuroanatomical regions, individual cell types (e.g., neuronal phenotypes and glia), severity of chronic alcohol exposure, as well as across differing stress types may prove useful in understanding differential mechanisms of induction and for targeting select systems for pharmacotherapeutic intervention in alcoholism.

Keywords: restraint stress; chronic ethanol withdrawal; cytokine mRNAs; CRF; alcohol; CP154,526

1. Introduction

Acute withdrawal from chronic ethanol (WCE) exposure is associated with increased anxiety-like behavior [1–3]. Breese et al. [4] also found in a three-withdrawal protocol that stress substituted for the initial two withdrawals such that withdrawal from a single five-day cycle of chronic ethanol induced anxiety. Subsequently, Breese et al. [5] found that the anxiety-like response to restraint stress was facilitated when the stress was applied after WCE—a finding in agreement with other reports that stress after WCE can enhance negative effects [6,7].

Breese et al. [8] and Knapp et al. [9] also reported that administration of lipopolysaccharide (LPS) or a cytokine into the brain substituted for the initial intermittent ethanol exposures applied prior to a single CE exposure to induce negative effects. This latter outcome was comparable to the change observed with prior exposure to stress [4,5] or after WCE [2,3,10]. More recently, Whitman et al. [9] reported that WCE increased cytokine mRNAs in the cortex—a cytokine immune response that was not related to infection [11–13]. Whitman et al. [9] also observed increases in mRNAs for toll-like receptor 4 (TLR4) and High Mobility Group Box 1 Protein (HMGB1) which serve as an endogenous system that activates neuroimmune function [11,12,14–16]. The induction of cytokine mRNAs increases after WCE was blocked by a CRF1 receptor (CRF1R) antagonist [9]—a finding possibly linking the cytokine mRNA changes to CRF involvement in the anxiety-like behavior that accompanies WCE and stress [3–5].

Various studies have linked stress to increases in cytokine mRNAs in various brain sites [17–25]. Collectively, these reports provided new information about the effects of various stressors (social stress/defeat, footshock or tailshock, restraint, forced swim, glucose/insulin challenge, or cold stress) on neuroimmune mRNA responses of the hypothalamus, hippocampus, cerebellum, posterior cortex, and nucleus of the solitary tract. Relatedly, work from our group had shown that restraint stress could substitute for the initial repeated exposures to chronic alcohol to induce a negative emotional state following a future withdrawal as inferred from anxiety-like behavior, (e.g., [4]). To explore the potential relevance of stress effects on neuroimmune responses in a chronic ethanol and withdrawal model, Breese et al. [8] administered LPS or a pro-inflammatory cytokine into brain to substitute for the initial intermittent ethanol withdrawals or mild stress to induce anxiety-like behavior following a single ethanol withdrawal that otherwise would be incapable of eliciting anxiety [4,5]. Missing from this strategy was an assessment of whether the restraint stress itself induced neuroimmune changes consistent with functional effects on behavior. Thus, a key new component of the current studies was to assess whether stress, which by itself has been shown in some studies to increase brain cytokines (e.g., [18,20,21,26]), produced changes comparable to those triggered by WCE. Additionally, comparisons were made of cytokine mRNA in different brain regions after stress or WCE. Finally, to complement earlier studies with WCE and cortical cytokines, the present study explored whether a corticotrophin-releasing factor receptor antagonist would attenuate stress-induced cytokines in the cortex. This line of inquiry is pertinent to understanding the relative overlap of neuroimmune effects of stress and the WCE model in relation to alcohol abuse, drug addiction, and several psychiatric disorders (see [6–8,27–35]).

2. Materials and Methods

2.1. Animals

Adult male Sprague–Dawley (S–D) rats or Wistar Rats (Charles-River, Raleigh, NC, USA) weighing 180–200 g upon arrival were group housed and fed RMH3000 rat chow (Test Diets, Richmond, IN, USA) for 2–3 days prior to study to acclimate them to the new environment (temperatures 70–72 °F; humidity 40%–60%; and light/dark cycle 12 h:12 h with lights from 7:00 a.m. to 7:00 p.m.).

Subsequently, all rats were singly housed for the duration of experimental procedures. Methods used in this study were approved by Institutional Animal Care and Use Committee (IACUC, protocol number: 14-125) at the University of North Carolina (Chapel Hill, NC, USA).

2.2. *Liquid Diet for Controls and for Chronic Ethanol Exposure*

In the initial experiment, rats that received an acute restraint stress were on chow diet before the stress challenge. For other experiments, a nutritionally-complete and calorically-balanced liquid diet was used for the rats that received a continuous 7% (*w*/*v*) ethanol diet followed by 24 h of withdrawal (WCE)—an approach previously utilized by our laboratory (e.g., [1,36,37]; see Figure 1) to administer daily ethanol doses of 9–13 g/kg. The liquid control diet (CD) was calorically balanced to the WCE diet by adjustments of the amount of dextrose. Rats were fed either control diet or the ethanol diet with a modified pair-feeding strategy [1].

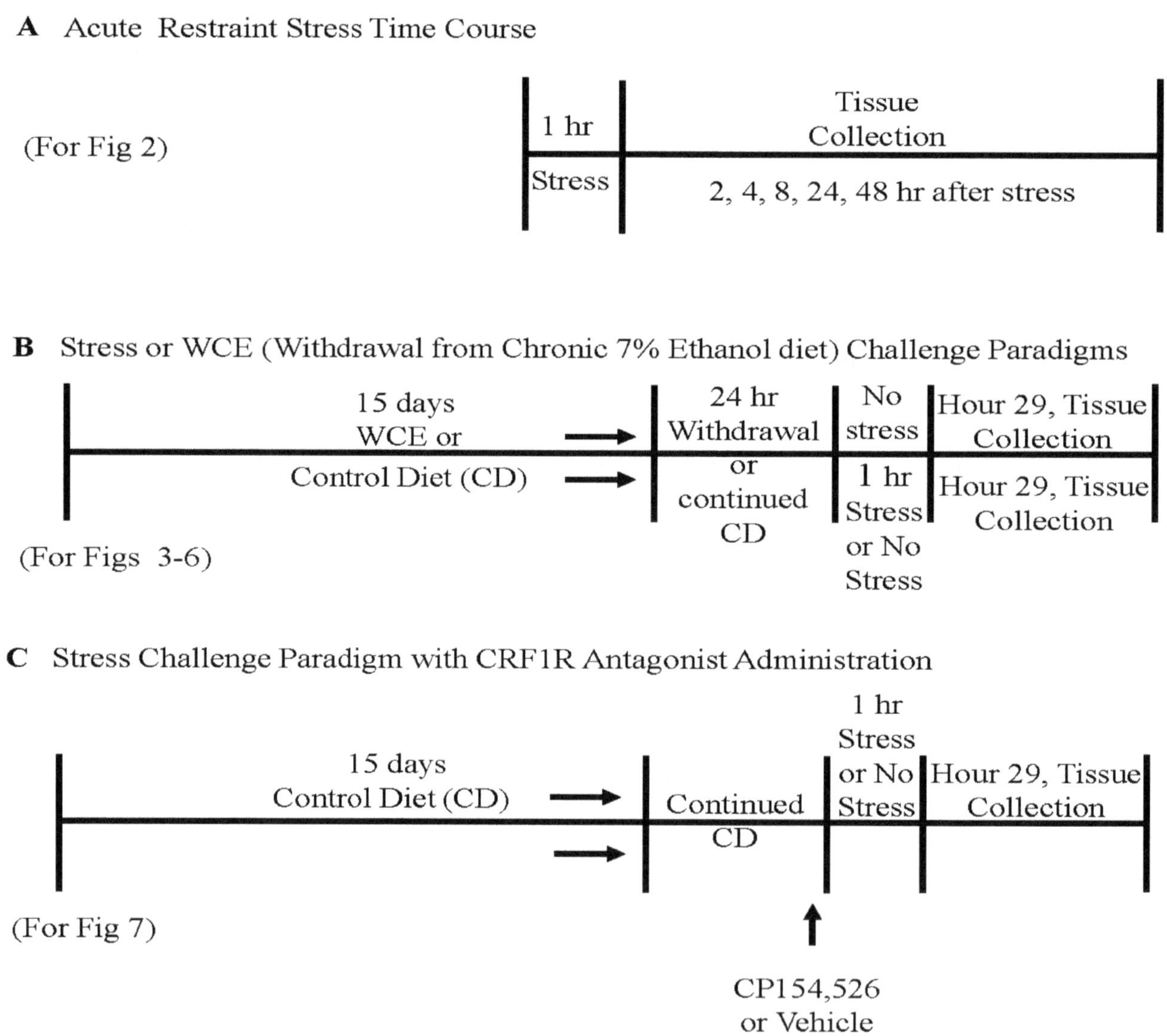

Figure 1. Schematics depicting experimental protocols. **A**: represents the acute restraint stress time course, while **B**: represents the stress and withdrawal from chronic alcohol and **C**: represents the CRF1R antagonist study.

2.3. Restraint Stress in Controls and after Withdrawal from Chronic Ethanol Exposure

Initial efforts determined the time course of stress effects on brain cytokine mRNAs. Stress consisted of 60 min of restraint in plastic decapicones. These rats were sacrificed 2, 4, 8, 24, or 48 h following the stress (see schematic in Figure 1A).

2.4. Brain Tissue Collection and Real-Time PCR Analysis for Tissue mRNA

Following experimental procedures, rats were rapidly decapitated and brain tissue stored at −80 °C for subsequent extractions for PCR. To initiate PCR procedures, total RNA was extracted with Trizol (Invitrogen, Carlsbad, CA, USA) from homogenized dissected brain regions from control and ethanol-treated experimental brain sections followed by use of the SV total RNA isolation system (Promega, Madison, WI, USA). This tissue was then used for reverse transcription PCR using the Superscript First Strand or Superscript III First Strand Synthesis Super mix (Life Technologies, Grand Island, NY, USA) [38]. The primer sequences used for the cortex were chemokine (C–C motif) ligand 2 (CCL2) = 5′-TCACGCTTCTGGGCCTGTTG-3′ (forward) and 5′-CAGCCGACTCATTGGGATC ATC-3′ (reverse); Interleukin-1β (IL-1β) = 5′-GAAACAGCAATGGTCGGGAC-3′ (forward) and 5′-AA GACACGGGTTCCATGGTG-3′ (reverse); tumor necrosis factor-α (TNFα) = 5′-ATGTGGAACTGGCAG AGGAG-3′ (forward) and 5′-ACGAGCAGGAATGAGAAGAGG-3′(reverse); Toll-like-receptor-4 (TLR4) = 5′-GCCGGAAAGTTATTGTGGTGGT-3′ (forward) and 5′-ATGGGTTTTAGGCGCAGAGTT T-3′ (reverse); β-actin, 5′-ATGGTGGGTATGGGTCAGAAGG-3′ (forward) and 5′-GCTCATTGTAG AAAGTGTGGTGCC-3′ (reverse). SYBR green PCR master mix (Applied Biosystems, Foster City, CA, USA) was used for real-time PCR analysis of the cortex on the Bio-Rad MyiQ (Bio-Rad, Hercules, CA, USA). For other brain regions (and the CP154,526 study), mRNA analyses were optimized with TaqMan® (Thermo Fisher Scientific, Waltham, MA, USA) expression assays—CCL2 (Rn00580555_m1), TNFα (Rn01525859_g1), IL-1β (Rn00580432_m1), TLR4 (Rn00569848_m1), and β-actin (Rn00667869_m1)—and samples were run on a StepOnePlus real time PCR machine (Life Technologies, Grand Island, NY, USA). For all data, the cycle time (Ct) values were normalized with β-actin to assess the relative differences in expression between groups. Ct values of β-actin never differed across groups therefore β-actin was an appropriate choice as a housekeeping gene. Calculated values were expressed as relative change to a designated control set as 100%.

2.5. Enzyme-linked Immunosorbent Assay (ELISA) for Cytokines

Because changes in levels of cytokine proteins in the S–D rats have been found to correlate poorly with mRNA changes (see [38,39]) initially only expression of mRNAs for cytokines was assessed. Nonetheless, because of interest in the relationship between mRNA and proteins induced by stress, ELISA assays for cytokine proteins in cortex were first performed 4 h after stress in the time course determination in the S–D rats (Figure 2). Subsequently, assays of cytokine proteins were performed 4 h after an acute restraint stress to Wistar rats (Charles River, Raleigh, NC, USA). Each cortical sample was homogenized in Iscove's Modified Dulbecco Medium (Invitrogen, #12440046, Carlsbad, CA, USA) containing 1 tablet per 50 mL of the complete protease inhibitor cocktail (Roche Diagnostics #11697498001, Indianapolis, IN, USA). Homogenized specimens were then centrifuged at 12,000× g for 10 min at 4 °C and the supernatants collected and stored at −80 °C until the ELISA determination was made. ELISA kits were purchased for IL-1β and TNFα from R & D Systems, (Minneapolis, MN, USA), and for the CCL2 from BD Bio-Sciences (San Jose, CA, USA). ELISA procedures were performed according to the manufacturer's instructions. Standards for IL-1β and TNFα were serially diluted 4 times to concentrations of 1.95 pg/mL and 0.78 pg/mL, respectively, and the standard for CCL2 was used as supplied. All tissue cytokine levels were corrected for protein using Pierce® BCA Protein assay (Thermo Scientific, Rockford, IL, USA).

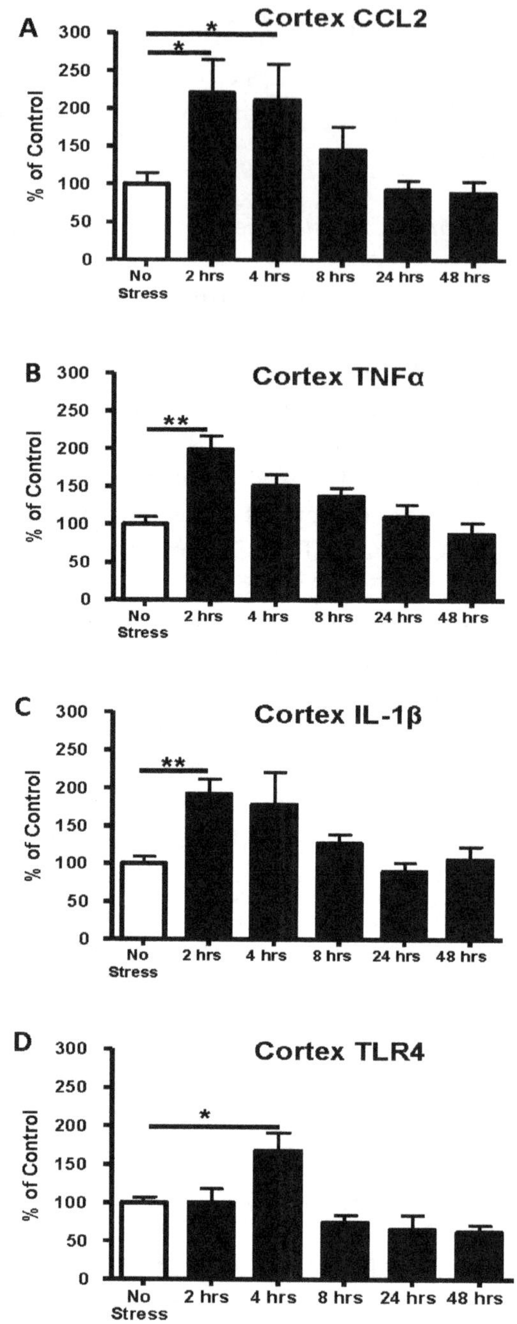

Figure 2. Time course of changes in cerebro-cortical mRNAs for CCL2, IL-1β, TNFα, and TLR4 following 1 h of restraint stress. Stress elevated CCL2 mRNA in cortex ($F(5,32) = 3.82$, $p = 0.008$), an effect that peaked at 2 and 4 h. A similar effect was found for IL-1β mRNA ($F(5,48) = 5.13$, $p < 0.01$) and TNFα ($F(5,53) = 8.51$, $p < 0.0001$). TLR4 mRNA was elevated at 4 h ($F(5,38) = 8.5$, $p < 0.0001$). In all cases, the cytokine mRNA levels gradually returned to control levels by 24 h. ** $p < 0.01$ * $p < 0.05$ compared with controls that received no stress (open bars). **A**, **B**, **C**, and **D** delineate data for CCL2, TNFα, IL-1β and TLR4 mRNAs, respectively, ($n = 5$–8 per time point)

2.6. CRF Receptor Antagonist Administration

Subgroups of CD rats were injected once with the CRF1R antagonist CP154,526 [38,40] or vehicle 15 min prior to the start of stress (Figure 1C). The drug was prepared as a microfine suspension in 0.5% carboxymethylcelluose and administered intraperitoneally at a dose of 15 mg/kg in a volume of 2 mL/kg.

2.7. Statistical Analysis

Data (expressed as mean ± standard error of mean (SEM)) were evaluated for statistical significance with ANOVA with Fisher's least significant difference (LSD) tests for individual comparisons of group pairs as appropriate. Individual data points that were three standard deviations from their respective group means were removed from the group prior to analysis. p-values < 0.05 were considered statistically significant.

3. Results

3.1. Time Course of Expression of Cytokine and TLR4 mRNAs in Cortex Following 1-Hour of Restraint Stress in Sprague–Dawley (S–D) Rats

Previous studies have shown that acute stress can affect neuroimmune function in brain [13,14,18–22,24–26,41]. Therefore, our initial investigation was to determine if the restraint stress utilized in previous behavioral studies [5] would induce a neuroimmune response. Figure 1A shows the experimental protocol for determining cytokine mRNA changes after 60 min of restraint stress in the absence of WCE. As shown in Figure 2, each mRNA assayed was increased 2–4 h after the restraint stress. The expression of CCL2 mRNA after stress was significantly increased above control by 121% at 2 h and by 111% at 4 h ($p < 0.05$). The expression of TNFα mRNA after stress was increased above control by 2 h (99%) ($p < 0.01$). Likewise, IL-1β mRNA was elevated by 92% above control by 2 h ($p < 0.01$). Cytokine mRNAs gradually returned to control levels by 8 h and remained there for up to 48 h after the acute-stress exposure (Figure 2). Because TLR4 has been implicated in induction of cytokines [11,15,41–45], we also examined whether mRNA for TLR4 would be altered by the acute restraint-stress. Figure 2D shows that TLR4 mRNA expression was significantly elevated by 68% above control 4 h following the stress challenge ($p < 0.05$) with return to control levels by 8 h.

3.2. Determination of Cytokine Protein Levels in Cortex after Restraint Stress

To determine whether increases in cytokine proteins accompanied the increases in CCL2, IL-1β, and TNFα mRNAs induced by restraint stress, proteins were measured in cortex 4 h after the restraint stress challenge to the S–D rats (Table 1). Cytokine protein levels, unlike cytokine mRNAs, in the controls were not statistically altered in the S–D rats (Table 1). Subsequently, this same assessment was performed for Wistar rats to determine if this rat strain might express a change in cytokine proteins following the 60 min of restraint stress. In the Wistar rats, as in the S–D rats, cytokine proteins were not increased by stress ($p > 0.05$). Because increases in cytokine protein levels were not observed in either rat strain [38], only S–D rats were used in the experiments assessing expression of cytokine mRNAs induced by stress or WCE.

Table 1. Effect of acute stress on cytokine proteins in brain.

Group	CCL2	IL-1β	TNFα
S-D Non-Stressed	12.9 (0.3)	0.37 (0.05)	ND
S-D Stressed	13.7 (0.6)	0.28 (0.02)	ND
Wistar Non-Stressed	42.2 (2.3)	1.48 (0.22)	0.11 (0.03)
Wistar Stressed	58.1 (15.4)	1.05 (0.84)	0.12 (0.03)

Data are mean +/− standard error of mean (SEM) protein/mg total protein from cerebral cortex of rats that were restrained for 1 h and sacrificed 4 h later. CCL2: Chemokine (C–C motif) ligand 2; IL-1β: Interleukin-1-beta; TNFα: Tumor Necrosis Factor alpha; ND: not detectable; S–D: Sprague–Dawley.

3.3. Effect of Stress or WCE on Selected Cytokine and TLR4 mRNAs in Cortex

In prior work, WCE increased anxiety-like behavior [46] and elevated cortical cytokines [38]. This study directly compared the magnitude of the WCE effect on cytokine mRNA with that produced by stress. Figure 3 shows that an acute 60 min restraint stress increased cortical cytokine mRNAs

4 h later to a degree comparable to that observed in Figure 2. Likewise, in accord with previous work [38], Figure 3 confirms that CCL2, IL-1β, TNFα, and TLR4 mRNAs were significantly increased over controls in cortex 29 h after WCE ($p < 0.05$). These cytokine mRNA increases following WCE were comparable in magnitude (80%–150% over control) to the increases induced by stress (Figure 2).

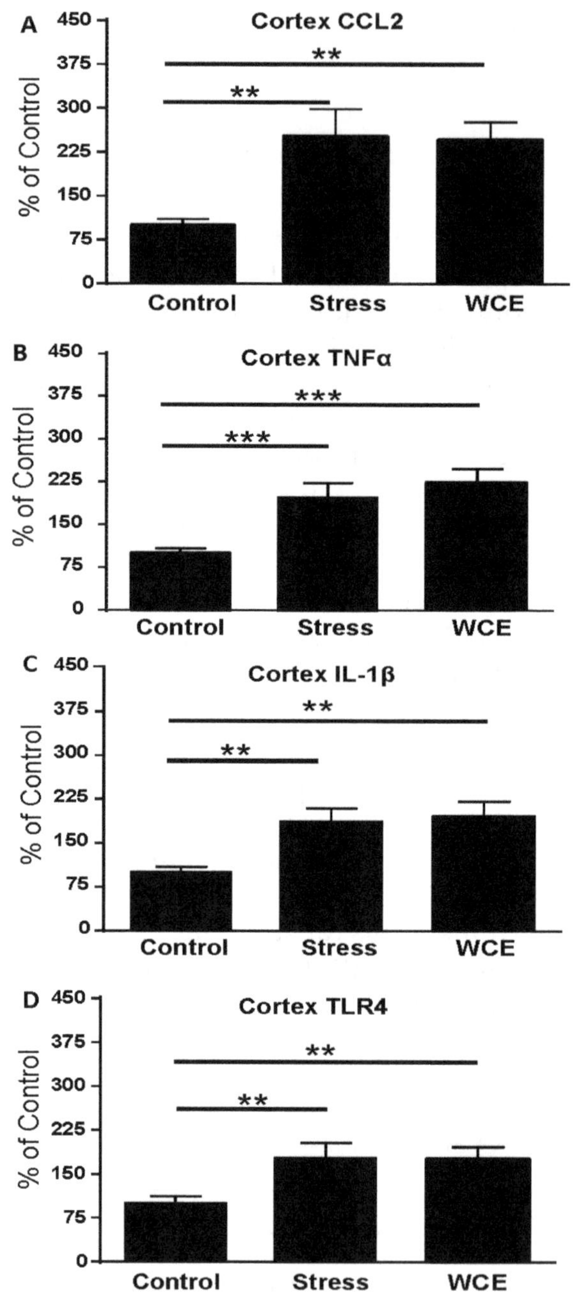

Figure 3. Effects of restraint stress or withdrawal from chronic ethanol (WCE) on cerebro-cortical neuroimmune mRNAs. Control and stress rats received non-ethanol containing liquid diets and 1 h restraint stress or no stress, respectively. WCE rats received chronic ethanol liquid diet for 15 days followed by 29 h of withdrawal. Overall, a significant effect was also noted across the groups for CCL2 ($F(2,23) = 6.47$, $p < 0.01$) with individual comparison of groups revealing significant effects of stress or WCE relative to controls. A similar profile was noted for TNFα ($F(2,32) = 10.2$, $p < 0.001$), IL-1β ($F(2,27) = 7.00$, $p < 0.01$), and TLR4 ($F(2,31) = 4.97$, $p < 0.05$) and individual group comparisons to the respective controls. * $p < 0.05$, ** $p < 0.01$, ** $p < 0.001$ versus Controls. **A**, **B**, **C**, and **D** delineate data for CCL2, TNFα, IL-1β and TLR4 mRNAs, respectively, ($n = 8–12$ per group).

3.4. Effect of Stress or WCE on Selected Cytokine mRNAs in Hypothalamus, Hippocampus, and Amygdala after WCE

To examine the generalizability of the cortical neuroimmune mRNA response, the effects of stress or WCE were studied in additional brain regions of known importance in chronic ethanol effects. Figure 4 illustrates that, whereas stress did not increase CCL2 or IL-1β mRNA in the hypothalamus ($p > 0.05$, Figure 4A,C), WCE increased both of these cytokine mRNAs significantly (by about 30%–45%, $p < 0.01$). Further, hypothalamic TLR4 and TNFα mRNAs were not significantly altered by either challenge ($p < 0.05$ vs. control).

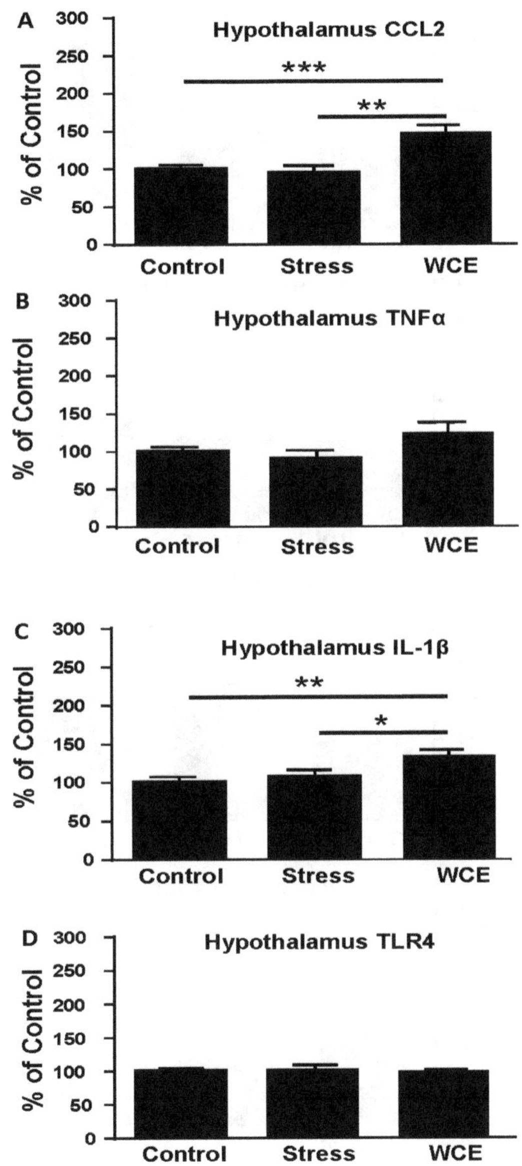

Figure 4. Effects of restraint stress or WCE on hypothalamic neuroimmune mRNAs. For CCL2, there was a significant overall effect of treatments ($F(2,35) = 9.13$, $p < 0.001$) with a significant group comparison relative to controls revealed only with the WCE treatment. For TNFα, there was no overall effect of treatment ($p > 0.05$) despite a trend toward a WCE effect. There was an overall effect of treatment on IL-1β ($F(2,38) = 4.59$, $p < 0.05$) with the WCE group being higher than controls or stressed rats. Finally, there were no effects on TLR4. Group designations are the same as those in Figure 3. * $p < 0.05$, ** $p < 0.01$, ** $p < 0.001$ versus controls. **A**, **B**, **C**, and **D** delineate data for CCL2, TNFα, IL-1β and TLR4 mRNAs, respectively, ($n = 8$–13 per group).

In the hippocampus, CCL2 (Figure 5A) increased with stress (by approximately 50%), but the effect of WCE was more dramatic (129% of control) and significantly higher than that for stress. In contrast, while WCE tended to increase TNFα in this region, no significant effects were found in response to stress (Figure 5B), with a similar result for TLR4 (Figure 5D). With regard to IL-1β (Figure 5C), both stress and WCE comparably induced this cytokine. Finally, in the amygdala (Figure 6), there was no effect of stress alone on any measure ($p > 0.05$), although WCE significantly increased CCL2 relative to stress levels.

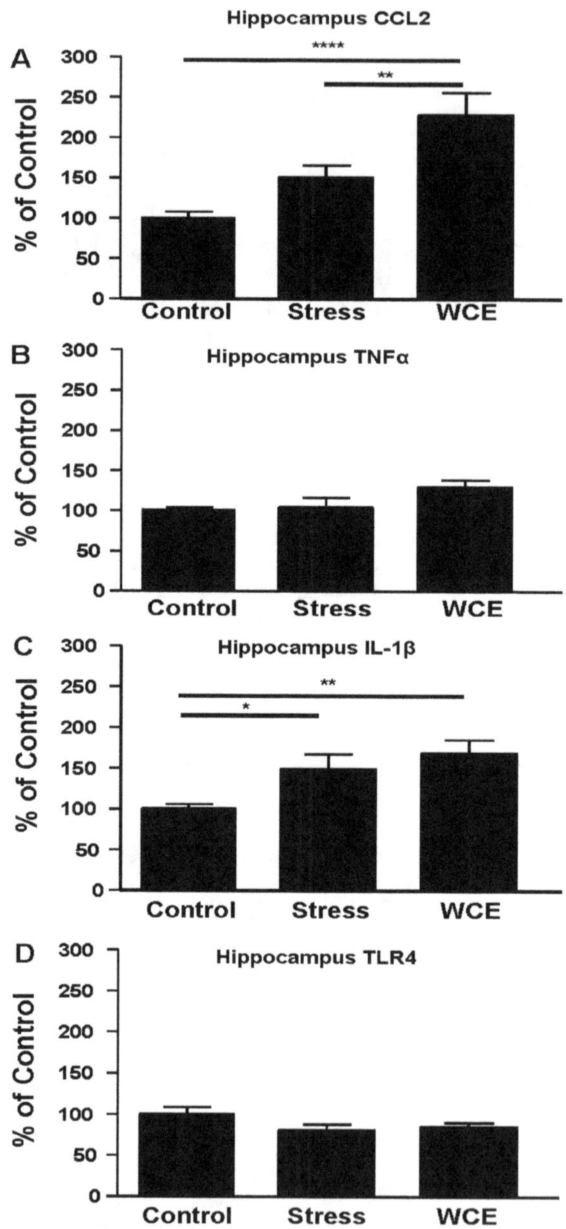

Figure 5. Effects of restraint stress or WCE for hippocampal neuroimmune mRNAs. For CCL2, there was an overall effect of the treatments ($F(2,34) = 10.54$, $p < 0.001$) and a significant effect of WCE relative to stress or control. The trend toward a stress effect was not significant. Similarly, an overall trend toward a significant effect of treatments for TNFα was not significant ($p = 0.07$). For IL-1β, there was an overall significant effect of treatments ($F(2,34) = 4.98$, $p < 0.05$) with significant effects of stress and WCE relative to controls. Finally, there were no significant effects found with TLR4 mRNA. * $p < 0.05$, ** $p < 0.01$, **** $p < 0.0001$ versus Controls. **A**, **B**, **C**, and **D** delineate data for CCL2, TNFα, IL-1β and TLR4 mRNAs, respectively, ($n = 9$–13 per group).

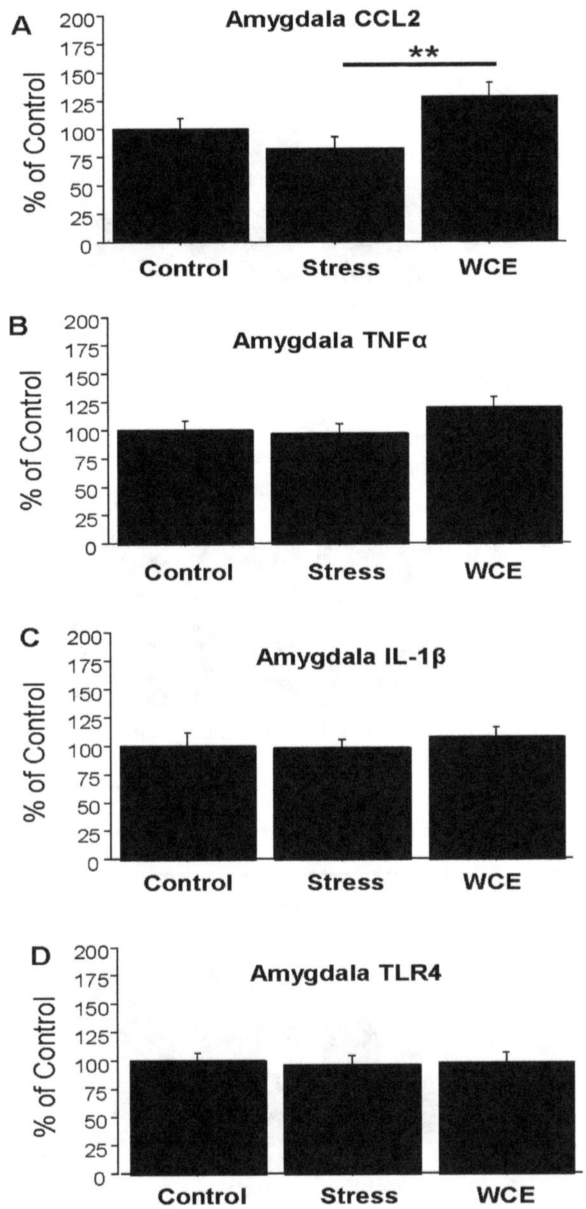

Figure 6. Effects of restraint stress or WCE on amygdala neuroimmune mRNAs. For CCL2, there was a modest, but significant, overall effect of treatments ($F(2,27) = 4.450$, $p < 0.05$) with a significant group difference between WCE and stress. There were no other effects of treatments for TNFα, IL-1β, or TLR4 mRNAs. ** $p < 0.01$ compared with the stressed group. **A**, **B**, **C**, and **D** delineate data for CCL2, TNFα, IL-1β and TLR4 mRNAs, respectively, ($n = 7$–11 per group).

3.5. Effect of the CRF1R Antagonist CP154,526 on Cortical Cytokine mRNAs Following Stress

Having twice shown previously that at CRF1R antagonist blocks cytokine induction arising during ethanol withdrawal in the cortex [38], the final experiment focused on determining whether the drug would also block the induction due to stress. Figure 7 illustrates the effect of CP154,526 on cytokine mRNAs in the cortex. Figure 7A shows that stress increased CCL2 (63%, $p < 0.05$) and this effect was not blocked by CP154,526. Similarly, Figure 7B shows that TNFα was increased by stress (41%, $p < 0.01$) and again the stress effect was unaltered by CP. Finally, the profile of action on IL-1β was similar as shown in Figure 7C which shows that IL-1β was significantly increased by stress (55%, $p < 0.05$) and CP154,526 failed to block this induction.

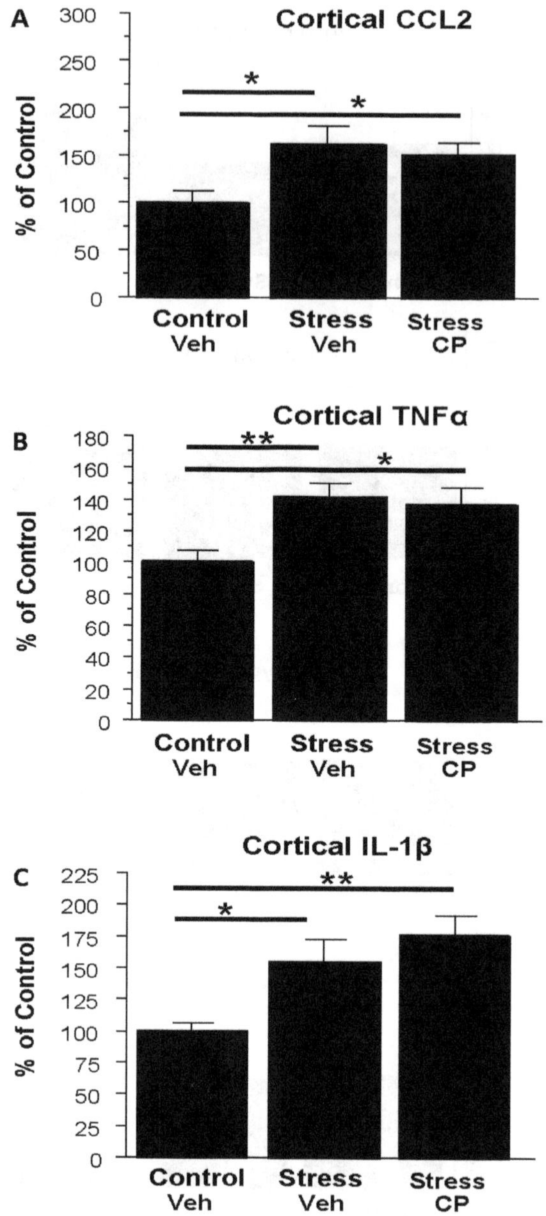

Figure 7. Effects of the corticotropin-releasing factor 1 (CRF1R) antagonist CP154,526 (CP) on cerebro-cortical neuroimmune mRNAs following restraint stress in rats. Overall there was a significant effect among the groups for CCL2 ($F(2,16) = 4.00$, $p < 0.05$) with CP failing to block stressed-induction. There also was an effect of treatments for TNFα ($F(2,16) = 4.87$, $p < 0.05$) with stress inducing and CP failing to block induction. Finally, as with CCL2 and TNFα, cortical IL-1β effects were significant overall ($F(2,16) = 6.34$, $p < 0.01$), but there was no blockade of the stress effect by the drug. * $p < 0.05$, ** $p < 0.01$ versus control-vehicle treated rats. Veh = 0.5% carboxymethylcellulose. **A**, **B**, and **C** delineate data for CCL2, TNFα, IL-1β and TLR4 mRNAs, respectively, (n = 5–7 per group).

4. Discussion

In the present investigation, restraint stress increased the mRNAs for CCL2, IL-1β, and TNFα and the receptor TLR4 in cortex of S–D rats (Figures 2 and 3)—a result supporting a growing body of reports of acute stressor-induced increases in neuroimmune mRNAs in various brain sites [19,20,23,24,26,47]. The restraint stress-associated increase in cytokine and TLR4 mRNAs in cortex peaked by around 4 h after exposure and then returned to control levels within 1 day. However, stress did not always affect these mRNAs in other brain sites. Even though mRNAs were increased

4 h after stress exposure in controls, corresponding cytokine proteins were not altered at this time point in either S–D or Wistar Rats (Table 1). Neuroimmune responses to WCE sometimes followed the response to stress and sometimes did not. While CCL2, TNFα, IL-1β, and TLR4 responses in the cortex were generally comparably high with either challenge, responses in the amygdala were comparably minimal. However, in the hippocampus, responses varied by type of challenge and across neuroimmune markers with a robust CCL2 response to withdrawal and a comparable IL-1β response to either challenge. In the hypothalamus, stress was inactive while withdrawal elevated CCL2 and IL-1β. Finally, the results showed that CRF1R inhibition did not alter stress-induced neuroimmune responses in the cortex, a result inconsistent with the earlier findings that CRF1R inhibition blocked cytokine responses to chronic withdrawal [38].

The reason that stress increased select cytokine mRNAs but not corresponding cytokine proteins is unknown. This pattern of mRNA versus protein results is similar to that observed in studies in other areas of rat brain. For example, Hueston et al. [21] demonstrated an increase in IL-1β mRNA without an accompanying increase in IL-1β protein in the paraventricular nucleus (PVN) to restraint stress. Deak et al. [19] found that IL-1β protein did not increase in the hypothalamus of S–D rats after restraint stress alone but did observe an increase in IL-1β to stress in the hypothalamus after applying a combination of restraint and shaking (i.e., a more severe stress). Additionally, Porterfield et al. [39] found that 2 h of restraint increased expression of IL-1β mRNA in the hypothalamus and caused a corresponding increase in this cytokine protein in the more stress-responsive Fischer 344 rats, but not in S–D rats [39]. However, Whitman et al. [38] found that an acute LPS challenge increased both selected cytokine proteins and corresponding cytokine mRNAs in the cortex of S–D rats [38]. While a focus on the hypothalamus and IL-1 (e.g., [19,23]) has been a fruitful focus of prior research so far as consistent effects of stress are concerned, reports of combinations of stressors may be particularly worthy of follow up. In addition to the work of Deak et al. [19] and Porterfield et al. [39] noted above, prior cold stress rendered animals' neuroimmune systems responsive to future LPS treatment [20], as shown by elevated hypothalamic and prefrontal cortical neuroimmune markers). Considered in aggregate, such studies suggest that genetic background and/or the degree and combinations of stress or challenge to the neuroimmune system may be at least in part responsible for the presence of a neuroimmune response and possibly for differences in protein versus mRNA responses as well. It may be particularly interesting in this context to examine the possibility that differentially engaged molecular mechanisms of mRNA versus protein processing across time may account for asynchrony of these constructs. That is, the observation of a stress-associated increase in cytokine mRNAs without corresponding changes in cytokine proteins could also be explained by release, utilization, and degradation of the protein during the stress challenge. Relatedly, habituation or exhaustion of mRNA generation could also be a factor in some cases. In this context, Minami et al. [23] showed that the IL-1β mRNA response in the hypothalamus declined over four hours despite continued immobilization stress. Such an effect could conceivably have influenced our amygdala and hypothalamic findings, but would be harder to extend to our cortical and hippocampal results. Also relevant is the more recent report of Vecchiarelli et al. [26] who found that increasing the length of restraint stress in Sprague–Dawley rats to two hours elevated protein levels of amygdala TNFα, decreased IL-6, while monocyte chemoattractant protein-1 (MCP-1/CCL2) remained unchanged. Based on our data, it is unlikely that any such diminished cortical response would apply to the cortex globally. Differential responses across subregions of the cortex might be critical with the net effect of global cortical responses being an increased response that must be dependent on some region(s) being particularly sensitive. Extending this logic to the hippocampus or hypothalamus may be premature, as Vecchiarelli did not see changes in these regions. The single hour of restraint stress in the present work did not alter amygdala or hypothalamic TNFα mRNA but did increase cortical IL-1β, TNFα and CCL2, and hippocampal IL-1β. Perhaps the length or severity of stress, along with a focus on cortical subregions represent key prerequisites to examinations of either individual or combinatorial challenges. Further research to explore these various possibilities is warranted, including combinations of different intensities, times, and types of stress with chronic alcohol challenges, circadian rhythms, and genetic background.

To assess the possible contribution of other components to neuroimmune activation pathways that result in the effects observed here, TLR4 mRNA was also assessed after restraint stress. A significant increase in TLR4 mRNA, was observed only at 4 h in cortical tissue following stress, returned to control level by 8 h, and remained at this level through 48 h after the stress (Figure 2D). This fairly tight time-response relative to the other mRNAs was one of the reasons for focusing on 29 h of withdrawal (4 h post stress relative to non-stressed alcohol withdrawn rats) as the target for comparison. A consideration here is that prior assessments [38] focused mostly on alcohol withdrawal-derived mRNA data from the 24th hour of withdrawal although they showed that mRNAs can remain elevated for longer periods, thus it seems unlikely that mRNA levels would be meaningfully different across these two time points within the present study. Regardless, these results agree with Blandino et al. [18] who found no change in cortical TLR4 mRNA at their 2 h time point post footshock or LPS treatment. It is notable that stress or WCE elevated TLR4 mRNA only in the cortex. The reasons for this specific effect on TLR4 are unknown, but suggests differential neuroimmune regulation and possibly lower thresholds for activation across brain regions. The TLR4 receptor complex is a prominent driver in neuroimmune processes in general and in alcoholism (e.g., see [48]) and animal models in particular (e.g., [38,49,50]). In fact, the TLR4 receptor may play a role in a positive feedback loop that amplifies the intensity of overall neuroimmune activation in alcoholism [51]. Such reduced thresholds for neuroimmune activation may be represented most profoundly following endotoxin where activation progresses to neurodegeneration in the substantia nigra with corresponding behavioral deficits [52].

While WCE alone generally elevated cortical cytokines (and see [38]) and hippocampal CCL2 and IL-1β, WCE or stress alone did not consistently do so for some mRNAs in some regions (e.g., the hippocampus and hypothalamus, Figures 4 and 5). The limited TNFα response in these regions contrasts with the effects of pain-associated stress such as footshock reported by Blandino et al. [18] and thus supports the idea that the type of stress may be important in cytokine induction. Again, the pattern of results suggests that unique mechanisms are operating across brain regions and it would likely be productive to further examine neuroimmune mRNAs more generally on a region by region basis and thus speak to the relatively understudied yet critical issue of how neuroimmune changes across regions or networks could produce neuropathology. The potential differential induction of anti-inflammatory cytokines such as IL-10 could also be informative. These future studies should elucidate how stress induction of some cytokine mRNAs, but not others, contributes to the profile of neuroimmune activation in models of alcoholism [3–5,9].

One potentially important focus in identifying mechanisms of cytokine regulation in this experimental context relates to the corticotropin-releasing factor (CRF) system. The data herein show that the CRF1R antagonist CP154,526 was inactive against stress induction of neuroimmune mRNAs. This effect provides an interesting comparison with previous work [38] that focused on the effect of this drug on cytokine mRNAs elevated by WCE. The mechanisms that explain how the drug comes to exert an effect on one challenge and not the other are unknown, but differential engagement of adaptive mechanisms might be one possibility. That is, the drug may affect a recruited process unique to rats experiencing WCE. This interesting possibility is reminiscent of the work of Koob and colleagues who noted that CRF receptor antagonist effects were generally not manifest unless rats were dependent on alcohol (e.g., [53]). It is important to note that the CP154,526 study herein was limited in its scope and could be expanded in future studies to examine related questions. For example, the drug could be employed in examining the effect on cytokine mRNAs in the context of combined stress and WCE which is arguably a very relevant experience in some alcohol abusers.

While the current research corroborates the demonstration by Whitman et al. [38] that cytokine mRNAs are increased in the cortex 24 h after WCE and extends our inquiry into other brain sites and to the effects of stress, the studies do not address this potentially interesting combinatorial effects of the two challenges. What our results do show is that effects of these challenges are each themselves complex and perhaps more nuanced in their consequence on the neuroimmune system than may have previously been appreciated. Such findings prompt considerations of the work of others where it was shown that the neuroimmune system may respond differently to stress depending on the degree and nature of prior challenges [17,20]. In related research, Buck et al. [54] reported that a single dose of ethanol before foot-shock stress had no effect on immune function and did not enhance the stress-induced increase in IL-1β mRNA in the PVN. In general, a second challenge before or after the WCE would seem appropriate strategy to gain new evidence for the possibility that an initial challenge to the neuroimmune system may permit or alter induction of select neuroimmune mediators by a second challenge. Thus, sufficient previous activation of immune function by chronic ethanol exposure might render stress capable of further increasing cytokine mRNAs, as previously noted behaviorally [2,4,10,55]. Thus, identification of the conditions under which prior stress or chronic alcohol exposure alters future responses to either challenge would seem to be a productive avenue for research.

Whatever future combinatorial stress studies might reveal, the present results nonetheless do provide an interesting contrast with Whitman et al. [38], who demonstrated that a CRF1R antagonist prevented the cytokine mRNA increases induced by the WCE alone. It would also be of interest to identify differential physiological effects of the drug in context of the two challenges. For example, in considering the idea that cytokines may have specific neurophysiological and behavioral actions manifest in select brain regions (e.g., [9,56]), it would seem likely that broadening the neuroanatomical focus of these CRF/cytokine interactions would very likely be a productive endeavor (see also [57]). Collectively, these studies implicate CRF involvement in the increased expression of cytokine mRNAs during the 24 h withdrawal from the WCE and suggest that there may be functional consequences. In this regard, amygdala CRF-amplified CCL2 regulation of alcohol self-administration [58] and elevated CRF-dependent amygdala CCL2 in human alcoholics [48] are consistent with a role of cytokines and CRF interacting to regulate alcohol consumption. These findings considered in the context of chronic alcohol dependent CCL2 induction within the central amygdala and robust elevations of the TNF receptor (Tnfrsf1a) in rats, support the idea that neuroimmune mechanisms in the amygdala are potentially critical in the behavioral pathology in alcoholism [59]. Thus, a future experiment should be undertaken to further examine the interactions of stress and WCE across additional relevant brain regions and to further isolate relevant mechanisms. Likewise, based upon the report by Johnson et al. [22] that norepinephrine-receptor antagonists blocked the stress increase in hypothalamic IL-1β protein induced by inescapable tail shock (i.e., a severe stress), and the finding that the beta-adrenergic agonist isoproterenol can enhance IL-1 production in the amygdala following chronic stress (Porterfield et al., [39]), the effects of this drug class on the cytokine mRNA changes across different brain regions after restraint stress in the presence and absence of WCE should also be explored.

5. Conclusions

The present findings provide additional evidence for neuroimmune involvement in brain function associated with stress or WCE and the differential induction of neuroimmune mRNAs and adds the novel observation that a CRF1R antagonist is inactive against a mild stress. The results herein show that some neuroimmune components are readily inducible in a brain-region-dependent manner while others are not. Such evidence adds to a growing literature that implicates neuroimmune dysfunction in alcoholism, other substance abuse disorders, and other neurobehavioral disorders associated with stress [7,9,27,28,32,60,61]. Our findings and others prompt questions about how some challenges exert specific neuroimmune effects within neuroanatomically limited areas and suggest further studies should be done to examine combinations of challenges/conditions thought to impact on alcoholism and associated neuropsychiatric conditions. Moreover, our findings, considered in the context of the documented roles of the neuroimmune system and stress in alcohol consumption and negative emotional symptoms due to chronic ethanol consumption [9,58,62–65], support the idea that specific neuroimmune processes are engaged in neurobehavioral processes fundamental to alcohol abuse.

It may be productive to ask whether risk of relapse in alcoholics relates to differential neuroimmune responses to stress as a consequence of prior chronic ethanol exposure history and to further develop animal models around this concept. These findings also have potentially broader implications in that neuroimmune system dysfunction has been implicated in other neurobehavioral disorders as well including insomnia [33], depression [31,34,66–68], and anxiety [6,35,60,69]. In particular, neuroimmune system regulation of anxiety associated with chronic alcohol and withdrawal are notable [8,9,49]. Identifying overlapping and independent neuroimmune processes across these pathologies would be worthy of further study.

While the current studies document that neural mechanisms associated with stress may at least partially overlap with the mechanisms that drive cytokine mRNA expression after WCE, the profile of effects shown herein for the two challenges do not completely overlap across neuroimmune marker or brain region. Further, the responses reported herein were elicited with relatively limited challenges (i.e., just 1 h of stress or 15 days of exposure to ethanol). Thus, it may be valuable to examine similar endpoints following exposure to the more chronic and/or severe challenges/stressors that define many neurobehavioral disorders. Of these effects, one could ask which are transient (yet perhaps behaviorally relevant), and which induce long term maladaptations that influence behavioral pathology. By understanding how stress and WCE engage the neuroimmune system, and worsens symptoms, therapeutic options by which to mitigate stress-associated neuroimmune dysfunction in drug addiction and other central nervous system disorders could emerge [29,32].

Acknowledgments: The authors wish to thank A. Leslie Morrow for generous contribution of time, space and equipment to this project. We also acknowledge Bob Angel and Todd O'Buckley for their excellent technical assistance. This work was supported by the National Institutes of Health, National Institute on Alcohol Abuse and Alcoholism (AA11605, AA14949, AA17462, AA021275, AA007573), and the Bowles Center for Alcohol Studies.

Author Contributions: D.J.K. participated in all phases of the research, was lead writer on the manuscript and co-wrote the funding behind the project with G.R.B.; K.M.H., B.A.W., and Z.Z. assisted with dietary manipulations, assays and statistical summaries, while B.A.W. prepared an initial summary draft of the manuscript. All authors reviewed and edited multiple drafts of the manuscript.

Abbreviations

ANOVA	analysis of variance
CCL2	chemokine (C-C motif) ligand 2
CRF	corticotropin releasing hormone
IL-1β	interleukin-1 beta
mRNA	messenger ribonucleic acid
S-D	Sprague-Dawley
TLR4	toll-like receptor 4
TNFα	tumor necrosis factor-alpha
WCE	withdrawal from chronic ethanol
qPCR	quantitative polymerase chain reaction

References

1. Overstreet, D.H.; Knapp, D.J.; Breese, G.R. Accentuated decrease in social interaction in rats subjected to repeated ethanol withdrawals. *Alcohol. Clin. Exp. Res.* **2002**, *26*, 1259–1268. [CrossRef] [PubMed]
2. Rassnick, S.; Heinrichs, S.C.; Britton, K.T.; Koob, G.F. Microinjection of CRF antagonist into the central nucleus of the amygdala reverses anxiogenic-like effects of ethanol withdrawal. *Brain Res.* **1993**, *605*, 25–32. [CrossRef]
3. Valdez, G.R.; Zorrilla, E.P.; Roberts, A.J.; Koob, G.F. Antagonism of corticotropin releasing factor attenuates the enhanced responsiveness to stress observed during protracted ethanol abstinence. *Alcohol* **2003**, *29*, 55–60. [CrossRef]

4. Breese, G.R.; Knapp, D.J.; Overstreet, D.H. Stress sensitization of ethanol withdrawal-induced reduction in social interaction: Inhibition by CRF-1 and benzodiazepine receptor antagonists and a 5-HT1A receptor agonist. *Neuropsychopharmacology* **2004**, *29*, 470–482. [CrossRef] [PubMed]
5. Breese, G.R.; Overstreet, D.H.; Knapp, D.J.; Navarro, M. Prior multiple ethanol withdrawals enhance stress-induced anxiety-like behavior: Inhibition by CRF-1 and benzodiazepine-receptor antagonists and a 5-HT1A receptor antagonists. *Neuropsychopharmacology* **2005**, *30*, 1662–1669. [CrossRef] [PubMed]
6. Breese, G.R.; Sinha, R.; Heilig, M. Chronic ethanol neuroadaptation and stress contribute to susceptibility for ethanol craving and relapse. *Pharmacol. Ther.* **2011**, *129*, 149–171. [CrossRef] [PubMed]
7. Sinha, R. How does stress increase risk of drug abuse and relapse? *Psychopharmacology* **2001**, *158*, 343–359. [CrossRef] [PubMed]
8. Breese, G.R.; Knapp, D.J.; Overstreet, D.H.; Navarro, M.; Wills, T.A.; Angel, R.A. Repeated lipopolysaccharide (LPS) or cytokine treatments sensitize ethanol withdrawal-induced anxiety-like behavior. *Neuropsychopharmacology* **2008**, *33*, 867–876. [CrossRef] [PubMed]
9. Knapp, D.J.; Whitman, B.A.; Wills, T.A.; Angel, R.A.; Overstreet, D.H.; Criswell, H.E.; Ming, Z.; Breese, G.R. Cytokine involvement in stress may depend on corticotrophin releasing factor to sensitize ethanol withdrawal anxiety. *Brain Behav. Immun.* **2011**, *25*, S146–S154. [CrossRef] [PubMed]
10. Huang, M.M.; Overstreet, D.H.; Knapp, D.J.; Angel, R.; Wills, T.A.; Navarro, M.; Rivier, J.; Vale, W.; Breese, G.R. Corticotropin-releasing factor (CRF) sensitization of ethanol withdrawal-induced anxiety-like behavior is site specific and mediated by CRF-1 receptors: Relation to stress-induced sensitization. *J. Pharmacol. Exp. Ther.* **2010**, *332*, 298–307. [CrossRef] [PubMed]
11. Andersson, U.; Tracey, K.J. HMGB1 is a therapeutic target for sterile inflammation and infection. *Ann. Rev. Immunol.* **2011**, *29*, 139–162. [CrossRef] [PubMed]
12. Fleshner, M. Stress-evoked sterile inflammation, danger associated molecular patterns (DAMLPs), microbial associated molecular patterns (MAMPS) and the inflammasome. *Brain Behav. Immun.* **2013**, *27*, 1–7. [CrossRef] [PubMed]
13. Suzuki, E.; Shintani, F.; Kanba, S.; Asai, M.; Nakaki, T. Immobilization stress increases mRNA levels of interleukin-1 receptor antagonist in various rat brain regions. *Cell Mol. Neurobiol.* **1997**, *17*, 557–562. [CrossRef] [PubMed]
14. Park, J.S.; Svetkauskaite, D.; He, Q.; Kim, J.Y.; Strassheim, D.; Ishizaka, A.; Esward, A. Involvement of toll-like receptors 2 and 4 in cellular activation by high mobility group box 1 protein. *J. Biol. Chem.* **2004**, *279*, 7370–7377. [CrossRef] [PubMed]
15. Park, J.S.; Gamboni-Robertson, F.; He, Q.; Svetkauskaite, D.; Kim, J.Y.; Strassheim, D.; Sohn, J.W.; Yamada, S.; Maruyama, I.; Banerjee, A.; et al. High mobility group box 1 protein interacts with multiple Toll-like receptors. *Am. J. Physiol. Cell Physiol.* **2006**, *290*, C917–C924. [CrossRef] [PubMed]
16. Bianchi, M.E. HMGB1 Loves Company. *J. Leukoc. Biol.* **2009**, *86*, 573–576. [CrossRef] [PubMed]
17. Barnum, C.J.; Blandino, P., Jr.; Deak, T. Social status modulates basal IL-1 concentrations in the hypothalamus of pair-housed rats and influences certain features of stress reactivity. *Brain Behav. Immun.* **2008**, *22*, 517–527. [CrossRef] [PubMed]
18. Blandino, P.; Barnum, C.J.; Solomon, L.G.; Larish, Y.; Lankow, B.S.; Deak, T. Gene expression changes in the hypothalamus provide evidence for regionally-selective changes in IL-1 and microglial markers after acute stress. *Brain Behav. Immun.* **2009**, *23*, 958–968. [CrossRef] [PubMed]
19. Deak, T.; Bordner, K.A.; McElderry, N.K.; Barnum, C.J.; Blandino, P., Jr.; Deak, M.M.; Tammariello, S.P. Stress-induced increases in hypothalamic IL-1: A systematic analysis of multiple stressor paradigms. *Brain Res. Bull.* **2005**, *64*, 541–556. [CrossRef] [PubMed]
20. Girotti, M.; Donegan, J.J.; Morilak, D.A. Chronic intermittent cold stress sensitizes neuroimmune reactivity in the rat brain. *Psychoneuroendocrinology* **2011**, *36*, 1164–1174. [CrossRef] [PubMed]
21. Hueston, C.M.; Barnum, C.J.; Eberle, J.A.; Ferraioli, F.J.; Buck, H.M.; Deak, T. Stress-dependent changes in neuroinflammatory markers observed after common laboratory stressors are not seen following acute social defeat of the Sprague Dawley rat. *Physiol. Behav.* **2011**, *104*, 187–198. [CrossRef] [PubMed]
22. Johnson, J.D.; Campisi, J.; Sharkey, C.M.; Kennedy, S.L.; Nickerson, M.; Greenwood, B.N.; Fleshner, M. Catecholamines mediate stress-induced increases in peripheral and central inflammatory cytokines. *Neuroscience* **2005**, *135*, 1295–1307. [CrossRef] [PubMed]

23. Minami, M.; Kuraishi, Y.; Yamaguchi, T.; Nakai, S.; Hirai, Y.; Satoh, M. Immobilization stress induces interleukin-1 beta mRNA in the rat hypothalamus. *Neurosci. Lett.* **1991**, *123*, 254–256. [CrossRef]
24. Nguyen, K.T.; Deak, T.; Owens, S.M.; Kohno, T.; Fleshner, M.; Watkins, L.R.; Maier, S.F. Exposure to acute stress induces brain interleukin-1beta protein in the rat. *J. Neurosci.* **1998**, *18*, 2239–2246. [PubMed]
25. Nguyen, K.T.; Deak, T.; Will, M.J.; Hansen, M.K.; Hunsaker, B.N.; Fleshner, M.; Watkins, L.R.; Maier, S.F. Time course and corticosterone sensitivity of the brain, pituitary, and serum interleukin-1beta protein response to acute stress. *Brain Res.* **2000**, *859*, 193–201. [CrossRef]
26. Vecchiarelli, H.A.; Gandhi, C.P.; Gray, J.M.; Morena, M.; Hassan, K.I.; Hill, M.N. Divergent responses of inflammatory mediators within the amygdala and medial prefrontal cortex to acute psychological stress. *Brain Behav. Immun.* **2016**, *51*, 70–91. [CrossRef] [PubMed]
27. Crews, F.T.; Zou, J.; Qin, L. Induction of innate immune genes in brain create the neurobiology of addiction. *Brain Behav. Immun.* **2011**, *25*, S4–S12. [CrossRef] [PubMed]
28. Crews, F.T.; Qin, L.; Sheedy, D.; Vetreno, R.P.; Zou, J. High mobility group box 1/Toll-like receptor danger signaling increases brain neuroimmune activation in alcohol dependence. *Biol. Psychiatry* **2013**, *73*, 602–612. [CrossRef] [PubMed]
29. Dodd, S.; Maes, M.; Anderson, G.; Dean, O.M.; Moylan, S.; Berk, M. Putative neuroprotective agents in neuropsychiatric disorders. *Prog. Neuropsychopharm. Biol. Psychiatry* **2013**, *42*, 135–145. [CrossRef] [PubMed]
30. Felger, J.C.; Lotrich, F.E. Inflammatory cytokines in depression: Neurobiological mechanisms and therapeutic implications. *Neuroscience* **2013**, *246*, 199–229. [CrossRef] [PubMed]
31. Hammen, C. Stress and Depression. *Annu. Rev. Clin. Psychol.* **2005**, *1*, 293–319. [CrossRef] [PubMed]
32. Koob, G.F. Neurobiological substrates for the dark side of compulsivity in addiction. *Neuropharmacology* **2008**, *56*, 18–31. [CrossRef] [PubMed]
33. Krueger, J.M.; Rector, D.M.; Churchill, L. Sleep and cytokines. *Sleep Med. Clin.* **2007**, *2*, 161–169. [CrossRef] [PubMed]
34. Miller, A.H.; Maletic, V.; Raison, C.L. Inflammation and its discontents: The role of cytokines in the pathophysiology of major depression. *Biol. Psychiat.* **2009**, *65*, 732–741. [CrossRef] [PubMed]
35. Shin, L.M.; Liberzon, I. The neurocircuitry of fear, stress, and anxiety disorders. *Neuropsychopharmacology* **2010**, *35*, 169–191. [CrossRef] [PubMed]
36. Frye, G.D.; McCown, T.J.; Breese, G.R. Characterization of susceptibility to audiogenic seizures in ethanol-dependent rats after microinjection of gamma-aminobutyric acid (GABA) agonists into the inferior colliculus, substantia nigra or medial septum. *J. Pharmacol. Exp. Ther.* **1983**, *227*, 663–670. [PubMed]
37. McCown, T.J.; Breese, G.R. Multiple withdrawals from chronic ethanol "kindles" inferior collicular seizure activity: Evidence for kindling of seizures associated with alcoholism. *Alcohol. Clin. Exp. Res.* **1990**, *14*, 394–399. [CrossRef] [PubMed]
38. Whitman, B.A.; Knapp, D.J.; Werner, D.F.; Crews, F.T.; Breese, G.R. The cytokine-mRNA Increase induced by withdrawal from chronic ethanol in the sterile environment of brain is mediated by CRF and HMGB1 Release. *Alcohol. Clin. Exp. Res.* **2013**, *37*, 2086–2097. [CrossRef] [PubMed]
39. Porterfield, V.M.; Zimomra, Z.R.; Caldwell, E.A.; Camp, R.M.; Gabella, K.M.; Johnson, J.D. Rat strain differences in restraint stress-induced brain cytokines. *Neuroscience* **2011**, *188*, 48–54. [CrossRef] [PubMed]
40. Overstreet, D.H.; Knapp, D.J.; Breese, G.R. Drug challenges reveal differences in mediation of stress facilitation of voluntary alcohol drinking and withdrawal-induced anxiety in alcohol-preferring P rats. *Alcohol Clin. Exp. Res.* **2007**, *31*, 1473–1481. [CrossRef] [PubMed]
41. Faraco, G.; Fossati, S.; Bianchi, M.E.; Patrone, M.; Pedrazzi, M.; Sparatore, B.; Moroni, F.; Chiarugi, A. High mobility group box 1 protein is released by neural cells upon different stresses and worsens ischemic neurodegeneration in vitro and in vivo. *J. Neurochem.* **2007**, *103*, 590–603. [CrossRef] [PubMed]
42. Akira, S.; Takeda, K. Toll-like receptor signaling. *Nat. Rev. Immunol.* **2004**, *4*, 499–511. [CrossRef] [PubMed]
43. Yamada, S.; Maruyama, I. HMGB1, a novel inflammatory cytokine. *Clin. Chim. Acta* **2007**, *375*, 36–42. [PubMed]
44. Yang, H.; Wang, H.; Czura, C.J.; Tracey, K.J. The cytokine activity of HMGB1. *J. Leukoc. Biol.* **2005**, *78*, 1–8. [CrossRef] [PubMed]
45. Yu, M.; Wang, H.; Ding, A.; Golenbock, D.T.; Latz, E.; Czura, C.J.; Fenton, M.J.; Tracey, K.J.; Yang, H. HMGB1 signals through toll-like receptor (TLR) 4 and TLR2. *Shock* **2006**, *26*, 174–179. [CrossRef] [PubMed]

46. Knapp, D.J.; Overstreet, D.H.; Breese, G.R. Modulation of ethanol withdrawal-induced anxiety-like behavior during later withdrawals by treatment of early withdrawals with benzodiazepine/gamma-aminobutyric acid ligands. *Alcohol Clin. Exp. Res.* **2005**, *29*, 553–563. [CrossRef] [PubMed]
47. Shizuya, K.; Komori, T.; Fujiwara, R.; Miyahara, S.; Ohmori, M.; Nomura, J. The influence of restraint stress on the expression of mRNAs for IL-6 and the IL-6 receptor in the hypothalamus and midbrain of the rat. *Life Sci.* **1997**, *61*, 135–140. [CrossRef]
48. He, J.; Crews, F.T. Increased MCP-1 and microglia in various regions of the human alcoholic brain. *Exp. Neurol.* **2008**, *210*, 349–358. [CrossRef] [PubMed]
49. Pascual, M.; Baliño, P.; Aragón, C.M.; Guerri, C. Cytokines and chemokines as biomarkers of ethanol-induced neuroinflammation and anxiety-related behavior: Role of TLR4 and TLR2. *Neuropharmacology* **2015**, *89*, 352–359. [CrossRef] [PubMed]
50. Crews, F.T.; Vetreno, R.P. Neuroimmune basis of alcoholic brain damage. *Int. Rev. Neurobiol.* **2014**, *118*, 315–357. [PubMed]
51. Crews, F.T.; Vetreno, R.P. Mechanisms of neuroimmune gene induction in alcoholism. *Psychopharmacology (Berl.)* **2016**, *333*, 1543–1547. [CrossRef] [PubMed]
52. Liu, Y.; Qin, L.; Wilson, B.; Wu, X.; Qian, L.; Granholm, A.C.; Crews, F.T.; Hong, J.S. Endotoxin induces a delayed loss of TH-IR neurons in substantia nigra and motor behavioral deficits. *Neurotoxicology* **2008**, *29*, 864–870. [CrossRef] [PubMed]
53. Funk, C.K.; O'Dell, L.E.; Crawford, E.F.; Koob, G.F. Corticotropin-releasing factor within the central nucleus of the amygdala mediates enhanced ethanol self-administration in withdrawn, ethanol-dependent rats. *J. Neurosci.* **2006**, *26*, 11324–11332. [CrossRef] [PubMed]
54. Buck, H.M.; Hueston, C.M.; Bishop, C.; Deak, T. Enhancement of the hypothalamic-pituitary-adrenal axis but not cytokine responses to stress challenges imposed during withdrawal from acute alcohol exposure in Sprague-Dawley rats. *Psychopharmacology* **2011**, *218*, 203–215. [CrossRef] [PubMed]
55. Baldwin, H.A.; Rassnick, S.; Rivier, J.; Koob, G.F.; Britton, K.T. CRF antagonist reverses the "anxiogenic" response to ethanol withdrawal in the rat. *Psychopharmacology* **1991**, *103*, 227–232. [CrossRef] [PubMed]
56. Ming, Z.; Criswell, H.E.; Breese, G.R. Evidence for TNFα action on excitatory and inhibitory neurotransmission in the central amygdala: A brain site influenced by stress. *Brain Behav. Immun.* **2013**, *33*, 102–111.
57. Breese, G.R.; Knapp, D.J. Persistent adaptation by chronic alcohol is facilitated by neuroimmune activation linked to stress and CRF. *Alcohol* **2016**, *52*, 9–23. [CrossRef] [PubMed]
58. June, H.L.; Liu, J.; Warnock, K.T.; Bell, K.A.; Balan, I.; Bollion, D.; Puche, A.; Aurelian, L. CRF-amplified neuronal TLR4/MCP-1 signaling regulates alcohol self-administration. *Neuropsychopharmacology* **2015**, *40*, 1549–1559. [CrossRef] [PubMed]
59. Freeman, K.; Brureau, A.; Vadigepalli, R.; Staehle, M.M.; Brureau, M.M.; Gonye, G.E.; Hoek, J.B.; Hooper, D.C.; Schwaber, J.S. Temporal changes in innate immune signals in a rat model of alcohol withdrawal in emotional and cardiorespiratory homeostatic nuclei. *J. Neuroinflamm.* **2012**, *9*, 97. [CrossRef] [PubMed]
60. Breese, G.R.; Overstreet, D.H.; Knapp, D.J. Conceptual framework for the etiology of alcoholism: A "kindling"/stress hypothesis. *Psychopharmacology* **2005**, *178*, 367–380. [CrossRef] [PubMed]
61. Heilig, M.; Koob, G.F. A key role of corticotropin-releasing factor in alcohol dependence. *Trends Neurosci.* **2007**, *30*, 399–406. [CrossRef] [PubMed]
62. Blednov, Y.A.; Bergeson, S.E.; Walker, D.; Ferreira, V.M.M.; Kuziel, W.A.; Harris, R.A. Perturbation of chemokine networks by gene deletion alters the reinforcing actions of ethanol. *Behav. Brain Res.* **2005**, *165*, 110–125. [CrossRef] [PubMed]
63. Blednov, Y.A.; Ponomarev, I.; Geil, C.; Bergeson, S.; Koob, G.F.; Harris, R.A. Neuroimmune regulation of alcohol consumption: Behavioral validation of genes obtained from genomic studies. *Addict. Biol.* **2012**, *17*, 108–120. [CrossRef] [PubMed]
64. Robinson, G.; Most, D.; Ferguson, L.B.; Mayfield, J.; Harris, R.A.; Blednov, Y.A. Neuroimmune pathways in alcohol consumption: Evidence from behavioral and genetic studies in rodents and humans. *Int. Rev. Neurobiol.* **2014**, *118*, 13–39. [PubMed]
65. Valenta, J.P.; Gonzales, R.A. Chronic Intracerebroventricular Infusion of Monocyte Chemoattractant Protein-1 leads to a persistent increase in sweetened ethanol consumption during operant self-administration but does not influence sucrose consumption in Long-Evans rats. *Alcohol. Clin. Exp. Res.* **2016**, *40*, 187–195. [CrossRef] [PubMed]

66. Lotrich, F.E. Psychiatric clearance for patients started on interferon-alpha-based therapies. *Am. J. Psychiatry* **2013**, *170*, 592–597. [CrossRef] [PubMed]
67. Raison, C.L.; Miller, A.H. Malaise, melancholia and madness: The evolutionary legacy of an inflammatory bias. *Brain Behav. Immun.* **2013**, *31*, 1–8. [CrossRef] [PubMed]
68. Iwata, M.; Ota, K.T.; Duman, R.S. The inflammasome: Pathways linking psychological stress, depression, and systemic illnesses. *Brain Behav. Immun.* **2013**, *31*, 105–114. [CrossRef] [PubMed]
69. Sinha, R.; Fox, H.C.; Hong, K.I.; Hansen, J.; Tuit, K.; Kreek, M.J. Effects of adrenal sensitivity, stress- and cue-induced craving, and anxiety on subsequent ethanol relapse and treatment outcomes. *Arch. Gen. Psychiat.* **2011**, *68*, 942–952. [CrossRef] [PubMed]

14

Neuroimmunology of the Interleukins 13 and 4

Simone Mori [1], Pamela Maher [2] and Bruno Conti [1,*]

[1] Department of Chemical Physiology, The Scripps Research Institute, 10550 North Torrey Pines Road, La Jolla, CA 92037, USA; smori@scripps.edu

[2] Cellular Neurobiology Laboratory, Salk Research Institute, La Jolla, CA 92037, USA; pmaher@salk.edu

[*] Correspondence: bconti@scripps.edu

Academic Editor: Donna Gruol

Abstract: The cytokines interleukin 13 and 4 share a common heterodimeric receptor and are important modulators of peripheral allergic reactions. Produced primarily by T-helper type 2 lymphocytes, they are typically considered as anti-inflammatory cytokines because they can downregulate the synthesis of T-helper type 1 pro-inflammatory cytokines. Their presence and role in the brain is only beginning to be investigated and the data collected so far shows that these molecules can be produced by microglial cells and possibly by neurons. Attention has so far been given to the possible role of these molecules in neurodegeneration. Both neuroprotective or neurotoxic effects have been proposed based on evidence that interleukin 13 and 4 can reduce inflammation by promoting the M2 microglia phenotype and contributing to the death of microglia M1 phenotype, or by potentiating the effects of oxidative stress on neurons during neuro-inflammation. Remarkably, the heterodimeric subunit IL-13Rα1 of their common receptor was recently demonstrated in dopaminergic neurons of the ventral tegmental area and the substantia nigra pars compacta, suggesting the possibility that both cytokines may affect the activity of these neurons regulating reward, mood, and motor coordination. In mice and man, the gene encoding for IL-13Rα1 is expressed on the X chromosome within the PARK12 region of susceptibility to Parkinson's disease (PD). This, together with finding that IL-13Rα1 contributes to loss of dopaminergic neurons during inflammation, indicates the possibility that these cytokines may contribute to the etiology or the progression of PD.

Keywords: Interleukin 13; Interleukin 4; neuron; microglia; Parkinson; brain; neurodegeneration; neuroinflammation; neurotoxic; neuroprotection

---

1. Introduction

In this review we summarize the current body of knowledge on the role of IL-13 in the central nervous system. Although the study of this subject is in its infancy and only a limited amount of work has been done at this stage, it is likely that this will change in the near future. In fact, one of the interesting aspects of investigating the biology of IL-13 in the central nervous system (CNS) is that its canonical receptor, alpha type I (IL-13Rα1), appears to be expressed not only in glial cells during pathological conditions, but also in specific subsets of neurons in the healthy brain. Specifically, IL-13Rα1 has, so far, been found on dopaminergic neurons of the Substantia Nigra pars compacta (SNc) and the Ventral Tegmental Area (VTA) [1]. This finding indicates that its ligands, IL-13 and IL-4, could be important regulators of dopaminergic function and cell survival, and may provide a direct link between the immune system and the neurobiology of reward, addiction, or motor coordination.

2. What We Know about IL-13 Comes from Studies of Its Biology in the Immune System

The cytokines Interleukin 13 (IL-13) and interleukin-4 (IL-4) are two secreted proteins recognized for their role in promoting T-helper type 2 (Th2) lymphocyte-mediated allergic inflammation and atopy in the periphery [2–17]. IL-13 and IL-4 also have the ability to downregulate the synthesis of T-helper type 1 (Th1) lymphocyte pro-inflammatory cytokines: for this reason they are normally listed as anti-inflammatory interleukins [8–10,15,18–20]. Both cytokines are produced by Th2, as well as by other cell types, including eosinophils and basophils [2,5,6,9,11–13] and IL-13 production is also stimulated in mast cells by lipopolysaccharides (LPS) [21–24].

IL-13 and IL-4 are often investigated together because they partially share a common receptor type: the IL-13 receptor alpha 1 chain (IL-13Rα1). IL-13Rα1 heterodimerizes with the IL-4R alpha chain (IL-4Rα) forming a complex capable of binding IL-13 or IL-4 (Figure 1) [25–32]. To date, this complex is the only known signal transducer for IL-13, while IL-4 can also signal through an IL-4Rα/gamma chain complex. A high-affinity IL-13-binding protein (IL-13Rα2) also exists and is a specific inhibitor of IL-13 signaling, likely by functioning as a decoy receptor [28,33–36]. IL-13Rα2 is not found in the healthy brain and, so far, has only been shown to be expressed in the CNS on glioblastoma cells [37] making it one of the major targets of immunotherapy. Work on IL-13Rα2 in the CNS and its role as a therapeutic target will not be discussed here and is covered by recent excellent reviews [38].

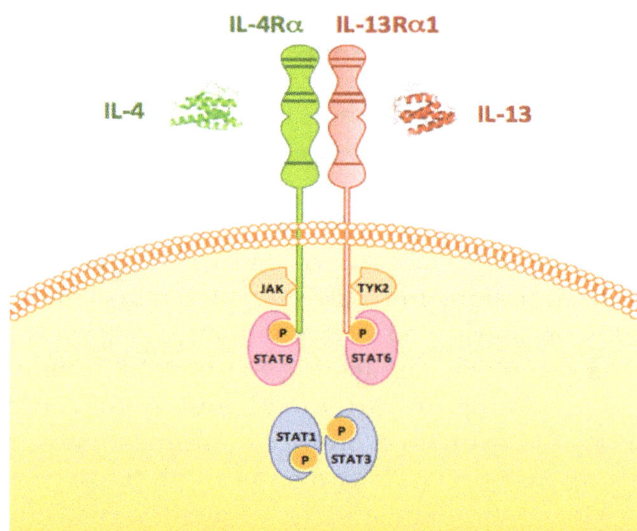

Figure 1. Schematic representation of the heterodimeric receptor for IL-13 and IL-4 and its signaling. Interleukins 13 (IL-13) and 4 (IL-4) can bind to the same heterodimeric receptor composed of the IL-13 Receptor alpha 1 (IL-13Rα1) and the Interleukin 4 Receptor alpha (IL-4Rα). Binding of the receptor activates the Janus kinase (JAK) and leads to phosphorylation of members of the Signal Transducer and Activator of Transcription (STAT) family. The tyrosine-protein kinase 2 (TYK2) is a member of the JAK family. See the text for more details.

Binding of IL-13 to its cognate functional receptor allows the trans-phosphorylation of a specific tyrosine residue located in the Janus Kinase (JAK) activation segment [31,39] which promotes the kinase activity required for the phosphorylation of downstream substrates in its signaling cascades [39,40]. IL-13 activates two intracellular signaling cascades: the JAK-STAT and the insulin receptor substrate (IRS)-phosphatidylinositol 3′-kinase pathways [26,28,31]. While the IRS-phosphatidylinositol 3′-kinase pathway leads to cell proliferation, the JAK-STAT pathway induces the transcription of genes that contain the Stat6-responsive enhancer element N6-GAS located in their promoter [41–43]. Upon activation of IL-13Rα1, Stat1, 3, and 6 are phosphorylated and form a homodimer that migrates to the nucleus and binds to N6-GAS to drive transcription [31,42,44,45]. Reactive oxygen species (ROS) also play a role in the IL-13/IL-4 cellular transduction signaling. In intestinal epithelial cells upon IL-13Rα1 activation both the JAK-STAT pathway and Mitogen Activated Protein Kinase (MAPK) stimulate nicotinamide adenine dinucleotide phosphate oxydase to produce intracellular ROS that, in a positive feedback loop, facilitate the phosphorylation of STAT6 and ERK [46]. Moreover, IL-13/IL-4-driven

ROS production has been recently shown in alternatively-activated monocytes/macrophages through activation of monoamino oxydase A (MAO-A) [44].

3. Expression of IL-13 and IL-4 in the CNS

As mentioned above, IL-13 and IL-4 were demonstrated to be produced peripherally. To date, there is no evidence that these two proteins, both with molecular weights in the range of 15 kDa, can cross the blood-brain barrier. However, experimental work shows, instead, their local production in the CNS. Expression of IL-13 in the rodent brain was described in microglia, where its production was enhanced by peripheral injection of LPS or the neurotoxin 1-metil-4-fenil-1,2,3,6-tetraidropiridina (MPTP) [47–51].

Evidence also exists that both IL-13 and IL-4 can be produced by neuronal cells of the hippocampus and the cortex in experimental models of ischemic insult [52,53]. In this context it has speculated that the production of IL-4 and IL-13, inducing alternative activation of microglia—known as the M2 state—can exert a protective effect against neuronal damage [53–55]. Neuronal production of IL-4 has been described lately in the noradrenergic neurons of the locus coeruleus, in which its release appears to be sensitive to behavioral stress [56]. Preliminary work in our laboratory also showed that IL-13 can be produced in neurons [57].

4. What Is the Role of IL-13 and IL-4 in the CNS?

Few studies have tested the effects of IL-13 and IL-4 in the CNS. Most of these have investigated a possible action on neuronal survival with some studies finding that IL-13 and/or IL-4 potentiate the effects of LPS and Interferon gamma (IFN-y), increasing oxidative damage and contributing to neuronal death [47–50,58–61]. On the other hand, other studies indicated that IL-13 and/or IL-4 could be neuroprotective either by directly reducing inflammation or by inducing the death of microglia cells that are considered to be cellular mediators of neuronal damage [47–50,59–65]. Notably, both IL-13 and IL-4 can potentiate LPS-induced sickness behavior when co-injected centrally with LPS, whereas only IL-4, and not IL-13, attenuates LPS-induced sickness behavior when administered several hours before LPS [47,66]. Recently, our laboratory collected evidence that IL-13 and IL-4 are not toxic when administered alone but can greatly increase the susceptibility of neurons to oxidative damage and contribute to their demise if they express IL-13Rα1 [1].

5. IL-13 and IL-4 in Multiple Sclerosis

Multiple sclerosis (MS) is an autoimmune disorder affecting the CNS with a relapsing-remitting time course. IL-13 seems to exert a protective role in this context, as it is believed that in the development of the disease, a crucial role is played by the imbalance between pro-inflammatory cytokines (IL-1β; TNF; INF-γ; IL-17) and anti-inflammatory cytokines (IL-4, IL-5, IL-10 and IL-13) [67,68]. IL-13 polymorphisms are associated with autoimmune diseases and also increase susceptibility to MS [69].

A study in humans with MS found that high levels of IL-13 in the cerebral spinal fluid (CSF) might exert a neuroprotective effect by enhancing Gamma Aminobuthirric Acid (GABA) over glutamate transmission [64]. Interestingly, an earlier report describes IL-4 having the same neural effect of increasing the GABA-induced inward current in neurons in a dose-dependent and reversible manner [70]. Moreover, the copolymer glatiramer acetate, an immunomodulatory drug currently used to treat MS, has shown to significantly increase the TH_2- lymphocyte production of IL-13 in patients [71].

Consistently, using the mouse experimental model of MS, experimental autoimmune encephalomyelitis (EAE), Cash and colleagues showed that IL-13 exerts its anti-inflammatory action by inactivating macrophages and reducing oxidative stress [72]. In the same model, an increase in circulating and spleen IL-13 prevented axonal injury [73] alone or in synergy with IL-4 [74], whereas IL-13 reduction was associated with loss of protection [75].

Sex difference can play a role in affecting the role of IL-13 in the MS model. While autoimmune diseases, including MS, are more common in women [76], the incidence and severity of EAE in mice, null for IL-13, was lower in females compared to males, suggesting the possibility that the contribution of IL-13 to EAE/MS may be gender specific [77]. To this end, it is interesting to note that the expression of IL-13 mRNA can be decreased by estrogen in a mouse model of inflammatory intestine disease [78] and that the gene encoding for IL-13Rα1 is located on the X chromosome in both humans and mice.

Together, these studies suggest that IL-13 may have a neuroprotective role in MS. Although this may be different in other neurodegenerative diseases that, unlike MS, are not characterized by a severely-compromised blood-brain barrier, and are not primarily mediated by peripheral immune cells, IL-13 and IL-4 also showed protection in a mouse model of Alzheimer's disease (AD). Specifically, intracerebral injection of a mixture of IL-13 and IL-4 reduced amyloid deposition and improved spatial learning and memory in an AD transgenic mouse model when applied to young mice but did not show protective effects when administered in adult animals [79].

6. Parkinson's Disease

The IL-13 system may have a specific role in the pathogenesis and/or the progression of Parkinson's disease (PD). Data mining using the Online Mendelian Inheritance in Man (OMIM) database [80] showed that IL-13Rα1 lies within the PARK12 region of susceptibility to PD. Although PARK12 comprises a large portion of DNA, it is located on the X chromosome, an observation that may be of interest in that PD has a higher incidence in men than in women. Even more intriguing was the finding that expression of IL-13Rα1 in the brain appeared to be specific to the dopaminergic neurons of the VTA and of the SNc, the region affected by PD. Double-immunostaining studies also revealed that approximately 80% of the SNc neurons expressing the dopaminergic marker tyrosine hydroxylase also expressed IL-13Rα1 [1].

The possible contribution of IL-13Rα1 to neuronal fate was measured using a pro-inflammatory experimental mouse model of PD. Animals received periodic peripheral intraperitoneal injections of bacterial LPS over a period of six months, a regimen previously demonstrated to induce central loss of dopaminergic SNc neurons [81]. Comparative analysis showed that mice lacking IL-13Rα1 were protected from neuronal loss when compared to their wild-type littermates, suggesting a neurotoxic action of its ligands, IL-13 and/or IL-4. *In vitro* experiments using a dopaminergic cell line showed, however, that neither IL-13 nor IL-4 had cytotoxic effects when administered alone. However, both cytokines increased the toxicity of non-toxic doses of oxidants in a dose-dependent manner.

Thus, activation of IL-13Rα1 may be one of the mechanisms whereby the vulnerability of dopaminergic neurons is increased during inflammation, when both cytokines and ROS are produced. On the other hand, the lack of neurotoxicity of IL-13 or IL-4 in the absence of ROS suggests that these cytokines may be capable of regulating neuronal function by affecting the neurobiology of those neurons that participate in reward, addiction, and motor control.

Investigating these phenomena is likely to provide important information on the mechanisms of how IL-13 and IL-4 and, more generally, the immune system, may be capable of influencing behavior or can contribute to neurodegeneration.

7. Conclusions

Although in its infancy, the investigation of the central role of the interleukins 13 and 4 has is an exciting area of research. What makes it so attractive is that these two cytokines can be produced locally in the CNS and are active on both microglia and neuronal cells. Of special interest is the fact that they act through a common heterodimeric receptor that is expressed in dopaminergic neurons.

Although these two Th2 cytokines are considered anti-inflammatory, studies conducted so far show that they can have cytotoxic effects on both glia and neurons. Interestingly these actions are not due to an intrinsic toxicity of IL-13 and IL-4 but rather to their ability to increase the cellular susceptibility to oxidative stress. This suggest that under pathological conditions, such as neuroinflammation when reactive oxygen species are produced, IL-13 and IL-4 can participate to tissue damage and thus to Parkinson's disease or other neurodegenerative disorders. Instead, under physiological conditions, these two cytokines can contribute to the regulation of neuronal function via direct action through neuronal IL-13Rα1. Thus, they have the requisites of being potential neuromodulators.

Acknowledgments: Supported by the NIH (NS085155) and by The Michael J. Fox Foundation.

References

1. Morrison, B.E.; Marcondes, M.C.; Nomura, D.K.; Sanchez-Alavez, M.; Sanchez-Gonzalez, A.; Saar, I.; Kim, K.S.; Bartfai, T.; Maher, P.; Sugama, S.; *et al.* Cutting edge: IL-13Rα1 expression in dopaminergic neurons contributes to their oxidative stress-mediated loss following chronic peripheral treatment with lipopolysaccharide. *J. Immunol.* **2012**, *189*, 5498–5502. [CrossRef] [PubMed]
2. Gibbs, B.F.; Haas, H.; Falcone, F.H.; Albrecht, C.; Vollrath, I.B.; Noll, T.; Wolff, H.H.; Amon, U. Purified human peripheral blood basophils release interleukin-13 and preformed interleukin-4 following immunological activation. *Eur. J. Immunol.* **1996**, *26*, 2493–2498. [CrossRef] [PubMed]
3. Haas, H.; Falcone, F.H.; Holland, M.J.; Schramm, G.; Haisch, K.; Gibbs, B.F.; Bufe, A.; Schlaak, M. Early interleukin-4: Its role in the switch towards a Th2 response and IgE-mediated allergy. *Int. Arch. Allergy Immunol.* **1999**, *119*, 86–94. [CrossRef] [PubMed]
4. Howard, M.; Paul, W.E. Interleukins for B lymphocytes. *Lymphokine Res.* **1982**, *1*, 1–4. [PubMed]
5. Jaffe, J.S.; Raible, D.G.; Post, T.J.; Wang, Y.; Glaum, M.C.; Butterfield, J.H.; Schulman, E.S. Human lung mast cell activation leads to IL-13 mRNA expression and protein release. *Am. J. Respir. Cell Mol. Biol.* **1996**, *15*, 473–481. [CrossRef] [PubMed]
6. Kim, E.Y.; Battaile, J.T.; Patel, A.C.; You, Y.; Agapov, E.; Grayson, M.H.; Benoit, L.A.; Byers, D.E.; Alevy, Y.; Tucker, J.; *et al.* Persistent activation of an innate immune response translates respiratory viral infection into chronic lung disease. *Nat. Med.* **2008**, *14*, 633–640. [CrossRef] [PubMed]
7. Lee, Y.C.; Lee, K.H.; Lee, H.B.; Rhee, Y.K. Serum levels of interleukins (IL)-4, IL-5, IL-13, and interferon-gamma in acute asthma. *J. Asthma* **2001**, *38*, 665–671. [CrossRef] [PubMed]
8. McKenzie, A.N.; Culpepper, J.A.; de Waal Malefyt, R.; Briere, F.; Punnonen, J.; Aversa, G.; Sato, A.; Dang, W.; Cocks, G.B.; Menon, S.; *et al.* Interleukin 13, a T-cell-derived cytokine that regulates human monocyte and B-cell function. *Proc. Natl. Acad. Sci. USA* **1993**, *90*, 3735–3739. [CrossRef] [PubMed]
9. Minty, A.; Chalon, P.; Derocq, J.M.; Dumont, X.; Guillemot, J.C.; Kaghad, M.; Labit, C.; Leplatois, P.; Liauzun, P.; Miloux, B.; *et al.* Interleukin-13 is a new human lymphokine regulating inflammatory and immune responses. *Nature* **1993**, *362*, 248–250. [CrossRef] [PubMed]
10. Morgan, J.G.; Dolganov, G.M.; Robbins, S.E.; Hinton, L.M.; Lovett, M. The selective isolation of novel cDNAs encoded by the regions surrounding the human interleukin 4 and 5 genes. *Nucleic Acids Res.* **1992**, *20*, 5173–5179. [CrossRef] [PubMed]
11. Ochensberger, B.; Daepp, G.C.; Rihs, S.; Dahinden, C.A. Human blood basophils produce interleukin-13 in response to IgE-receptor-dependent and -independent activation. *Blood* **1996**, *88*, 3028–3037. [PubMed]
12. Reglier, H.; Arce-Vicioso, M.; Fay, M.; Gougerot-Pocidalo, M.A.; Chollet-Martin, S. Lack of IL-10 and IL-13 production by human polymorphonuclear neutrophils. *Cytokine* **1998**, *10*, 192–198. [CrossRef] [PubMed]
13. Schmid-Grendelmeier, P.; Altznauer, F.; Fischer, B.; Bizer, C.; Straumann, A.; Menz, G.; Blaser, K.; Wuthrich, B.; Simon, H.U. Eosinophils express functional IL-13 in eosinophilic inflammatory diseases. *J. Immunol.* **2002**, *169*, 1021–1027. [CrossRef] [PubMed]
14. Silvestri, M.; Bontempelli, M.; Giacomelli, M.; Malerba, M.; Rossi, G.A.; Di Stefano, A.; Rossi, A.; Ricciardolo, F.L. High serum levels of tumour necrosis factor-α and interleukin-8 in severe asthma: Markers of systemic inflammation? *Clin. Exp. Allergy* **2006**, *36*, 1373–1381. [CrossRef] [PubMed]
15. Wills-Karp, M.; Luyimbazi, J.; Xu, X.; Schofield, B.; Neben, T.Y.; Karp, C.L.; Donaldson, D.D. Interleukin-13: Central mediator of allergic asthma. *Science* **1998**, *282*, 2258–2261. [CrossRef] [PubMed]

16. Wong, C.K.; Ho, C.Y.; Ko, F.W.; Chan, C.H.; Ho, A.S.; Hui, D.S.; Lam, C.W. Proinflammatory cytokines (IL-17, IL-6, IL-18 and IL-12) and Th cytokines (IFN-gamma, IL-4, IL-10 and IL-13) in patients with allergic asthma. *Clin. Exp. Immunol.* **2001**, *125*, 177–183. [CrossRef] [PubMed]
17. Wynn, T.A. IL-13 effector functions. *Annu. Rev. Immunol.* **2003**, *21*, 425–456. [CrossRef] [PubMed]
18. Brown, K.D.; Zurawski, S.M.; Mosmann, T.R.; Zurawski, G. A family of small inducible proteins secreted by leukocytes are members of a new superfamily that includes leukocyte and fibroblast-derived inflammatory agents, growth factors, and indicators of various activation processes. *J. Immunol.* **1989**, *142*, 679–687. [PubMed]
19. Kuperman, D.A.; Schleimer, R.P. Interleukin-4, interleukin-13, signal transducer and activator of transcription factor 6, and allergic asthma. *Curr. Mol. Med.* **2008**, *8*, 384–392. [CrossRef] [PubMed]
20. Wills-Karp, M. Interleukin-13 in asthma pathogenesis. *Immunol. Rev.* **2004**, *202*, 175–190. [CrossRef] [PubMed]
21. Chiba, N.; Masuda, A.; Yoshikai, Y.; Matsuguchi, T. Ceramide inhibits LPS-induced production of IL-5, IL-10, and IL-13 from mast cells. *J. Cell. Physiol.* **2007**, *213*, 126–136. [CrossRef] [PubMed]
22. Galli, S.J.; Gordon, J.R.; Wershil, B.K. Cytokine production by mast cells and basophils. *Curr. Opin. Immunol.* **1991**, *3*, 865–872. [CrossRef]
23. Masuda, A.; Yoshikai, Y.; Aiba, K.; Matsuguchi, T. Th2 cytokine production from mast cells is directly induced by lipopolysaccharide and distinctly regulated by c-Jun N-terminal kinase and p38 pathways. *J. Immunol.* **2002**, *169*, 3801–3810. [CrossRef] [PubMed]
24. Supajatura, V.; Ushio, H.; Nakao, A.; Okumura, K.; Ra, C.; Ogawa, H. Protective roles of mast cells against enterobacterial infection are mediated by Toll-like receptor 4. *J. Immunol.* **2001**, *167*, 2250–2256. [CrossRef] [PubMed]
25. Aman, M.J.; Tayebi, N.; Obiri, N.I.; Puri, R.K.; Modi, W.S.; Leonard, W.J. cDNA cloning and characterization of the human interleukin 13 receptor α chain. *J. Biol. Chem.* **1996**, *271*, 29265–29270. [PubMed]
26. Callard, R.E.; Matthews, D.J.; Hibbert, L. IL-4 and IL-13 receptors: Are they one and the same? *Immunol. Today* **1996**, *17*, 108–110. [CrossRef]
27. Hilton, D.J.; Zhang, J.G.; Metcalf, D.; Alexander, W.S.; Nicola, N.A.; Willson, T.A. Cloning and characterization of a binding subunit of the interleukin 13 receptor that is also a component of the interleukin 4 receptor. *Proc. Natl. Acad. Sci. USA* **1996**, *93*, 497–501. [CrossRef] [PubMed]
28. Jiang, H.; Harris, M.B.; Rothman, P. IL-4/IL-13 signaling beyond JAK/STAT. *J. Allergy Clin. Immunol.* **2000**, *105 Pt 1*, 1063–1070. [CrossRef] [PubMed]
29. Leonard, W.J.; O'Shea, J.J. Jaks and STATs: Biological implications. *Annu. Rev. Immunol.* **1998**, *16*, 293–322. [CrossRef] [PubMed]
30. Lin, J.X.; Migone, T.S.; Tsang, M.; Friedmann, M.; Weatherbee, J.A.; Zhou, L.; Yamauchi, A.; Bloom, E.T.; Mietz, J.; John, S.; *et al.* The role of shared receptor motifs and common Stat proteins in the generation of cytokine pleiotropy and redundancy by IL-2, IL-4, IL-7, IL-13, and IL-15. *Immunity* **1995**, *2*, 331–339. [CrossRef]
31. Nelms, K.; Keegan, A.D.; Zamorano, J.; Ryan, J.J.; Paul, W.E. The IL-4 receptor: Signaling mechanisms and biologic functions. *Annu. Rev. Immunol.* **1999**, *17*, 701–738. [CrossRef] [PubMed]
32. Orchansky, P.L.; Ayres, S.D.; Hilton, D.J.; Schrader, J.W. An interleukin (IL)-13 receptor lacking the cytoplasmic domain fails to transduce IL-13-induced signals and inhibits responses to IL-4. *J. Biol. Chem.* **1997**, *272*, 22940–22947. [CrossRef] [PubMed]
33. Caput, D.; Laurent, P.; Kaghad, M.; Lelias, J.M.; Lefort, S.; Vita, N.; Ferrara, P. Cloning and characterization of a specific interleukin (IL)-13 binding protein structurally related to the IL-5 receptor α chain. *J. Biol. Chem.* **1996**, *271*, 16921–16926. [PubMed]
34. Donaldson, D.D.; Whitters, M.J.; Fitz, L.J.; Neben, T.Y.; Finnerty, H.; Henderson, S.L.; O'Hara, R.M., Jr.; Beier, D.R.; Turner, K.J.; Wood, C.R.; *et al.* The murine IL-13 receptor α 2: Molecular cloning, characterization, and comparison with murine IL-13 receptor α 1. *J. Immunol.* **1998**, *161*, 2317–2324. [PubMed]
35. Feng, N.; Lugli, S.M.; Schnyder, B.; Gauchat, J.F.; Graber, P.; Schlagenhauf, E.; Schnarr, B.; Wiederkehr-Adam, M.; Duschl, A.; Heim, M.H.; *et al.* The interleukin-4/interleukin-13 receptor of human synovial fibroblasts: Overexpression of the nonsignaling interleukin-13 receptor α2. *Lab. Investig.* **1998**, *78*, 591–602. [PubMed]

36. Liu, H.; Jacobs, B.S.; Liu, J.; Prayson, R.A.; Estes, M.L.; Barnett, G.H.; Barna, B.P. Interleukin-13 sensitivity and receptor phenotypes of human glial cell lines: Non-neoplastic glia and low-grade astrocytoma differ from malignant glioma. *Cancer Immunol. Immunother.* **2000**, *49*, 319–324. [CrossRef] [PubMed]
37. Debinski, W.; Gibo, D.M.; Hulet, S.W.; Connor, J.R.; Gillespie, G.Y. Receptor for interleukin 13 is a marker and therapeutic target for human high-grade gliomas. *Clin. Cancer Res.* **1999**, *5*, 985–990. [PubMed]
38. Sengupta, S.; Thaci, B.; Crawford, A.C.; Sampath, P. Interleukin-13 receptor α 2-targeted glioblastoma immunotherapy. *Biomed. Res. Int.* **2014**, *2014*, 952128. [CrossRef] [PubMed]
39. Haque, S.J.; Wu, Q.; Kammer, W.; Friedrich, K.; Smith, J.M.; Kerr, I.M.; Stark, G.R.; Williams, B.R. Receptor-associated constitutive protein tyrosine phosphatase activity controls the kinase function of JAK1. *Proc. Natl. Acad. Sci. USA* **1997**, *94*, 8563–8568. [CrossRef] [PubMed]
40. Johnson, L.N.; Noble, M.E.; Owen, D.J. Active and inactive protein kinases: Structural basis for regulation. *Cell* **1996**, *85*, 149–158. [CrossRef]
41. Hou, J.; Schindler, U.; Henzel, W.J.; Ho, T.C.; Brasseur, M.; McKnight, S.L. An interleukin-4-induced transcription factor: IL-4 Stat. *Science* **1994**, *265*, 1701–1706. [CrossRef] [PubMed]
42. Mikita, T.; Campbell, D.; Wu, P.; Williamson, K.; Schindler, U. Requirements for interleukin-4-induced gene expression and functional characterization of Stat6. *Mol. Cell. Biol.* **1996**, *16*, 5811–5820. [CrossRef] [PubMed]
43. Schindler, U.; Wu, P.; Rothe, M.; Brasseur, M.; McKnight, S.L. Components of a Stat recognition code: Evidence for two layers of molecular selectivity. *Immunity* **1995**, *2*, 689–697. [CrossRef]
44. Bhattacharjee, A.; Shukla, M.; Yakubenko, V.P.; Mulya, A.; Kundu, S.; Cathcart, M.K. IL-4 and IL-13 employ discrete signaling pathways for target gene expression in alternatively activated monocytes/macrophages. *Free Radic. Biol. Med.* **2013**, *54*, 1–16. [CrossRef] [PubMed]
45. Darnell, J.E., Jr.; Kerr, I.M.; Stark, G.R. Jak-STAT pathways and transcriptional activation in response to IFNs and other extracellular signaling proteins. *Science* **1994**, *264*, 1415–1421. [CrossRef] [PubMed]
46. Mandal, D.; Fu, P.; Levine, A.D. REDOX regulation of IL-13 signaling in intestinal epithelial cells: Usage of alternate pathways mediates distinct gene expression patterns. *Cell. Signal.* **2010**, *22*, 1485–1494. [CrossRef] [PubMed]
47. Bluthe, R.M.; Bristow, A.; Lestage, J.; Imbs, C.; Dantzer, R. Central injection of interleukin-13 potentiates LPS-induced sickness behavior in rats. *Neuroreport* **2001**, *12*, 3979–3983. [CrossRef] [PubMed]
48. Shin, W.H.; Lee, D.Y.; Park, K.W.; Kim, S.U.; Yang, M.S.; Joe, E.H.; Jin, B.K. Microglia expressing interleukin-13 undergo cell death and contribute to neuronal survival *in vivo*. *Glia* **2004**, *46*, 142–152. [CrossRef] [PubMed]
49. Yang, M.-S.; Ji, K.-A.; Jeon, S.-B.; Jin, B.-K.; Kim, S.U.; Jou, N.; Joe, E. Interleukin-13 enhances cyclooxygenase-2 expression in activated rat brain microglia: Implications for death of activated microglia. *J. Immunol.* **2006**, *177*, 1323–1329. [CrossRef] [PubMed]
50. Yang, M.S.; Park, E.J.; Sohn, S.; Kwon, H.J.; Shin, W.H.; Pyo, H.K.; Jin, B.; Choi, K.S.; Jou, I.; Joe, E.H. Interleukin-13 and -4 induce death of activated microglia. *Glia* **2002**, *38*, 273–280. [CrossRef] [PubMed]
51. Yasuda, Y.; Shimoda, T.; Uno, K.; Tateishi, N.; Furuya, S.; Yagi, K.; Suzuki, K.; Fujita, S. The effects of MPTP on the activation of microglia/astrocytes and cytokine/chemokine levels in different mice strains. *J. Neuroimmunol.* **2008**, *204*, 43–51. [CrossRef] [PubMed]
52. Yu, J.T.; Lee, C.H.; Yoo, K.Y.; Choi, J.H.; Li, H.; Park, O.K.; Yan, B.; Hwang, I.K.; Kwon, Y.G.; Kim, Y.M.; *et al.* Maintenance of anti-inflammatory cytokines and reduction of glial activation in the ischemic hippocampal CA1 region preconditioned with lipopolysaccharide. *J. Neurol. Sci.* **2010**, *296*, 69–78. [CrossRef] [PubMed]
53. Zhao, X.; Wang, H.; Sun, G.; Zhang, J.; Edwards, N.J.; Aronowski, J. Neuronal interleukin-4 as a modulator of microglial pathways and ischemic brain damage. *J. Neurosci.* **2015**, *35*, 11281–11291. [CrossRef] [PubMed]
54. Latta, C.H.; Sudduth, T.L.; Weekman, E.M.; Brothers, H.M.; Abner, E.L.; Popa, G.J.; Mendenhall, M.D.; Gonzalez-Oregon, F.; Braun, K.; Wilcock, D.M. Determining the role of IL-4 induced neuroinflammation in microglial activity and amyloid-β using BV2 microglial cells and APP/PS1 transgenic mice. *J. Neuroinflamm.* **2015**, *12*, 41. [CrossRef] [PubMed]
55. Xiong, X.; Xu, L.; Wei, L.; White, R.E.; Ouyang, Y.B.; Giffard, R.G. IL-4 is required for sex differences in vulnerability to focal ischemia in mice. *Stroke* **2015**, *46*, 2271–2276. [CrossRef] [PubMed]
56. Lee, H.J.; Park, H.J.; Starkweather, A.; An, K.; Shim, I. Decreased interleukin-4 release from the neurons of the Locus Coeruleus in response to immobilization stress. *Med. Inflamm.* **2016**, *2016*, 3501905. [CrossRef] [PubMed]
57. Conti, B. The Scripps Research Institute, CA, USA. Unpublished work, 2016.

58. Nam, J.H.; Park, K.W.; Park, E.S.; Lee, Y.B.; Lee, H.G.; Baik, H.H.; Kim, Y.S.; Maeng, S.; Park, J.; Jin, B.K. Interleukin-13/-4-induced oxidative stress contributes to death of hippocampal neurons in aβ1-42-treated hippocampus *in vivo*. *Antioxid. Redox Signal.* **2012**, *16*, 1369–1383. [CrossRef] [PubMed]
59. Park, K.W.; Baik, H.H.; Jin, B.K. Interleukin-4-induced oxidative stress via microglial NADPH oxidase contributes to the death of hippocampal neurons *in vivo*. *Curr. Aging Sci.* **2008**, *1*, 192–201. [CrossRef] [PubMed]
60. Park, K.W.; Baik, H.H.; Jin, B.K. IL-13-induced oxidative stress via microglial NADPH oxidase contributes to death of hippocampal neurons *in vivo*. *J. Immunol.* **2009**, *183*, 4666–4674. [CrossRef] [PubMed]
61. Yadav, M.C.; Burudi, E.M.; Alirezaei, M.; Flynn, C.C.; Watry, D.D.; Lanigan, C.M.; Fox, H.S. IFN-gamma-induced IDO and WRS expression in microglia is differentially regulated by IL-4. *Glia* **2007**, *55*, 1385–1396. [CrossRef] [PubMed]
62. Clarke, R.M.; Lyons, A.; O'Connell, F.; Deighan, B.F.; Barry, C.E.; Anyakoha, N.G.; Nicolaou, A.; Lynch, M.A. A pivotal role for interleukin-4 in atorvastatin-associated neuroprotection in rat brain. *J. Biol. Chem.* **2008**, *283*, 1808–1817. [CrossRef] [PubMed]
63. Deboy, C.A.; Xin, J.; Byram, S.C.; Serpe, C.J.; Sanders, V.M.; Jones, K.J. Immune-mediated neuroprotection of axotomized mouse facial motoneurons is dependent on the IL-4/STAT6 signaling pathway in CD4(+) T cells. *Exp. Neurol.* **2006**, *201*, 212–224. [CrossRef] [PubMed]
64. Rossi, S.; Mancino, R.; Bergami, A.; Mori, F.; Castelli, M.; De Chiara, V.; Studer, V.; Mataluni, G.; Sancesario, G.; Parisi, V.; *et al.* Potential role of IL-13 in neuroprotection and cortical excitability regulation in multiple sclerosis. *Mult. Scler. J.* **2011**, *17*, 1301–1312. [CrossRef] [PubMed]
65. Won, S.Y.; Kim, S.R.; Maeng, S.; Jin, B.K. Interleukin-13/Interleukin-4-induced oxidative stress contributes to death of prothrombinkringle-2 (pKr-2)-activated microglia. *J. Neuroimmunol.* **2013**, *265*, 36–42. [CrossRef] [PubMed]
66. Bluthe, R.M.; Lestage, J.; Rees, G.; Bristow, A.; Dantzer, R. Dual effect of central injection of recombinant rat interleukin-4 on lipopolysaccharide-induced sickness behavior in rats. *Neuropsychopharmacology* **2002**, *26*, 86–93. [CrossRef]
67. Linker, R.A.; Sendtner, M.; Gold, R. Mechanisms of axonal degeneration in EAE—Lessons from CNTF and MHC I knockout mice. *J. Neurol. Sci.* **2005**, *233*, 167–172. [CrossRef] [PubMed]
68. Zeis, T.; Graumann, U.; Reynolds, R.; Schaeren-Wiemers, N. Normal-appearing white matter in multiple sclerosis is in a subtle balance between inflammation and neuroprotection. *Brain* **2008**, *131*, 288–303. [CrossRef] [PubMed]
69. Seyfizadeh, N.; Kazemi, T.; Farhoudi, M.; Reza Aliparasti, M.; Sadeghi-Bazargani, H.; Almasi, S.; Babaloo, Z. Association of IL-13 single nucleotide polymorphisms in Iranian patients to multiple sclerosis. *Am. J. Clin. Exp. Immunol.* **2014**, *3*, 124–129. [PubMed]
70. Rozsa, K.S.; Rubakhin, S.S.; Szucs, A.; Hughes, T.K.; Stefano, G.B. Opposite effects of interleukin-2 and interleukin-4 on GABA-induced inward currents of dialysed lymnaea neurons. *Gen. Pharmacol.* **1997**, *29*, 73–77. [CrossRef]
71. Sanna, A.; Fois, M.L.; Arru, G.; Huang, Y.M.; Link, H.; Pugliatti, M.; Rosati, G.; Sotgiu, S. Glatiramer acetate reduces lymphocyte proliferation and enhances IL-5 and IL-13 production through modulation of monocyte-derived dendritic cells in multiple sclerosis. *Clin. Exp. Immunol.* **2006**, *143*, 357–362. [CrossRef] [PubMed]
72. Cash, E.; Minty, A.; Ferrara, P.; Caput, D.; Fradelizi, D.; Rott, O. Macrophage-inactivating IL-13 suppresses experimental autoimmune encephalomyelitis in rats. *J. Immunol.* **1994**, *153*, 4258–4267. [PubMed]
73. Offner, H.; Subramanian, S.; Wang, C.; Afentoulis, M.; Vandenbark, A.A.; Huan, J.; Burrows, G.G. Treatment of passive experimental autoimmune encephalomyelitis in SJL mice with a recombinant TCR ligand induces IL-13 and prevents axonal injury. *J. Immunol.* **2005**, *175*, 4103–4111. [CrossRef] [PubMed]
74. Young, D.A.; Lowe, L.D.; Booth, S.S.; Whitters, M.J.; Nicholson, L.; Kuchroo, V.K.; Collins, M. IL-4, IL-10, IL-13, and TGF-β from an altered peptide ligand-specific Th2 cell clone down-regulate adoptive transfer of experimental autoimmune encephalomyelitis. *J. Immunol.* **2000**, *164*, 3563–3572. [CrossRef] [PubMed]
75. Ochoa-Repáraz, J.; Rynda, A.; Ascón, M.A.; Yang, X.; Kochetkova, I.; Riccardi, C.; Callis, G.; Trunkle, T.; Pascual, D.W. IL-13 production by regulatory T cells protects against experimental autoimmune encephalomyelitis independently of autoantigen. *J. Immunol.* **2008**, *181*, 954–968. [CrossRef] [PubMed]
76. Compston, A.; Coles, A. Multiple sclerosis. *Lancet* **2008**, *372*, 1502–1517. [CrossRef]

77. Sinha, S.; Kaler, L.J.; Proctor, T.M.; Teuscher, C.; Vandenbark, A.A.; Offner, H. IL-13-mediated gender difference in susceptibility to autoimmune encephalomyelitis. *J. Immunol. (Baltim. Md. 1950)* **2008**, *180*, 2679–2685. [CrossRef]
78. Verdu, E.F.; Deng, Y.; Bercik, P.; Collins, S.M. Modulatory effects of estrogen in two murine models of experimental colitis. *Am. J. Physiol. Gastrointest. Liver Physiol.* **2002**, *283*, 27–36. [CrossRef] [PubMed]
79. Kawahara, K.; Suenobu, M.; Yoshida, A.; Koga, K.; Hyodo, A.; Ohtsuka, H.; Kuniyasu, A.; Tamamaki, N.; Sugimoto, Y.; Nakayama, H. Intracerebral microinjection of interleukin-4/interleukin-13 reduces β-amyloid accumulation in the ipsilateral side and improves cognitive deficits in young amyloid precursor protein 23 mice. *Neuroscience* **2012**, *207*, 243–260. [CrossRef] [PubMed]
80. Man (OMIM) database. Available online: http://www.omim.org (accessed on 9 June 2016).
81. Frank-Cannon, T.C.; Tran, T.; Ruhn, K.A.; Martinez, T.N.; Hong, J.; Marvin, M.; Hartley, M.; Trevino, I.; O'Brien, D.E.; Casey, B.; *et al.* Parkin deficiency increases vulnerability to inflammation-related nigral degeneration. *J. Neurosci.* **2008**, *28*, 10825–10834. [CrossRef] [PubMed]

15

Relation of Structural and Functional Changes in Auditory and Visual Pathways after Temporal Lobe Epilepsy Surgery

Margarita Minou Báez-Martín [1,*], Lilia Maria Morales-Chacón [1], Iván García-Maeso [1], Bárbara Estupiñán-Díaz [1], María Eugenia García-Navarro [1], Yamila Pérez Téllez [1], Lourdes Lorigados-Pedre [1], Nelson Quintanal-Cordero [1], Ricardo Valdés-Llerena [1], Judith González González [1], Randis Garbey-Fernández [1], Ivette Cabrera-Abreu [1], Celia Alarcón-Calaña [1], Juan E. Bender del Busto [1], Rafael Rodríguez Rojas [2], Karla Batista García-Ramó [2] and Reinaldo Galvizu Sánchez [3]

1 Epilepsy Surgery Program, International Center for Neurological Restoration, 25th Ave, No 15805, PC 11300 Havana, Cuba; lily@neuro.ciren.cu (L.M.M.-C.); ivangarciamaeso@gmail.com (I.G.-M.); baby@neuro.ciren.cu (B.E.-D.); marugeniagarcian@gmail.com (M.E.G.-N.); yamilaperez86@yahoo.es (Y.P.T.); lourdesl@neuro.ciren.cu (L.L.-P.); nquintanal@neuro.ciren.cu (N.Q.-C.); rvaldes@neuro.ciren.cu (R.V.-L.); judith@neuro.ciren.cu (J.G.G.); randis0770@gmail.com (R.G.-F.); ivettec@neuro.ciren.cu (I.C.-A.); calarcon@neuro.ciren.cu (C.A.-C.); jebender@infomed.sld.cu (J.E.B.d.B.)

2 Imaging Department, International Center for Neurological Restoration, 25th Ave, No 15805, PC 11300 Havana, Cuba; rrguezrojas@gmail.com (R.R.R.); kbatista@neuro.ciren.cu (K.B.G.-R.)

3 Clinical Department, International Center for Neurological Restoration, 25th Ave, No 15805, PC 11300 Havana, Cuba; rgalvizu@infomed.sld.cu

* Correspondence: minou@neuro.ciren.cu

Abstract: Auditory and visual pathways may be affected as a consequence of temporal lobe epilepsy surgery because of their anatomical relationships with this structure. The purpose of this paper is to correlate the results of the auditory and visual evoked responses with the parameters of tractography of the visual pathway, and with the state of connectivity between respective thalamic nuclei and primary cortices in both systems after the surgical resection of the epileptogenic zone in drug-resistant epileptic patients. Tractography of visual pathway and anatomical connectivity of auditory and visual thalamus-cortical radiations were evaluated in a sample of eight patients. In general, there was a positive relationship of middle latency response (MLR) latency and length of resection, while a negative correlation was found between MLR latency and the anatomical connection strength and anatomical connection probability of the auditory radiations. In the visual pathway, significant differences between sides were found with respect to the number and length of tracts, which was lower in the operated one. Anatomical connectivity variables and perimetry (visual field defect index) were particularly correlated with the latency of P100 wave which was obtained by quadrant stimulation. These results demonstrate an indirect functional modification of the auditory pathway and a direct traumatic lesion of the visual pathway after anterior temporal lobectomy in patients with drug resistant epilepsy.

Keywords: auditory evoked responses; connectivity; drug-resistant epilepsy; temporal lobectomy; tractography; visual evoked potentials

---

1. Introduction

The natural history of mesial temporal lobe epilepsy (mTLE) is variable; among 20% and 40% of patients have pharmacologically intractable seizures despite more than ten new antiepileptic drugs being added to the market in recent years [1–4]. This refractoriness to medication leads to a progressive deterioration from the neurobiological, psychological and social point of view of the patients. Hence, surgical resection of the epileptogenic zone continues to be an important and effective therapeutic option for people with mTLE, with seizures totally disappearing in around 70–85% of cases [3,5,6]. However, due to the morbidity of the procedure, the risk-benefit balance, as well as secondary effects, should be considered. Particularly, the surgery of the temporal lobe may involve structures related to sensory processing. From the anatomical and functional point of view, the temporal lobe is closely related to the auditory and visual pathways before its projection to the temporal operculum and the calcarine sulcus, respectively [7]. Thus, these pathways can be directly or indirectly affected as a consequence of surgical treatment.

Visual field defects may appear as a consequence of direct injury of the optic radiations during the surgical procedure (superior quadrantanopia contralateral to the side of resection), particularly the Meyer's loop which runs in the vicinity of the temporo-mesial structures [8–13]. However, less is known about possible modifications that may occur in the auditory pathway [6,14].

In previous papers, we studied the variations of auditory and visual evoked potentials in patients with temporal lobe epilepsy that were submitted to surgical resection of the epileptogenic area [15,16]. Auditory brainstem response, auditory middle latency response and partial field visual evoked potentials were evaluated in particular. Additionally, some anatomical characteristics of the resected tissue and its relationship with the auditory and visual pathways were evaluated in a sample of these patients. A high coincidence rate between quadrant visual evoked potentials and perimetry was found, particularly in the superior quadrant that was contralateral to surgery. The volumetric study also showed that the injury of structures were probably related to the visual field defect. However, the results of the auditory evoked potentials and their relation to the volumetric findings pointed towards indirect damage of the auditory pathway, secondary to surgery. The aim of this paper is to correlate the results of the quadrant visual evoked potentials with the parameters of tractography of the visual pathway, and the results of the auditory and visual evoked responses with the state of connectivity between respective thalamic nuclei and primary cortices in both systems after the surgical resection of the epileptogenic zone.

2. Materials and Methods

2.1. Subjects

The study sample consisted of twenty-seven patients who were evaluated at the Telemetric Unit of the International Center for Neurological Restoration in Havana, Cuba in a prospective study. These patients were referred to this Unit from specialized consultations throughout the country once their intractability to medications was defined. They had crisis for at least two years with the use of at least two major antiepileptic drugs (Carbamazepine, Diphenylhydantoin, Valproate, Phenobarbital, Primidone) at the maximum tolerated doses for adequate periods of time. The inclusion criteria were:

- Patients with mTLE evaluated according to the institution's protocols and who were candidates for resective surgery according to agreed criteria.
- Patients who met the drug-resistance criteria.
- Patients who gave their informed consent to participate in the investigation.

Presurgical evaluation was performed, including the localization of the ictal zone by combining Electroencephalogram-video, ictal and interictal SPECT (Single Photon Emission Computed Tomography), qualitative and quantitative MRI and neuropsychological tests. Clinical and demographical data of the patients and controls are shown in Table 1.

The most frequently used drugs for treatment before and after surgical procedure were carbamazepine, clonazepam and valproate, and this did not change for at least two years after the surgical procedure. By the time the study began, 88.8% of patients had taken more than one medication.

Table 1. Clinical and demographical characteristics of the sample.

	N	Sex		Age Years μ (SD)	Duration of Illness Years μ (SD)	Temporo-Mesial Sclerosis N	Focal Cortical Dysplasia		
		M	F				IIIa	IIIb	No
Patients									
Left lobectomy	14	5	9	33.07 (9.06)	21.14 (9.08)	14	8	2	4
Right lobectomy	13	7	6	34.69 (5.28)	22.53 (12.14)	13	9	1	3
Healthy subjects	16	8	8	33.68 (7.96)	-	-		-	

μ: mean value; SD: standard deviation.

All patients underwent standard anterior temporal lobectomy guided by electrocorticography. Tissue samples that were obtained during surgery were histopathologically studied. Also, focal cortical dysplasias were classified according to Blumcke's criteria [17] (Table 1).

Refraction defects were tested and corrected in every subject before the evaluation of the visual system. Additionally, hearing threshold level was evaluated.

All subjects were right-handed and gave their consent to participate in the study.

2.2. Electrophysiological Tests

Auditory brainstem response (ABR), middle latency response (MLR) and partial field visual evoked potentials were measured in all of the patients and healthy subjects.

The recording conditions of the auditory and visual electrophysiological tests are summarized in Table 2.

The records were obtained with a Neuropack four-mini and a Neuropack M1 device (Nihon Khoden, Tokyo, Japan).

Table 2. Recording conditions of auditory responses and visual evoked potentials.

Parameters	ABR	MLR	VEP
Analysis time (ms)	10	100	300
Filters (Hz)	100–3000	20–1000	1–100
Stimulus frequency (Hz)	10	5	1
Maximal intensity (dBnHL)	105	90	-
Average responses	2000	500	30
Sensibility (μV/div)	5	20	20
Recording electrodes	A1, A2	Cz	O1, Oz, O2
Reference electrode	Cz	A1-A2	Fz
Ground electrode	Fpz	Fpz	A1
Stimulation mode	Monoaural	Binaural	Quadrants

ABR: auditory brainstem response; MLR: middle latency response; VEP: visual evoked potentials.

The auditory stimuli were 0.1 ms alternating clicks that were delivered through a headphone (DR-531B-7, Elegas Acous Co. Ltd., Tokyo, Japan).

The visual stimuli consisted of a pattern-reversal checkerboard (black and white checks) with a fixation center-point, 16′ size and high contrast. They were presented on a VD-401A monitor.

2.3. Resection Measure

The absolute length of the lateral and mesial resected tissue was measured by the neurosurgeon using slices of MRI in T1, T2 and FLAIR (Fluid-Attenuated Inversion Recovery) six months after surgery. The lateral (neocortical) aspect included the distance (in mm) between the posterior edge of the internal table and the anterior limit of the resected area, considering the middle temporal gyrus in the axial slices of the MRI, whereas the mesial aspect was calculated from axial slices in parallel with the preserved hippocampus. Two tangential lines were drawn: one between the posterior border of the resection and the contralateral hippocampus, and the other between the anterior limit of the preserved hippocampus and the side of resection. The distance between these tangential lines was the mesial longitude.

2.4. Perimetry

The requirements for the perimetric evaluation can be reviewed in Báez Martín et al. 2010 (16). Moreover, the area of the superior quadrant that was ipsilateral to the resection was used as a reference of the subject itself [18], and the calculation of the visual field defect index (VFD-I) was carried out using the following expression:

VFD-I = 1 − (preserved area in the contralateral superior quadrants/preserved area in the ipsilateral superior quadrants), so that a high index corresponded to a greater visual defect.

2.5. Diffusion Tensor Imaging (DTI)

The diffusion neuroimaging studies were performed in eight patients, six with right lobectomy and two with left. By using the standard gradient direction scheme (twelve weighted diffusion images and one b = 0 image), the diffusion images were acquired by an echo-planar sequence (EPI) with the following parameters: b = 1200 s/mm^2; FOV = 256 × 256 mm^2; acquisition matrix = 128 × 128 mm^2; corresponding to a spatial resolution 2 × 2 mm^2; TE/TR = 160 ms/7000 ms.

For the processing of the images, the diffusion spectrum imaging (DSI) Studio software (dsi-studio.labsolver.org/dsi-studio-download) was used and the DTI method that was proposed by Basser et al. which characterizes the main direction of fiber diffusion in the brain [19].

2.6. Tractography

Quantitative measurements, such as fractional anisotropy (FA), apparent diffusion coefficient (ADC) as well as axial and radial diffusivity values were obtained. These measures were analyzed through predetermined areas, according to regions of interest (ROIs) that were positioned following anatomical guides. In the case of optic radiation, the ROI was drawn on the FA map of each subject individually, also evaluating the occipital cortex (area 17 of Brodmann) as an independent ROI. This analysis was not possible for the auditory pathway due to the poor visualization of the thalamus-cortical segment, which did not allow drawing the ROI on the FA map.

2.7. Brain Anatomical Connectivity

The condition of the connections between the thalamus and the cortex for the visual and auditory pathways was evaluated. In the case of the visual pathway, anatomical connectivity was measured between the lateral geniculate body and the primary visual cortex (area 17 of Brodmann). For the auditory pathway, the same analysis was performed between the medial geniculate body and the primary auditory cortex (area 41 of Brodmann). A methodology that was based on graph theory that was proposed by Iturria et al. (2007) was implemented to describe the specific connections between the different regions of gray matter. The method consists of three essential steps: (1) definition of a Brain Graph model in which each voxel is considered as a node of a non-directed weighted graph; (2) use of an iterative algorithm to find the route of maximum probability between two nodes and the subsequent definition of the anatomical connectivity measure between them; (3) definition of three anatomical connectivity measures between different gray matter regions: anatomical connection strength (ACS), anatomical connection probability (ACP) and anatomical connection density (ACD) [20].

2.8. Statistics

Data analysis included the comparison between hemispheres for tractography and connectivity six months after surgery (t test for dependent samples). Normalization of the electrophysiological data was carried out using the mean and standard deviation values of the control group for correlation studies. The relationship among electrophysiological tests, perimetry, length of resection, tractography and anatomical connectivity was measured by the Pearson correlation test. Differences were considered significant if $p < 0.05$ for all tests (Statistica 8.0.360 Copyright StatSoft. Inc., Tulsa, OK, USA, 1984–2011).

2.9. Ethical Considerations

All the procedures followed the rules of the Declaration of Helsinki of 1975 for human research, and the study was approved by the scientific and ethics committee from the International Center for Neurological Restoration (CIREN37/2012).

3. Results

3.1. Auditory Pathway

As already noted, it was not possible to evaluate the tracts corresponding to the auditory radiations, however it was possible to study their connections. The results (mean and standard deviation) of the variables that were considered for this study are summarized in Table 3.

Table 3. Auditory radiations variables of DTI (Diffusion Tensor Imaging).

Variables	Ipsilateral Auditory Radiation		Contralateral Auditory Radiation		
	μ	SD	μ	SD	p
Density of connection	0.193	0.0773	0.251	0.0660	0.026 *
Density of connection (FA)	0.068	0.0293	0.093	0.0189	0.0800
Density of connection (MD)	0.080	0.0306	0.112	0.0261	0.0652
Anatomical Connection probability	0.422	0.1613	0.498	0.1172	0.3981
Anatomical Connection probability (FA)	0.181	0.0992	0.210	0.0372	0.4783
Anatomical Connection probability (MD)	0.193	0.0965	0.230	0.0565	0.4317
Anatomical connection strength	726.900	402.7487	1214.176	330.9955	0.0346 *
Anatomical connection strength (FA)	257.677	149.3024	449.342	100.6329	0.020 *
Anatomical connection strength (MD)	302.172	161.8940	542.212	135.5526	0.0214 *

FA: fractional anisotropy MD: media diffusivity. μ: media; SD: standard deviation. * Statistically significant differences between sides (t test for dependent samples, $p < 0.05$).

Structure-Function Relationships

For the correlation analysis with the anatomical variables, using the normalized data, both groups of patients were united, considering whether the pathway to be evaluated was ipsi or contralateral to the resection.

ABR: There were no statistically significant correlation between the variables of the ABR and the length of resection (Pearson correlation test, $p > 0.05$). There was a negative correlation between the connection density and the latency of the wave III that was ipsilateral to the resection (Pearson correlation test, $p < 0.05$, $r = -0.76$) only in the analysis of the connectivity in the auditory radiations. This showed a significant prolongation of latency in the group with right lobectomy.

MLR: As a whole, we found a positive relationship between the latency of the MLR components and the length of the resection; whereas a negative one was observed with the connectivity of the auditory thalamus-cortical radiation.

Table 4 summarizes the results of the correlation analysis between the electrophysiological variables of the MLR and the anatomical studies (Pearson correlation test, $p < 0.05$).

Table 4. Correlations between middle latency response and anatomical variables.

	Na Latency	Pa Latency	Nb Latency	Na Amplitude
Mesial length of resection	+0.13	+0.51 *	+0.48 *	−0.39
Neocortical length of resection **	+0.61 *	+0.31	+0.21	+0.16
Anatomical connection probability (FA) **	−0.88 *	−0.86	−0.89 *	+0.92 *
Anatomical connection strength (FA) *	−0.87	−0.89 *	−0.89 *	0.83

Note: The table refers to the correlation of the anatomical variables that were ipsilateral to the resection with the normalized values of middle latency response recorded in Cz. The + and − signs indicate whether the relationship is positive or negative, and the numbers correspond to the r of each correlation (Pearson correlation test, $p < 0.05$). FA: fractional anisotropy. ** Patients with right temporal lobectomy. * Statistically significant values.

The latency of Na correlated positively with the length of neocortical resection, however only in the group of patients with right lobectomy (Pearson correlation test, $p < 0.05$, r = 0.61). This group is precisely the one that showed a prolongation of latency of this component after resection, which reached statistical significance twelve months after surgery (t test, $p < 0.05$). It was also the group that showed the most extensive resection in the temporal neocortex (average 42.81 mm). The latency of the components Pa and Nb correlated positively with the mesial length of the resection in the whole group of operated patients (Pearson correlation test, $p < 0.05$, r = 0.51 and r = 0.48, respectively).

In a previous report, it described the positive correlation between the amplitude of Na and Pa waves and the resected volume in the middle temporal pole (Pearson correlation test $p < 0.05$, r = 0.84 and r = 0.65, respectively), especially in left temporal lobectomy patients. On the contrary, negative correlations were previously observed between the amplitude of these components and the residual indexes of the middle temporal pole (Pearson correlation test, $p < 0.05$, Na: r = −0.89 y Pa: r = −0.79), inferior temporal gyrus and amygdala (Pearson correlation test, $p < 0.05$, only Pa: r = −0.67 y r = −0.59, respectively) [15].

3.2. *Visual Pathway*

The results (mean and standard deviation) of the variables that were considered for the white matter tracts of optic radiation in both hemispheres are summarized in Table 5.

Table 5. DTI values in optic radiation and occipital cortex. Tractography.

		Ipsilateral		Contralateral		
		μ	SD	μ	SD	p
OR	Number of tracts **	356.625	185.997	578.500	155.902	0.0041 *
	Length of tracts	19.671	7.139	26.870	7.557	0.0307 *
	Volume of tracts	3167.500	1339.976	4368.750	1462.917	0.1988
	FA	0.403	0.127	0.499	0.031	0.0587
	ADC	0.001	0.000	0.001	0.000	0.1448
	AD	0.001	0.000	0.001	0.000	0.3502
	RD	0.001	0.000	0.001	0.000	0.1228
OC	Number of tracts	1961.87	832.04	2971.25	661.71	0.0017 *
	Length of tracts	14.986	4.748	18.190	2.669	0.1127
	Volume of tracts	7396.25	3425.97	9145.00	2655.12	0.0499 *
	FA	0.348	0.083	0.388	0.099	0.0026 *
	ADC	0.001	0.000	0.001	0.000	0.1062
	AD	0.001	0.000	0.001	0.000	0.7131
	RD	0.001	0.000	0.001	0.000	0.0741

OR: optic radiation; OC: occipital cortex. FA: fractional anisotropy; ADC: apparent diffusion coefficient; AD: axial diffusivity; RD: radial diffusivity. μ: average; SD: standard deviation. ** Right lobectomy patients. (t test for dependent samples, $p < 0.05$). * Statistically significant differences between sides. When comparing the optic radiations of both sides, statistically significant differences were evidenced for the whole group of patients with respect to the length of the tracts (t test for dependent samples, $p = 0.0307$) being smaller on the operated side. When we limited the analysis to the group with right lobectomy, the number of tracts was also significantly different (t test for dependent samples, $p = 0.0041$).

The comparative analysis of the tracts that were related to the occipital cortex showed differences between the sides that were statistically significant for the number of tracts, volume of tracts and fractional anisotropy (*t* test for dependent samples), which was also lower on the operated side.

Table 6 shows the results (mean and standard deviation) of the variables that were considered in the study of anatomical connectivity. The comparisons between the sides showed lower values of density, probability and strength of the anatomical connection on the side of the resection. However, these differences did not reach statistical significance (*t* test for dependent samples, $p > 0.05$).

Table 6. DTI values in optic radiation. Anatomical connectivity.

	Ipsilateral		**Contralateral**		
	μ	**SD**	**μ**	**SD**	***p***
Anatomical connection density	0.155	0.0733	0.174	0.0757	0.6104
Anatomical connection density (FA)	0.050	0.0271	0.069	0.0323	0.2115
Anatomical connection density (MD)	0.059	0.0306	0.075	0.0305	0.3426
Anatomical connection probability	0.387	0.1810	0.404	0.1292	0.8029
Anatomical connection probability (FA)	0.134	0.0711	0.174	0.0512	0.2581
Anatomical connection probability (MD)	0.178	0.0885	0.181	0.0537	0.9418
Anatomical connection strength	890.987	450.569	1239.440	610.7670	0.2174
Anatomical connection strength (FA)	290.970	171.595	487.988	260.4703	0.0958
Anatomical connection strength (MD)	342.933	188.255	531.343	253.9019	0.1243

FA: fractional anisotropy; MD: medium diffusivity. μ: average; SD: standard deviation (*t* test for dependent samples, $p > 0.05$).

Structure-Function Relationships

For the analysis of correlation with the anatomical studies, both groups of patients were united considering whether the quadrant to be evaluated was ipsi or contralateral to the resection, and standardized data of the quadrant-visual evoked potentials was used. The longest latency (maximum latency) and the smallest amplitude (minimum amplitude) of the P100 wave were taken from the pair of affected quadrants.

Table 7 summarizes the results of the correlation analysis that had statistical significance among the electrophysiological variables, the perimetry and the anatomical studies (Pearson correlation test, $p < 0.05$).

Table 7. Correlations with statistical significance between the anatomical variables, quadrant visual evoked potentials and the perimetry.

(A) Optic Radiations	**P100 Latency**			**P100 Amplitude**			**Perimetry (VFD-I)**
Electrodes	**O1**	**Oz**	**O2**	**O1**	**Oz**	**O2**	
Perimetry	+0.53	+0.50	+0.50				
Neocortical length of resection	+0.61	+0.60	+0.59				+0.72
FA *	−0.96	−0.98	−0.97				−0.73
ADC *	+0.98	+0.97	+0.98				
Axial diffusivity *	+0.99	+0.99	+0.99				
Radial diffusivity *	+0.99	+0.99	+0.99				
Connection density	−0.79	−0.78	−0.78			+0.76	
Connection probability	−0.89	−0.87	−0.86				
Connection strength	−0.88	−0.88	−0.89			+0.74	

Table 7. *Cont.*

(B) Occipital Cortex	P100 Latency			P100 Amplitude			Perimetry (VFD-I)
Electrodes	O1	Oz	O2	O1	Oz	O2	
Number of tracts						+0.86	
Volume of tracts				+0.87	+0.94	+0.80	
FA					+0.82		−0.71

Note: The table refers to the correlation of the anatomical variables with the normalized values of the visual evoked potential by quadrants (maximum latency and minimum amplitude) in the contralateral superior quadrant to the resection. The + and − signs indicate whether the relationship is positive or negative, and the numbers correspond to the r of each correlation (Pearson correlation test, $p < 0.05$). * Patients with right lobectomy, right eye. VFD-I: visual field defect index. FA: fractional anisotropy; ADC: apparent diffusion coefficient.

Figure 1 shows an example of the tractography of optic radiation in a patient with right lobectomy, where the reduction in the number of fibers on that side is appreciated and whose perimetry showed a superior left quadrantanopia.

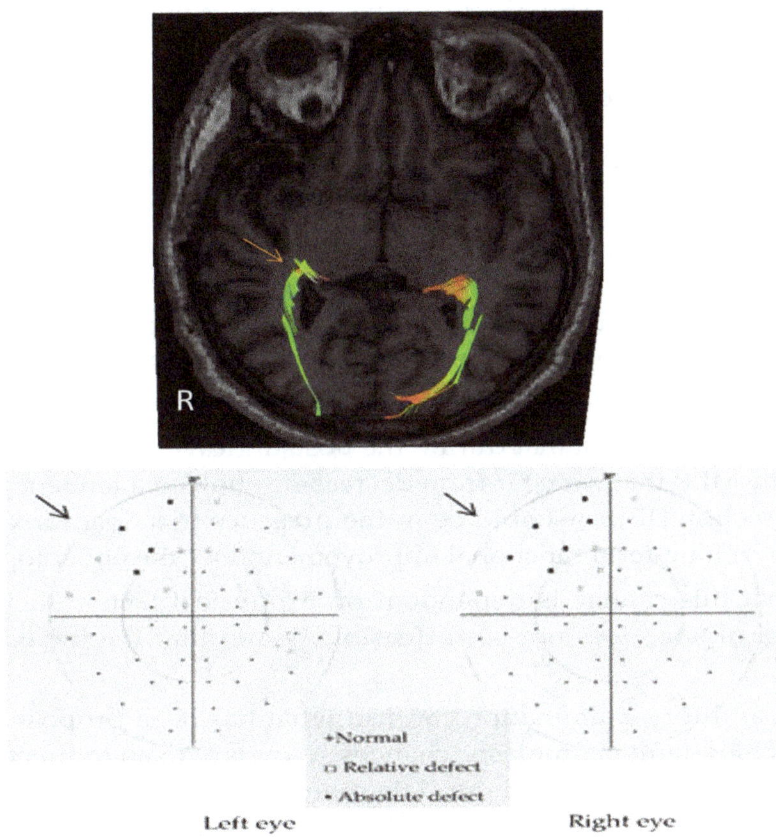

Figure 1. Tractography of optic radiations and perimetry of a patient with right lobectomy. Arrows indicate the pathological optic radiation (tractography) and the affected quadrants (perimetry). R: right side of the image.

4. Discussion

Epilepsy surgery as a therapeutic option for patients with drug-resistant mTLE produced structural and functional changes in the auditory and visual sensory systems, which were detected by the use of electrophysiological techniques and in correspondence with the structural variations that were evidenced with neuroimaging techniques.

The relationships that were found between the brainstem exploration (ABR) on the same side of the resection and the density of the connection in the auditory pathway could correspond to the known fact that the fibers which participate in the efferent control that are exerted by the cortex on the lower levels of the auditory pathway (mesencephalon-pons-cochlear receptor) are mostly ipsilateral [21].

It is known that the primary auditory cortex, preserved during this surgery, inhibits the conduction of the ascending impulses by means of the sensory control system, modifying the activity in the relay stations of the pathway (inferior colliculi and olive-cochlear complex) ipsilaterally, while the stimulation of secondary auditory areas enhances the ascending impulses [21]. These latter areas could be influenced by the removed zone, especially in patients with right lobectomy where the resection is wider. As a result of this excitatory-inhibitory imbalance, the inhibition of the aference on the same side of the surgery dominates, which is expressed by a delay in conduction at the subcortical levels of the pathway.

The magnitude of the resection of mesial structures, which is greater in the group with left temporal lobectomy, had greater repercussions on the thalamus-cortical components of the MLR (Pa, Nb), while the extension of the resection in its neocortical lateral aspect exerted a greater influence on the most caudal component (Na), especially in the group with right lobectomy. All these results speak in favor of a possible functional relationship between the resected structures and the generators of these components, with a variable behavior depending on whether the operated hemisphere is right or left.

The study of the anatomical connectivity showed an inverse relationship of the probability and strength of connection (particularly its FA) with the latency of Pa and Nb for the auditory radiation of the operated hemisphere. Interestingly, the Na component was related to the connection probability: the higher the latency and the lower the amplitude, the lower the connection probability (see Table 4).

These results suggest the existence of a modification of the functional state in the auditory pathway, which is given by a lower speed of propagation of the nerve impulse in correspondence with a reduction in the flow of information from the medial geniculate body to the auditory cortex and a lower functional relationship among these structures, with repercussion to other lower levels in the neuroaxis (inferior colliculi-superior olive complex).

However, if we take into account that during the postsurgical evaluation, the amplitude analysis of the components of the MLR that were far from decreasing showed a tendency to increase at 12 and 24 months after the resection [15], we could be in the presence of a "paradoxical" phenomenon of release, characterized by a long-term functional improvement once the epileptogenic zone is removed.

The possibility that this change is dependent on a physical factor, such as the reduction of impedance at the surgical site, does not seem feasible, given that the increase in amplitude was progressive over time.

The results of the auditory examination confirm what has been proposed in previous studies about the occurrence of long-term neuroplastic changes secondary to an indirect effect of the resection of temporal lobe structures [15]. Although our data seem to point to a possible effect of the surgery in the auditory pathway, these measures are not fully independent. In summary, there are functional implications of mTLE surgery on auditory processing. Concerning the visual pathway, the damage of Meyer's loop after temporal lobectomy [9,10,22–30] is well known, with the consequent visual field defect (homonymous superior quadrantanopia contralateral to the resected side) that can limit activities of daily life like driving [28,31].

Unlike the postulates that were used in the evaluation of the auditory pathway, in the case of the visual pathway, the sequelae of the anterior temporal lobectomy do constitute, a consequence of the direct aggression of the optical radiation fibers, dependent on the surgical procedure employed [32] and the distance between the tip of the Meyer loop and the posterior edge of the temporal pole [33]. Its anatomical disposition predisposes for this type of affectation to occur, especially in patients with right lobectomy where there is no risk of damaging eloquent areas for language, with which more generous removals from the epileptogenic zone can be carried out guided by trans-operative electrocorticography.

However, none of these studies have considered the relationship between functional variations and anatomical changes of the visual pathway.

The latency of the P100 wave that was obtained with quadrant stimulation correlated with the fiber damage in optic radiation, which was demonstrated by the effect of the extension of the resection in the neocortex of the temporal lobe (positive) and the value of the connectivity between the lateral geniculate body and the occipital cortex (negative) on this electrophysiological variable. This relationship was also evident between the latency of the P100 wave and the results of the perimetry (positive) for the three recording electrodes.

The amplitude of P100 correlated with the volume of the tracts that were related to the occipital cortex. The density and strength of the connection between the regions of interest had a positive relationship with this variable, selectively for the O2 electrode (right occipital cortex), which seems to be congruent given that most of the patients that were included in the anatomical study of the tracts had resection of the anterior temporal lobe of the right side (6 of 8). Furthermore, subjects with the higher volume of resected tissue showed the most delayed latencies and the lowest P100 amplitude [16].

Note that perimetry, classically considered the "gold standard" for the evaluation of visual field defects, also had a statistically significant relationship with the neocortical length of the resection and with the values of fractional anisotropy, both from the optic radiation and the occipital cortex (See Table 7).

When evaluating the tractography variables in optic radiation, we found no statistically significant relationship with the remaining measurements in the studied subjects (Pearson correlation test, $p > 0.05$).

However, when considering the side of the resection and the responses of each eye separately, a negative correlation of the P100 latency in the contralateral superior quadrant of the ipsilateral eye was found with the values of fractional anisotropy, and a positive correlation with the ADC and diffusivity (axial and radial) in patients with right lobectomy. This result suggests, as it did with visual potential and perimetry, that there is a higher probability of damaging fibers from the eye on the same side of the resection that derive from the temporal retina (nasal visual field) and that run more ventrally in the Meyer's loop, causing the incongruous visual field defects [8].

Finally, it is worth noting that we found a statistically significant negative correlation of the tract volume and the fractional anisotropy of the occipital cortex of the operated side with the P100 latency in the contralateral superior quadrant (Pearson correlation test, $p < 0.05$, $r = -0.87$ and $r = -0.89$ respectively), and with the amplitude of P100 in the same quadrant (Pearson's correlation test, $p < 0.05$, $r = 0.94$ and $r = 0.92$, respectively). The above was valid only when the analysis of the patients with right temporal lobectomy was performed. Once again, the results point to a greater anatomical and functional compromise of optic radiation when it comes to the non-dominant hemisphere for language.

In summary, the highest values of P100 latency in the contralateral superior quadrant indicate probable myelin damage in the optic radiation, which is supported by neuroimaging studies of diffusion (tractography and connectivity) and in correspondence with the perimetric results [16]. All of these findings confirm the existence of a partial and selective dysfunction of the visual pathway, in particular of the optic radiations on the side of the temporal lobectomy, which is expressed as a superior homonymous quadrantanopia contralateral to the resection, which is imperceptible for most patients with epilepsy that are resistant to medication and subjected to this surgical procedure.

These visual sequels could be minimized with transoperative monitoring guided by tractography of optic radiations, a method that is not available today in all groups that perform this type of surgery.

Among the limitations of this study is the absence of presurgical references of the magnetic resonance images in both pathways, as well as the difficulties to evaluate the images of the auditory radiations.

5. Conclusions

Taken as a whole, these results demonstrate an indirect functional modification of the auditory pathway and a direct traumatic lesion of the visual pathway after anterior temporal lobectomy in patients with pharmaco-resistant epilepsy.

The novelty of our study lies in the combined use of electrophysiological and imaging techniques to evaluate sensory pathways that are related to resected tissue in patients undergoing this surgical procedure. Undoubtedly, the results of tractography and structural connectivity are in line with the findings of the functional tests, which further strengthens our study.

Author Contributions: M.M.B.-M. and L.M.M.-C. conceived and designed the experiments and wrote the paper; I.G.-M. and N.Q.-C. made the surgical procedures; R.V.-L. and R.G.-F. made the anesthetics procedures; Y.P.T., I.C.-A. and C.A.-C. performed the electrophysiological tests; J.G.G., J.E.B.d.B., and R.G.S. made the clinical evaluation; M.E.G.-N. performed the neuropsychological evaluation; K.B.G.-R. and R.R.R. made the image processing; B.E.-D. and L.L.-P. performed the anatomopathological procedures.

Acknowledgments: We thank Odalys Morales-Chacon for the English revision of the manuscript and Jorge Bergado-Rosado for his contributions.

References

1. Gronich, G.; Arno, L.; Dualib, K. Neurofisiologia nao-invasiva (EEG) das diferentes síndromes epilépticas. In *Tratamento clínico e cirúrgico das epilepsias de dificil controle*; Cukiert, A., Ed.; Lemos: Sao Paulo, Brazil, 2002; p. 157.
2. Hauser, W. The natural history of temporal lobe epilepsy. In *Epilepsy Surgery*; Luders, H., Ed.; Raven Press: New York, NY, USA, 2000; pp. 133–141.
3. Viera, O., Jr. Tratamento cirúrgico da epilepsia do lobo temporal. In *Tratamento Clínico e Cirúrgico das Epilepsias de Difícil Controle*; Cukiert, A., Ed.; Lemos: Sao Paulo, Brazil, 2002; pp. 269–289.
4. Bonilha, L.; Marzt, G.U.; Glazier, S.S.; Edwards, J.C. Subtypes of medial temporal lobe epilepsy: Influence on temporal lobectomy outcomes? *Epilepsia* **2012**, *53*, 1–6. [CrossRef] [PubMed]
5. Bazil, C.; Morrell, M.J.; Peddley, T. Epilepsy. In *Merritt's Neurology*; Rowland, L., Ed.; Lippincott Williams & Wilkins: Philadelphia, PA, YSA, 2005; pp. 990–1008.
6. Karceski, S.; Morrell, M. Principles of epilepsy management: Diagnosis and treatment. In *Neurological Therapeutics: Principles and Practice*; Noseworthy, J.H., Ed.; Informa Healthcare: Rochester, NY, USA, 2006; pp. 341–354.
7. Sindou, M.; Guenot, M. Surgical anatomy of the temporal lobe for epilepsy surgery. *Adv. Tech. Stand. Neurosurg.* **2003**, *28*, 315–343. [PubMed]
8. Hughes, T.S.; Abou-Khalil, B.; Lavin, P.J.; Fakhoury, T.; Blumenkopf, B.; Donahue, S.P. Visual field defects after temporal lobe resection: A prospective quantitative analysis. *Neurology* **1999**, *53*, 167–172. [CrossRef] [PubMed]
9. James, J.S.; Radhakrishnan, A.; Thomas, B.; Madhusoodanan, M.; Kesavadas, C.; Abraham, M.; Menon, R.; Rathore, C.; Vilanilam, G. Diffusion tensor imaging tractography of Meyer's loop in planning resective surgery for drug-resistant temporal lobe epilepsy. *Epilepsy Res.* **2015**, *110*, 95–104. [CrossRef] [PubMed]
10. Jeelani, N.U.; Jindahra, P.; Tamber, M.S.; Poon, T.L.; Kabasele, P.; James-Galton, M.; Stevens, J.; Duncan, J.; McEvoy, A.W.; Harkness, W.; et al. 'Hemispherical asymmetry in the Meyer's Loop': A prospective study of visual-field deficits in 105 cases undergoing anterior temporal lobe resection for epilepsy. *J. Neurol. Neurosurg. Psychiatry* **2010**, *81*, 985–991. [CrossRef] [PubMed]
11. Nilsson, D.; Malmgren, K.; Rydenhag, B.; Frisen, L. Visual field defects after temporal lobectomy—Comparing methods and analysing resection size. *Acta Neurol. Scand.* **2004**, *110*, 301–307. [CrossRef] [PubMed]
12. Pathak-Ray, V.; Ray, A.; Walters, R.; Hatfield, R. Detection of visual field defects in patients after anterior temporal lobectomy for mesial temporal sclerosis-establishing eligibility to drive. *Eye (Lond.)* **2002**, *16*, 744–748. [CrossRef] [PubMed]

13. Mandelstam, S.A. Challenges of the Anatomy and Diffusion Tensor Tractography of the Meyer Loop. *AJNR Am. J. Neuroradiol.* **2012**, *33*, 1204–1210. [CrossRef] [PubMed]
14. Japaridze, G.; Kvernadze, D.; Geladze, T.; Kevanishvili, Z. Auditory brain-stem response, middle-latency response, and slow cortical potential in patients with partial epilepsy. *Seizure* **1997**, *6*, 449–456. [CrossRef]
15. Baez-Martin, M.M.; Morales Chacon, L.M.; Garcia-Maeso, I.; Estupiñan-Diaz, B.; Lorigados-Pedre, L.; Garcia, M.E.; Galvizu, R.; Bender, J.E.; Cabrera-Abreu, I.; Perez-Tellez, Y.; et al. Temporal lobe epilepsy surgery modulates the activity of auditory pathway. *Epilepsy Res.* **2014**, *108*, 748–754. [CrossRef] [PubMed]
16. Baez Martin, M.M.; del Carmen Perez, T.Y.; Morales Chacon, L.M.; Diaz, B.E.; Trapaga-Quincoses, O.; Maeso, I.G.; Bender, J.E.; Galvizu, R.; Garcia, M.E.; Abreu, I.C.; et al. Innovative evaluation of visual field defects in epileptic patients after standard anterior temporal lobectomy, using partial field visual evoked potentials. *Epilepsy Res.* **2010**, *90*, 68–74. [CrossRef] [PubMed]
17. Blumcke, I.; Aronica, E.; Urbach, H.; Alexopoulos, A.; Gonzalez-Martinez, J.A. A neuropathology-based approach to epilepsy surgery in brain tumors and proposal for a new terminology use for long-term epilepsy-associated brain tumors. *Acta Neuropathol.* **2014**, *128*, 39–54. [CrossRef] [PubMed]
18. Daga, P.; Winston, G.; Modat, M.; White, M.; Mancini, L.; Cardoso, M.J.; Symms, M.; Stretton, J.; McEvoy, A.W.; Thornton, J.; et al. Accurate localization of optic radiation during neurosurgery in an interventional MRI suite. *IEEE Trans. Med. Imaging* **2012**, *31*, 882–891. [CrossRef] [PubMed]
19. Basser, P.J.; Mattiello, J.; LeBihan, D. Estimation of the effective self-diffusion tensor from the NMR spin echo. *J. Magn. Reson. B* **1994**, *103*, 247–254. [CrossRef] [PubMed]
20. Iturria-Medina, Y.; Canales-Rodriguez, E.J.; Melie-Garcia, L.; Valdés-Hernández, P.A.; Martínez-Montes, E.; Alemán-Gómez, Y.; Sánchez-Bornot, J.M. Characterizing brain anatomical connections using diffusion weighted MRI and graph theory. *Neuroimage* **2007**, *36*, 645–660. [CrossRef] [PubMed]
21. Khalfa, S.; Bougeard, R.; Morand, N.; Veuillet, E.; Isnard, J.; Guenot, M.; Ryvlin, P.; Fischer, C.; Collet, L. Evidence of peripheral auditory activity modulation by the auditory cortex in humans. *Neuroscience* **2001**, *104*, 347–358. [CrossRef]
22. Chen, X.; Weigel, D.; Ganslandt, O.; Buchfelder, M.; Nimsky, C. Prediction of visual field deficits by diffusion tensor imaging in temporal lobe epilepsy surgery. *Neuroimage* **2009**, *45*, 286–297. [CrossRef] [PubMed]
23. Egan, R.A.; Shults, W.T.; So, N.; Burchiel, K.; Kellogg, J.X.; Salinsky, M. Visual field deficits in conventional anterior temporal lobectomy versus amygdalohippocampectomy. *Neurology* **2000**, *55*, 1818–1822. [CrossRef] [PubMed]
24. Guenot, M.; Krolak-Salmon, P.; Mertens, P.; Isnard, J.; Ryvlin, P.; Fischer, C.; Vighetto, A.; Mauguiere, F.; Sindou, M. MRI assessment of the anatomy of optic radiations after temporal lobe epilepsy surgery. *Stereotact. Funct. Neurosurg.* **1999**, *73*, 84–87. [CrossRef] [PubMed]
25. Hervas-Navidad, R.; Altuzarra-Corral, A.; Lucena-Martin, J.A.; Castaneda-Guerrero, M.; Vela-Yebra, R.; Sanchez, A. Defects in the visual field in resective surgery for temporal lobe epilepsy. *Rev. Neurol.* **2002**, *34*, 1025–1030. [PubMed]
26. McDonald, C.R.; Hagler, D.J., Jr.; Girard, H.M.; Pung, C.; Ahmadi, M.E.; Holland, D.; Patel, R.H.; Barba, D.; Tecoma, E.S.; Iragui, V.J.; et al. Changes in fiber tract integrity and visual fields after anterior temporal lobectomy. *Neurology* **2010**, *75*, 1631–1638. [CrossRef] [PubMed]
27. Mengesha, T.; Abu-Ata, M.; Haas, K.F.; Lavin, P.J.; Sun, D.A.; Konrad, P.E.; Pearson, M.; Wang, L.; Song, Y.; Abou-Khalil, B.W. Visual field defects after selective amygdalohippocampectomy and standard temporal lobectomy. *J. Neuroophthalmol.* **2009**, *29*, 208–213. [CrossRef] [PubMed]
28. Manji, H.; Plant, G.T. Epilepsy surgery, visual fields, and driving: A study of the visual field criteria for driving in patients after temporal lobe epilepsy surgery with a comparison of Goldmann and Esterman perimetry. *J. Neurol. Neurosurg. Psychiatry* **2000**, *68*, 80–82. [CrossRef] [PubMed]
29. Taoka, T.; Sakamoto, M.; Nakagawa, H.; Nakase, H.; Iwasaki, S.; Takayama, K.; Taoka, K.; Hoshida, T.; Sakaki, T.; Kichikawa, K. Diffusion tensor tractography of the Meyer loop in cases of temporal lobe resection for temporal lobe epilepsy: Correlation between postsurgical visual field defect and anterior limit of Meyer loop on tractography. *AJNR Am. J. Neuroradiol.* **2008**, *29*, 1329–1334. [CrossRef] [PubMed]
30. Winston, G.P.; Daga, P.; Stretton, J.; Modat, M.; Symms, M.R.; McEvoy, A.W.; Ourselin, S.; Duncan, J.S. Optic radiation tractography and vision in anterior temporal lobe resection. *Ann. Neurol.* **2012**, *71*, 334–341. [CrossRef] [PubMed]

31. Winston, G.P. Epilepsy surgery, vision, and driving: What has surgery taught us and could modern imaging reduce the risk of visual deficits? *Epilepsia* **2013**, *54*, 1877–1888. [CrossRef] [PubMed]
32. Wu, W.; Rigolo, L.; O'Donnell, L.J.; Norton, I.; Shriver, S.; Golby, A.J. Visual pathway study using in vivo diffusion tensor imaging tractography to complement classic anatomy. *Neurosurgery* **2012**, *70*, 145–156. [CrossRef] [PubMed]
33. Wang, Y.X.; Zhu, X.L.; Deng, M.; Siu, D.Y.; Leung, J.C.; Chan, Q.; Chan, D.T.; Mak, C.H.; Poon, W.S. The use of diffusion tensor tractography to measure the distance between the anterior tip of the Meyer loop and the temporal pole in a cohort from Southern China. *J. Neurosurg.* **2010**, *113*, 1144–1151. [CrossRef] [PubMed]

16

Immunomodulators as Therapeutic Agents in Mitigating the Progression of Parkinson's Disease

Bethany Grimmig [1], Josh Morganti [2], Kevin Nash [3] and Paula C. Bickford [1,4,*]

1 Center of Excellence for Aging and Brain Repair, Department of Neurosurgery and Brain Repair, Morsani College of Medicine, University of South Florida, Tampa, FL 33612, USA; bgrimmig@health.usf.edu
2 Sanders-Brown Center on Aging, Department of Anatomy and Neurobiology, University of Kentucky, Lexington, KY 40508, USA; josh.morganti@uky.edu
3 Byrd Alzheimer's Institute, Department of Molecular Pharmacology and Physiology, Morsani College of Medicine, University of South Florida, Tampa, FL 33613, USA; Knash@health.usf.edu
4 James A Haley VA Hospital, 13000 Bruce B Downs Blvd, Tampa, FL 33612, USA
* Correspondence: pbickfor@health.usf.edu

Academic Editor: Donna Gruol

Abstract: Parkinson's disease (PD) is a common neurodegenerative disorder that primarily afflicts the elderly. It is characterized by motor dysfunction due to extensive neuron loss in the substantia nigra pars compacta. There are multiple biological processes that are negatively impacted during the pathogenesis of PD, and are implicated in the cell death in this region. Neuroinflammation is evidently involved in PD pathology and mitigating the inflammatory cascade has been a therapeutic strategy. Age is the number one risk factor for PD and thus needs to be considered in the context of disease pathology. Here, we discuss the role of neuroinflammation within the context of aging as it applies to the development of PD, and the potential for two representative compounds, fractalkine and astaxanthin, to attenuate the pathophysiology that modulates neurodegeneration that occurs in Parkinson's disease.

Keywords: Parkinson's disease; neuroinflammation; microglia; fractalkine; astaxanthin

1. Parkinson's Disease

Parkinson's disease (PD) is a debilitating condition that affects millions of people worldwide. With the development of drugs to treat complications associated with significant morbidity and mortality, patients are living up to 20 years after the diagnosis of PD. Although the use of medications has led to a relative improvement in quality of life, these patients are often substantially disabled, requiring significant health care and compensation for loss of wages. It has been projected that the prevalence of PD will double by 2040, indicating severe economic consequences to come as the incidence increases. There are currently no available medications that prevent or reverse the neurodegeneration that causes these disabilities [1].

Parkinson's disease is primarily characterized neuroanatomically by the degeneration of the neurons in the substantia nigra pars compacta (SN), resulting in a substantial loss of dopamine (DA) afferents to the striatum and subsequent motor impairment. It is estimated that nearly 50% of dopaminergic cells in the SN have been lost prior to clinical presentation of motor dysfunction. It is now understood that PD pathology extends to extra nigral regions including the locus coeruleus, nucleus basalis of Meynert, peduculopontine nucleus, intralaminar thalamus, and lateral hypothalamus suggesting dysfunction and neurodegeneration in many areas of the brain [2]. It is histopathologically characterized by the formation of Lewy bodies, intraneuronal protein inclusions comprised predominantly of α-synuclein (α-syn). These protein aggregates have been observed throughout the brain, and pathological α-syn deposition is thought to begin in the medulla and spread throughout the midbrain to cortical regions in a manner that corresponds to the onset of clinical symptoms [2]. These protein aggregates are associated with microgliosis [3], and impaired cellular physiology, although the precise mechanisms leading to cytotoxicity are currently unknown.

The vast majority of Parkinson's disease cases are classified as idiopathic, but approximately 5% of PD cases are genetically linked. There are several gene mutations that confer susceptibility or are associated with the development of PD, including mutations in leucine-rich repeat kinase 2 (LRRK), PTEN Induced putative kinase 1 (PINK1), and the protein deglycase (DJ1). However, α-syn has proven to have a very strong association and relevance to PD and similar disorders collectively known as synucleinopathies. Abnormalities in the SNCA gene that encodes the α-syn protein are strongly correlated with the development of an autosomal dominant familial form of PD [4]. Multiplications of the SNCA gene are known to increase the expression of the α-syn protein, whereas certain missense mutations of the gene (A53T, A30P, E46K) produce variants of α-syn, both of which have known pathological attributes related to the increased propensity to aggregate.

The physiological role of α-syn, along with the isoforms β- and γ-synuclein, is related to neurotransmission, and they are primarily located in the synapse. Increased concentrations of α-syn protein or mutated forms of α-syn make the protein susceptible to misfolding and polymerization by self-assembly. These misfolded aggregates have heterogeneous conformations that have not been clearly elucidated. These aggregates are associated with various deleterious biological activities including (1) the permeabilization of the cellular membranes [5], associated with an alteration of intracellular ion concentrations [6]; (2) disruption of energy production through interactions with the mitochondria [7]; and (3) interruption of intracellular transport via physical interference of motor proteins, or direct interaction with organelles and vesicles [8]. The formation of soluble oligomeric species is presumed to be relatively more toxic than fibrils, through the energetically favorable association within the phospholipids that forms pores in the cellular membrane [9]. The amount of LB formations throughout the brain reflects the severity of impairment [10]. However, it has been postulated that the organizing of fibrils into Lewy Bodies may serve as a protective mechanism to divert toxic aggregate species into less harmful formations to preserve normal cellular physiology [11].

2. The Interaction with Aging

Aging is a major risk factor for the development of PD [12], evidenced by the fact that the incidence increases for every decade over 50 years of age. While aging contributes to PD, it is also underrepresented in PD research, as it is common for the experimental models to be carried out using young animals. However, the impact of aging is essential to consider in terms of the disease process because many of the physiological changes that occur in aged animals can drive or exacerbate the pathological mechanisms that lead to PD and alter both the course and tempo of the disease.

The impact of aging on the incidence of PD is compounded by the fact that the dopaminergic neurons of the SN seem to have a unique vulnerability to cellular stressors in the microenvironment [12]. Although it is not completely understood what sets these cells apart from those of other DA pathways, the neurons of this nucleus are more susceptible to the homeostatic disturbances and degenerate significantly more compared to similar or adjacent regions [13]. This can be grossly attributed to high oxidative stress and inflammation. It is known that the SN is exposed to higher levels of oxidation compared to other dopaminergic centers [11]. This is partly due to an unusually high concentration of iron, which through the Fenton reaction, can generate free radicals, as well as nitric oxide released by microglia that densely populate this region [14,15]. In addition to the accumulation of reactive oxygen and nitrogen species, the SN is also ill-equipped to neutralize them, due to a low expression of glutathione, an important endogenous antioxidant molecule, leading to an inevitable increase in oxidative stress [16]. Aging is also associated with increased levels of oxidative stress and altered microglial function and this combined with the SN's reduced resilience to reactive oxygen species (ROS) could promote neurodegeneration.

The role of neuroinflammation in PD is also particularly important in the context of aging. Inflammation is known to increase with age. This is largely attributed to the age related changes in microglial physiology. Microglia, myeloid derived macrophages, are the resident immune cell of the CNS and constitute 10% of the cell population. Their highly ramified processes are highly motile and constantly survey parenchyma, facilitating the detection and the cellular response to infection and injury. However, microglia are also involved in many homeostatic functions and are now known to be highly active during post-natal synaptic pruning and synaptic plasticity [17,18]. Microglia are known to undergo a phenomenon known as priming with age. This describes a propensity for microglia to attain a pro-inflammatory state and is characterized by 4 principal features: (1) primed microglia will exhibit higher levels of inflammatory mediators and surface makers even in the absence of immune stimulation; (2) microglia also demonstrate hyperactivity upon subsequent activation where they release exaggerated amounts of cytokines and reactive oxygen/nitrogen species; (3) they are also resistant to regulatory mechanisms that typically restore microglia back to their inactivated state, causing them to remain in an aggravated state for a longer period of time [19]; and (4) they do not respond to stimuli, such as IL4, that promote anti-inflammatory factors, angiogenesis, and neurotrophic factor secretion [19,20]. For example, Lee, Ruiz et al. (2013) induced microglial activation in the brains of young and old mice with the application of a cytokine cocktail designed to elicit an M1, pro-inflammatory phenotype (IL1β + IL12) or an anti-inflammatory, M2 phenotype (IL-4 + IL-13). These authors demonstrated that M1 cocktail elicits an increased response microglia from the aged brain, while the same aged cells were less responsive to the M2 cocktail. This phenomenon has been reproduced with isolated microglia and has been termed priming [21].

In order to elucidate the molecular underpinnings of the age-related alterations in microglial function, numerous researchers have begun to assess the differential expression of genes and protein in primary microglia. A recent study using RNAseq comparing the transcriptional profiles of isolated microglia to whole brain has identified the microglial sensome [22]. These authors further assessed the sensome in microglia isolated from aged animals and demonstrated that many of the genes related to sensing endogenous ligands were down regulated, whereas genes pertaining to host defense were up-regulated. Furthermore, another recent study using gene microarrays of isolated microglia identified an up-regulation of NFκB related genes in these aged cells [23]. Sustained microglial activation and microglial priming can perpetuate neurodegeneration by increasing cellular stress both from enhanced release of cytotoxic substances, but also from the loss of trophic support as a result of impaired microglial homeostatic function.

3. Role of Neuroinflammation

The precise pathophysiology that precipitates the development of PD is unknown, although it is understood that a few key biological processes are often impacted in patients, including mitochondrial function, proteostaisis, immune function leading to oxidative stress and inflammation. Neuroinflammation is critical factor in the disease process that clearly contributes significantly to the neurodegeneration seen in PD. However, it is difficult to ascertain if inflammation initiates pathological features of PD, or is triggered by the widespread protein aggregation and neuronal death that occurs during disease progression. McGeer et al. (1988) described the presence of increased reactive gliosis and infiltrating T-cells around the SN in post mortem analysis of PD brains [24]. Their observations provided some of the first indications that increased neuroinflammation is associated with DA cell death. Many other studies have reported features of inflammation in post-mortem samples, such as increased levels of inflammatory mediators like iNos and Cox-2 [25], supporting the contribution of increased neuroinflammation during advanced stages of the disease. Similar patterns of activated microglia have been detected in the brain areas associated with clinical symptoms of the disease [26]. Interestingly, this distribution of gliosis was evident in both newly diagnosed patients and those with advanced pathology. Elevated levels of pro-inflammatory cytokines have also been detected in the cerebrospinal fluid and plasma of PD patients at early stages of the disease. These findings suggest that microglial activation may be initiated in early stages and remain an ongoing process throughout the disease. Furthermore, inflammatory insults and injuries are known to increase the risk of developing PD. Traumatic brain injuries (TBI) have been linked to an increased risk of developing the disease in a frequency and severity dependent manner; multiple injuries or injuries requiring hospitalization were more strongly correlated with PD onset [27]. This occurrence is largely attributed to the neuroinflammatory cascade that follows trauma. Certain infections causing neuroinflammation have been known to lead to a post-encephalitic Parkinsonism. This may be because the SN is densely populated by microglia [28], rendering it is especially susceptible to inflammatory stimuli. For example, intracranial injections of lipopolysaccharide (LPS), a bacterial antigen, dramatically activate microglia and leads to nigrostriatal degeneration and motor symptoms of PD [29]. Parkinsonism is a separate condition distinct from PD, but these observations of inflammatory insults leading to cell death may have important implications for PD itself. Taken together, these data suggest a potential role of neuroinflammation in ongoing cell death that occurs in PD.

Furthermore, pathological forms of α-syn are associated with microglial activation in the brains of PD patients and this is consistently recapitulated in animal models. The presence of α-syn aggregates modulates glial activity, often eliciting the release of inflammatory mediators. Codolo et al. (2013) treated monocytes with various species of α-syn to demonstrate that the aggregated and pathogenic forms of the protein can facilitate the secretion of IL-1β though stimulation of the inflammasome [30]. The nitration of α-syn is a common modification associated with pathology thought to be promoted in an oxidative environment. Stimulation of microglial cells with nitrated and aggregated α-syn alters the cellular morphology and transcriptional profile to a pro-inflammatory phenotype, with increased transcription of IL-1β, TNF-α, and IFN-γ as well as induction of NF-Kβ signaling [31]. Additionally, this α-syn activation of microglia seems to be related to phagocytic capacity, as inflammatory cascades and activation of NADPH oxidase are initiated after the glial cells take up the aggregates [3,32,33]. Zhang et al. (2005) demonstrated that impeding phagocytosis of primary microglia attenuates the release of superoxide from these cells when exposed to α-syn in vitro. This detection and engulfment of α-syn seems to be dependent on the FCγ receptor, as FCγ deficient mice are protected the resultant neurodegeneration from AAV driven over expression of α-syn [32,33]. It is thought that this inflammatory response to abnormal α-syn will perpetuate neural dysfunction through the release of cytotoxic compounds that leads to cell death. Many of these studies were done using either glial cell lines or in young animals, neglecting the impact of the pro-inflammatory actions of α-syn within the primed glial environment of an aging brain, thus causing even more damage. In fact, when α-syn is introduced into an aged animal it is more cytotoxic compared to the young controls [34].

4. Fractalkine as an Anti-Inflammatory Treatment

There is promising pre-clinical experimental evidence to support that reducing inflammation, specifically by suppressing microglial activity, can modify the progression of the loss of DA neurons [35–38]. Non-steroidal anti-inflammatory drugs have been suggested to reduce the risk of PD onset [39]. Also, the use of minocycline, a tetracycline with pharmaceutical actions that extend beyond the classical antimicrobial activity, has been shown to reduce cell death in a neurotoxic model of PD using 1-methyl-4-phenyl-1,2,3,6-tetrahydropyridine (MPTP). These researchers attributed the neuroprotective effect to the down-regulation of iNOS expression and glial activation [40]. Minocycline was also shown to inhibit apoptosis through a reduction of related inflammatory mediators [41]. Because glial activation is associated with the release of pro-inflammatory factors capable of damaging neurons, this data suggests that mediating the excessive inflammation in PD is a viable therapeutic strategy. There are several signals produced by neurons that have an anti-inflammatory action on microglia, including CD200, CD22, CD47 and fractalkine (FKN, CX3CL1), which could be potential therapeutic targets.

Fractalkine is a protein expressed constitutively by neurons in a membrane bound form that can be cleaved by disintegrin and metalloproteinase (ADAM) 10 and 17. This proteolysis releases a soluble form of the protein, but both isoforms are thought to ligate the cognate receptor, CX3CR1, located on the surface of microglia in the CNS [42]. This neuron-glia interaction serves as an important endogenous mechanism to suppress microglial activation and regulate the output of inflammatory mediators and other damaging molecules [42]. It has been shown that increasing fractalkine levels using an AAV9 gene therapy approach can be neuroprotective [35,36], while the absence of this FKN-CX3CR1 signaling cascade confers susceptibility to neurodegeneration in rodent models of PD. Cardona et al. (2006) demonstrated that CX3CR1 deficiency lead to increase neurotoxicity to both peripheral LPS and MPTP injections. In these experiments, both heterozygous and homozygous mice exhibited increased neurodegeneration and IL-1β expression compared to the intact wild-type controls [43]. There is evidence indicating that fractalkine can regulate microglial function and subsequently reduce inflammation in the CNS. Multiple in vitro studies have established that enhancing fractalkine signaling through application of the ligand or stimulation of the receptor can protect against cell death in culture; FKN-ligand decreases microglial apoptosis and protects against neurotoxicity by both LPS and TNF-α. It has been demonstrated that maintaining or enhancing communication of FKN/CX3CR1 is neuroprotective in multiple rodent models of PD. Pabon et al. (2011) [37] attenuated the neurotoxicity of 6 hydroxydopamine (6OHDA) by delivering a chronic intrastriatal infusion of recombinant fractalkine ligand. This preservation of dopaminergic terminals in the striatum was also associated with decreased microglial activation around the lesion site, indicated by a reduced expression of the MHCII surface marker. To further examine the action of fractalkine in a model of PD where synuclein is introduced in the SN via AAV, Nash et al. (2015) corroborated the neuroprotective effects of FKN by using a viral vector to over express the different isoforms of FKN; membrane-bound (mFKN) or the soluble portion (sFKN). In this study, sFKN reduced DA cell death in young rats with overexpression α-syn in the SN via AAV9. These findings may be due to altered FKN-CX3CR1 signaling [44] and a reduction in pro-inflammatory cytokines and modulation of microglial function into a more protective role (Figure 1). These results suggest that supraphysiological levels of the fractalkine are protective against the neurodegeneration occurring in two separate experimental models of PD. Morganti et al. (2012) [36] also illustrated the importance of neuron-glial communication by administering MPTP to animals deficient in the fractalkine ligand. These FKN knockouts were extremely susceptible to MPTP toxicity, and display both a dramatic loss of TH in the SN and the robust gliosis associated with the lesion site. Not only does this work indicate that FKN-CX3CR1 communication is necessary for moderating cell death and subsequent detrimental inflammatory events, but it also suggests that further enhancing or supplementing this signaling pathway above baseline activity is sufficient to achieve neuroprotection against these potent toxins (Figure 1). However, the action of fractalkine is quite complex; CX3CR1 knockout mice have been shown to increase phagocytosis of amyloid, but decrease phagocytosis of synuclein [44]. It is unclear if this action is mediated by membrane bound fractalkine or the cleaved, soluble form. Several studies have tried to clarify the roles of the differential processing of fractalkine and there does not appear to be a clear conclusion at this point. When an obligate soluble version of fractalkine is used, as described here with a gene therapy approach, it has been shown to be beneficial in models of PD and AD tau pathology [35,36,45]. However, in other models where an obligate soluble fractalkine mouse is used, opposite results have been observed, and this paper concludes that the membrane anchored fractalkine is associated with phagocytosis of Aβ [46].

Much of the current data regarding the therapeutic potential of FKN in the treatment of inflammatory and neurodegenerative conditions stems from studies involving young animals. However, it is essential to note that aged microglia have been shown to be resistant to their regulatory signals [20,47]. Furthermore, communication via the FKN/CX3CR1 axis becomes dysregulated with age and can also contribute to microglial priming and dysfunction. There are age associated changes affecting both the ligand and receptor. It has been has shown that FKN is reduced by in the aged hippocampus [48], although the extent of FKN downregulation in the SN has not yet been fully characterized. Additionally, immune challenges in the aged CNS lead to a prolonged down regulation of the fractalkine receptor that is associated with a sustained inflammatory response, further compromising this protective neuron glia interaction [49]. Therefore, it is imperative to investigate the therapeutic potential of FKN in the treatment of PD in aged animal models; future studies are needed to examine the efficacy of FKN on aged or primed microglia.

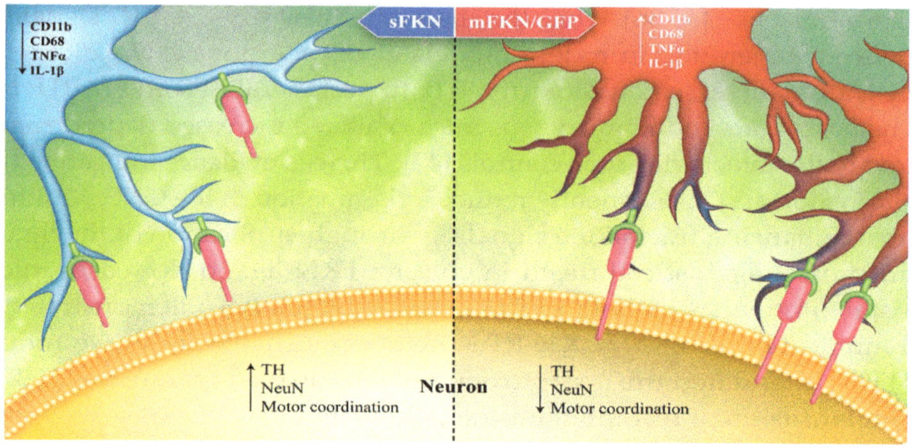

Figure 1. A depiction of ligand/receptor binding for both the soluble and membrane bound isoforms of CX3CL1 (FKN) and their respective influences on the release of inflammatory mediators in the substantia nigra. As discussed above, sFKN when delivered via AAV into CX3CL1-/- mice following MPTP is associated with the suppression of cytokine production. However, when we delivered an obligate membrane bound form of CX3CL1 or a vector with GFP there was no rescue of TH neurons or a reduction in inflammatory mediators.

5. Therapeutic Potential of Astaxanthin

As discussed above, the SN is exposed to high levels of oxidative stress relative to other areas of the brain due to innate features of the neurons that comprise this region [50]. For example, there are low levels of glutathione and high concentration of iron leads to the production of free radicals through the Fenton reaction [51]. Glutathione activity in this region declines with age, further reducing the capacity to manage the accumulation of ROS in the SN. Taken together, these characteristics create an environment of high oxidative stress that can impair neuronal function.

One natural compound of particular interest is astaxanthin, a naturally occurring xanthophyll carotenoid. It is produced by the marine algae *Heamatococcus Pluvialis* or synthetically derived from carotenoid precursors and used commercially to feed to farmed fish species to increase pigmentation. Astaxanthin has many suggested mechanisms of action that uniquely oppose pathophysiology that underlie Parkinson's disease including actions as an anti-inflammatory action and improvements in aspects of mitochondrial function, indicating a distinct and promising therapeutic potential in the treatment and management of symptoms in PD patients that are likely more important than its role to simply scavenge free radicals [52–54].

Astaxanthin has potent and diverse actions as an antioxidant and is reported to be several times more effective than other carotenoids in its class. The molecular structure of astaxanthin allows it to reduce free radicals in a variety of ways, including absorbing them into the carbon backbone, donating electrons and forming adducts with the reactive species. Although xanthophyll carotenoids are structurally similar, the presence of polar ionone rings at either end of the astaxanthin molecule makes it energetically favorable. The configuration allows the molecule to span across the phospholipid bilayer of cell membranes and protect the membrane against lipid peroxidation [55].

There is substantial evidence indicating that treatment with astaxanthin causes a reduction in the markers of cellular stress due to excess ROS production, such as 8-isoprostane, protein carbonyl moieties and 8OHdG [56]. Additionally, astaxanthin has been shown to increase the efficacy of endogenous antioxidant mechanisms in vivo including increasing the expression or activity of glutathione, catalase, thioredoxin reductase and superoxide dismutase (SOD) [57,58]. It has also been shown to upregulate heme-oxygenease 1 (HO-1) through increase in NRF [59,60]. These findings suggest that astaxanthin treatment may help alleviate some of the ongoing oxidative stress that occurs during the progression of PD as it contributes to cellular dysfunction.

However, in addition to oxidative damage, there are a number of physiological changes that occur with age that exacerbate the cellular stress in the SN. Mitochondrial dynamics, proteosomal efficiency [61] and levels of synuclein [62] are all altered with age, likely rendering the DA cells more vulnerable to neurodegeneration. Aging also leads to microglial priming and may facilitate PD disease progression. Chronic microglial activation results in prolonged exposure to cytotoxic, pro-inflammatory cytokines, increasing cellular stress and ultimately leading to neurodegeneration [33]. Age_induced primed microglia are hyperactive upon subsequent stimulation and release exaggerated amounts of cytokines. They are resistant to reversion back to a state of tissue repair and maintenance of homeostasis, as they are less responsive to regulatory mechanisms [20,63,64]. As stated above, synuclein aggregation may also directly facilitate the release of these inflammatory mediators. It is thought that this inflammatory response to abnormal α-syn will perpetuate neural dysfunction through the release of cytotoxic compounds that overwhelm the DA cells, inevitably leading to cell death.

Given the range of pathological mechanisms involved in neurodegeneration seen in PD, astaxanthin seems to have a unique potential for the treatment of this disorder. Many diverse biological activities have been described in the literature that are particular relevant to that pathophysiology of PD, as well as normal aging. Based on this knowledge, the interaction of aging and parkinsonian symptoms should be responsive to treatment with astaxanthin. For example, astaxanthin has also been implicated in modulating microglial activity. Experiments using astaxanthin to treat a transformed microglial cell line can reduce the expression of IL-6 and iNOS/NO in vitro when exposed to an immune stimulus such as LPS [65]. These results were corroborated by other studies using aged animals where astaxanthin reduced the release of nitric oxide [56]. These molecules are released in high amounts by activated microglia and are associated with neuronal damage; attenuating the output of inflammatory mediators with astaxanthin may offer some neuroprotection from the inflammatory cascades occurring in the SN.

Some authors have reported alterations in mitochondrial function after astaxanthin treatment. Although most of these studies were conducted in vitro, this is of great interest to the treatment of PD. Mitochondrial dysfunction has been implicated in the etiology of the disorder evidenced by the common toxins that induce Parkinsonism. Both MPTP and rotenone are used to produce Parkinson's models by selectively targeting mitochondria leading to the death of SN neurons. Multiple genetic mutations of proteins involved in mitochondrial dynamics have been clearly linked to the development of familial Parkinson's. Furthermore, some of these mitochondrial proteins are associated with a loss of function with age, and may contribute to the increased incidence of diagnosis over the lifespan.

Furthermore, it has been demonstrated recently that mitochondria are a significant source of oxidative stress not only in these DA neurons, but also in additional nuclei known to degenerate in PD. For example, both the locus coeruleus and SN express L-type calcium channels that allow for an extraneous calcium influx that taxes the mitochondria [66,67]. The presence of these channels and their associated calcium burden has been proposed to be a common physiological feature that contributes to the cellular vulnerability for the brain regions affected in PD. Attenuating this mitochondrial derived oxidative stress that results from calcium overload has led to the use of calcium channel antagonists for the treatment of PD [68]. These dihydropyrdines, specifically israpidine, have been shown to be tolerable and safe among PD patients are now in Phase III clinical trial [69].

The success of these drugs lends support for the therapeutic use of AXT as well. There is substantial evidence to suggest that astaxanthin works at the level of the mitochondria. According to HPLC analysis of cellular fractions, astaxanthin will accumulate in mitochondria, and has the capacity to increase mitochondrial activity as indicated by increased respiration and mitochondrial membrane potential (MMP) [70]. Mitochondrial dysfunction is a common pathophysiological observation in PD, and is recapitulated in the α-synuclein model. It has been shown that treating isolated mitochondria with α-synuclein oligomers induced mitochondrial dysfunction by inhibiting complex 1 and associated with reduced calcium retention time, release of ROS and induced mitochondrial swelling [7]. In specific studies related to PD, astaxanthin has been shown to protect SH-SY5Y cells from 6-OHDA [53]. In a similar experiment, astaxanthin treatment mitigated cytotoxicity in PC12 cells from MPP+ induced cytotoxicity. MPP+ is a toxic metabolite of the dopaminergic neurotoxin MPTP used in experimental animal models of PD [71]. These cell culture results were corroborated by an in vivo study using astaxanthin to prevent the neurodegeneration in the SN in response to dose of MPTP (1 i.p. dose 30 mg/kg daily for 28 days) [54]. This treatment regimen effectively protected against the loss of tyrosine hydroxylase in the SN and striatum after chronic exposure to the neurotoxin. However, it is important to understand that many drugs that have been successful in some pre-clinical models of PD have failed to translate to patients with PD. Developing and testing pre-clinical models involving disease relevant proteins such as α-synuclein and the impact of aging must be considered for future studies.

6. Conclusions

Parkinson's disease is primarily characterized by degeneration of the dopaminergic neurons of the substantia nigra. The pathophysiology underlying this cell death is not yet clearly understood, although it is evident that many biological processes are impaired in this vulnerable brain region, explaining the rapid deterioration of the SN with age. Neuroinflammation is an integral factor perpetuating cellular damage during progression of the disease, and efforts to mitigate the inflammatory cascade have been successful in experimental settings, suggesting that anti-inflammatory treatments are a viable therapeutic strategy to employ in managing Parkinson's disease. Fractalkine signaling has proven to be a critical pathway in inflammation-mediated cell death that occurs in animal models of PD. Astaxanthin has diverse biological activities that have been reported in the literature, many of which seem to directly oppose the pathological mechanisms involved in neurodegeneration of the SN. Both fractalkine and astaxanthin represent two promising novel therapeutic agents for the treatment and management of PD.

Acknowledgments: This work was supported by NIA grants AG04418 (PCB), AG044919 (PCB); VA IO1BX000231 (PCB), and the Michael J Fox foundation (KN/PCB). This work was supported by the federal government. The contents of this manuscript do not represent the views of the Department of Veterans Affairs or the United States Government.

Author Contributions: This is a review paper, but P.C.B., K.N., and J.M. conceived and designed the experiments from our lab that are cited within the document; B.G. and J.M. performed the previous experiments and analyzed the data discussed within the text; B.G., P.C.B., and K.N. wrote the paper.

References

1. Kowal, S.L.; Dall, T.M.; Chakrabarti, R.; Storm, M.V.; Jain, A. The current and projected economic burden of Parkinson's disease in the United States. *Mov. Disord.* **2013**, *28*, 311–318. [CrossRef] [PubMed]
2. Braak, H.; Ghebremedhin, E.; Rüb, U.; Bratzke, H.; Del Tredici, K. Stages in the development of Parkinson's disease-related pathology. *Cell Tissue Res.* **2004**, *318*, 121–134. [CrossRef] [PubMed]
3. Zhang, W.; Wang, T.; Pei, Z.; Miller, D.S.; Wu, X.; Block, M.L.; Wilson, B.; Zhang, W.; Zhou, Y.; Hong, J.-S.S.; Zhang, J. Aggregated alpha-synuclein activates microglia: A process leading to disease progression in Parkinson's disease. *FASEB J.* **2005**, *19*, 533–542. [CrossRef] [PubMed]
4. Stefanis, L. α-Synuclein in Parkinson's disease. *Cold Spring Harb. Perspect. Med.* **2012**, *2*, a009399. [CrossRef] [PubMed]

5. Stefanovic, A.N.; Stöckl, M.T.; Claessens, M.M.; Subramaniam, V. α-Synuclein oligomers distinctively permeabilize complex model membranes. *FEBS J.* **2014**, *281*, 2838–2850. [CrossRef] [PubMed]
6. Danzer, K.M.; Haasen, D.; Karow, A.R.; Moussaud, S.; Habeck, M.; Giese, A.; Kretzschmar, H.; Hengerer, B.; Kostka, M. Different species of alpha-synuclein oligomers induce calcium influx and seeding. *J. Neurosci.* **2007**, *27*, 9220–9232. [CrossRef] [PubMed]
7. Luth, E.S.; Stavrovskaya, I.G.; Bartels, T.; Kristal, B.S.; Selkoe, D.J. Soluble, prefibrillar α-synuclein oligomers promote complex I-dependent, Ca^{2+}-induced mitochondrial dysfunction. *J. Biol. Chem.* **2014**, *289*, 21490–21507. [CrossRef] [PubMed]
8. Volpicelli-Daley, L.A.; Gamble, K.L.; Schultheiss, C.E.; Riddle, D.M.; West, A.B.; Lee, V.M. Formation of α-synuclein Lewy neurite-like aggregates in axons impedes the transport of distinct endosomes. *Mol. Biol. Cell* **2014**, *25*, 4010–4023. [CrossRef] [PubMed]
9. Lashuel, H.A.; Petre, B.M.; Wall, J.; Simon, M.; Nowak, R.J.; Walz, T.; Lansbury, P.T. Alpha-synuclein, especially the Parkinson's disease-associated mutants, forms pore-like annular and tubular protofibrils. *J. Mol. Biol.* **2002**, *322*, 1089–1102. [CrossRef]
10. Hurtig, H.I.; Trojanowski, J.Q.; Galvin, J.; Ewbank, D.; Schmidt, M.L.; Lee, V.M.; Clark, C.M.; Glosser, G.; Stern, M.B.; Gollomp, S.M.; et al. Alpha-synuclein cortical Lewy bodies correlate with dementia in Parkinson's disease. *Neurology* **2000**, *54*, 1916–1921. [CrossRef] [PubMed]
11. Tanaka, M.; Kim, Y.M.; Lee, G.; Junn, E.; Iwatsubo, T.; Mouradian, M.M. Aggresomes formed by alpha-synuclein and synphilin-1 are cytoprotective. *J. Biol. Chem.* **2004**, *279*, 4625–4631. [CrossRef] [PubMed]
12. Reeve, A.; Simcox, E.; Turnbull, D. Ageing and Parkinson's disease: Why is advancing age the biggest risk factor? *Ageing Res. Rev.* **2014**, *14*, 19–30. [CrossRef] [PubMed]
13. Hirsch, E.; Graybiel, A.M.; Agid, Y.A. Melanized dopaminergic neurons are differentially susceptible to degeneration in Parkinson's disease. *Nature* **1988**, *334*, 345–348. [CrossRef] [PubMed]
14. Dias, V.; Junn, E.; Mouradian, M.M. The role of oxidative stress in Parkinson's disease. *J. Parkinsons Dis.* **2013**, *3*, 461–491. [PubMed]
15. Bharath, S.; Hsu, M.; Kaur, D.; Rajagopalan, S.; Andersen, J.K. Glutathione, iron and Parkinson's disease. *Biochem. Pharmacol.* **2002**, *64*, 1037–1048. [CrossRef]
16. Venkateshappa, C.; Harish, G.; Mythri, R.B.; Mahadevan, A.; Bharath, M.M.; Shankar, S.K. Increased oxidative damage and decreased antioxidant function in aging human substantia nigra compared to striatum: Implications for Parkinson's disease. *Neurochem. Res.* **2012**, *37*, 358–369. [CrossRef] [PubMed]
17. Paolicelli, R.C.; Gross, C.T. Microglia in development: Linking brain wiring to brain environment. *Neuron Glia Biol.* **2011**, *7*, 77–83. [CrossRef] [PubMed]
18. Schafer, D.P.; Lehrman, E.K.; Kautzman, A.G.; Koyama, R.; Mardinly, A.R.; Yamasaki, R.; Ransohoff, R.M.; Greenberg, M.E.; Barres, B.A.; Stevens, B. Microglia sculpt postnatal neural circuits in an activity and complement-dependent manner. *Neuron* **2012**, *74*, 691–705. [CrossRef] [PubMed]
19. Jurgens, H.A.; Johnson, R.W. Dysregulated neuronal-microglial cross-talk during aging, stress and inflammation. *Exp. Neurol.* **2012**, *233*, 40–48. [CrossRef] [PubMed]
20. Lee, D.C.; Ruiz, C.R.; Lebson, L.; Selenica, M.-L.B.L.; Rizer, J.; Hunt, J.B.; Rojiani, R.; Reid, P.; Kammath, S.; Nash, K.; et al. Aging enhances classical activation but mitigates alternative activation in the central nervous system. *Neurobiol. Aging* **2013**, *34*, 1610–1620. [CrossRef] [PubMed]
21. Norden, D.M.; Muccigrosso, M.M.; Godbout, J.P. Microglial priming and enhanced reactivity to secondary insult in aging, and traumatic CNS injury, and neurodegenerative disease. *Neuropharmacology* **2015**, *96*, 29–41. [CrossRef] [PubMed]
22. Hickman, S.E.; Kingery, N.D.; Ohsumi, T.K.; Borowsky, M.L.; Wang, L.C.; Means, T.K.; El Khoury, J. The microglial sensome revealed by direct RNA sequencing. *Nat. Neurosci.* **2013**, *16*, 1896–1905. [CrossRef] [PubMed]
23. Cho, S.-H.H.; Chen, J.A.; Sayed, F.; Ward, M.E.; Gao, F.; Nguyen, T.A.; Krabbe, G.; Sohn, P.D.; Lo, I.; Minami, S.; et al. SIRT1 deficiency in microglia contributes to cognitive decline in aging and neurodegeneration via epigenetic regulation of IL-1β. *J. Neurosci.* **2015**, *35*, 807–818. [CrossRef] [PubMed]
24. McGeer, P.L.; Itagaki, S.; Akiyama, H.; McGeer, E.G. Rate of cell death in parkinsonism indicates active neuropathological process. *Ann. Neurol.* **1988**, *24*, 574–576. [CrossRef] [PubMed]
25. Knott, C.; Stern, G.; Wilkin, G.P. Inflammatory regulators in Parkinson's disease: iNOS, lipocortin-1, and cyclooxygenases-1 and -2. *Mol. Cell. Neurosci.* **2000**, *16*, 724–739. [CrossRef] [PubMed]

26. Gerhard, A.; Trender-Gerhard, I.; Turkheimer, F.; Quinn, N.P.; Bhatia, K.P.; Brooks, D.J. In vivo imaging of microglial activation with [11C](R)-PK11195 PET in progressive supranuclear palsy. *Mov. Disord.* **2006**, *21*, 89–93. [CrossRef] [PubMed]
27. Goldman, S.M.; Tanner, C.M.; Oakes, D.; Bhudhikanok, G.S.; Gupta, A.; Langston, J.W. Head injury and Parkinson's disease risk in twins. *Ann. Neurol.* **2006**, *60*, 65–72. [CrossRef] [PubMed]
28. Lawson, L.J.; Perry, V.H.; Dri, P.; Gordon, S. Heterogeneity in the distribution and morphology of microglia in the normal adult mouse brain. *Neuroscience* **1990**, *39*, 151–170. [CrossRef]
29. Sharma, N.; Nehru, B. Characterization of the lipopolysaccharide induced model of Parkinson's disease: Role of oxidative stress and neuroinflammation. *Neurochem. Int.* **2015**, *87*, 92–105. [CrossRef] [PubMed]
30. Codolo, G.; Plotegher, N.; Pozzobon, T.; Brucale, M.; Tessari, I.; Bubacco, L.; de Bernard, M. Triggering of inflammasome by aggregated α-synuclein, an inflammatory response in synucleinopathies. *PLoS ONE* **2013**, *8*, e55375. [CrossRef] [PubMed]
31. Reynolds, A.D.; Glanzer, J.G.; Kadiu, I.; Ricardo-Dukelow, M.; Chaudhuri, A.; Ciborowski, P.; Cerny, R.; Gelman, B.; Thomas, M.P.; Mosley, R.L.; et al. Nitrated alpha-synuclein-activated microglial profiling for Parkinson's disease. *J. Neurochem.* **2008**, *104*, 1504–1525. [CrossRef] [PubMed]
32. Cao, S.; Theodore, S.; Standaert, D.G. Fcγ receptors are required for NF-κB signaling, microglial activation and dopaminergic neurodegeneration in an AAV-synuclein mouse model of Parkinson's disease. *Mol. Neurodegener.* **2010**, *5*, 42. [CrossRef] [PubMed]
33. Cao, S.; Standaert, D.G.; Harms, A.S. The gamma chain subunit of Fc receptors is required for alpha-synuclein-induced pro-inflammatory signaling in microglia. *J. Neuroinflamm.* **2012**, *9*, 259. [CrossRef] [PubMed]
34. Polinski, N.K.; Gombash, S.E.; Manfredsson, F.P.; Lipton, J.W.; Kemp, C.J.; Cole-Strauss, A.; Kanaan, N.M.; Steece-Collier, K.; Kuhn, N.C.; Wohlgenant, S.L.; et al. Recombinant adenoassociated virus 2/5-mediated gene transfer is reduced in the aged rat midbrain. *Neurobiol. Aging* **2015**, *36*, 1110–1120. [CrossRef] [PubMed]
35. Nash, K.R.; Moran, P.; Finneran, D.J.; Hudson, C.; Robinson, J.; Morgan, D.; Bickford, P.C. Fractalkine over expression suppresses α-synuclein-mediated neurodegeneration. *Mol. Ther.* **2015**, *23*, 17–23. [CrossRef] [PubMed]
36. Morganti, J.M.; Nash, K.R.; Grimmig, B.A.; Ranjit, S.; Small, B.; Bickford, P.C.; Gemma, C. The soluble isoform of CX3CL1 is necessary for neuroprotection in a mouse model of Parkinson's disease. *J. Neurosci.* **2012**, *32*, 14592–14601. [CrossRef] [PubMed]
37. Pabon, M.M.; Jernberg, J.N.; Morganti, J.; Contreras, J.; Hudson, C.E.; Klein, R.L.; Bickford, P.C. A spirulina-enhanced diet provides neuroprotection in an α-synuclein model of Parkinson's disease. *PLoS ONE* **2012**, *7*, e45256. [CrossRef] [PubMed]
38. Pabon, M.M.; Bachstetter, A.D.; Hudson, C.E.; Gemma, C.; Bickford, P.C. CX3CL1 reduces neurotoxicity and microglial activation in a rat model of Parkinson's disease. *J. Neuroinflamm.* **2011**, *8*, 9. [CrossRef] [PubMed]
39. Rees, K.; Stowe, R.; Patel, S.; Ives, N.; Breen, K.; Clarke, C.E.; Ben-Shlomo, Y. Non-steroidal anti-inflammatory drugs as disease-modifying agents for Parkinson's disease: Evidence from observational studies. *Cochrane Database Syst. Rev.* **2011**, *11*, CD008454. [PubMed]
40. Du, Y.; Ma, Z.; Lin, S.; Dodel, R.C.; Gao, F.; Bales, K.R.; Triarhou, L.C.; Chernet, E.; Perry, K.W.; Nelson, D.L.; et al. Minocycline prevents nigrostriatal dopaminergic neurodegeneration in the MPTP model of Parkinson's disease. *Proc. Natl. Acad. Sci. USA* **2001**, *98*, 14669–14674. [CrossRef] [PubMed]
41. Lee, S.M.; Yune, T.Y.; Kim, S.J.; Kim, Y.C.; Oh, Y.J.; Markelonis, G.J.; Oh, T.H. Minocycline inhibits apoptotic cell death via attenuation of TNF-alpha expression following iNOS/NO induction by lipopolysaccharide in neuron/glia co-cultures. *J. Neurochem.* **2004**, *91*, 568–578. [CrossRef] [PubMed]
42. Jones, B.A.; Beamer, M.; Ahmed, S. Fractalkine/CX3CL1: A potential new target for inflammatory diseases. *Mol. Interv.* **2010**, *10*, 263–270. [CrossRef] [PubMed]
43. Cardona, A.E.; Pioro, E.P.; Sasse, M.E.; Kostenko, V.; Cardona, S.M.; Dijkstra, I.M.; Huang, D.; Kidd, G.; Dombrowski, S.; Dutta, R.; et al. Control of microglial neurotoxicity by the fractalkine receptor. *Nat. Neurosci.* **2006**, *9*, 917–924. [CrossRef] [PubMed]
44. Thome, A.D.; Standaert, D.G.; Harms, A.S. Fractalkine signaling regulates the inflammatory response in an α-synuclein model of Parkinson disease. *PLoS ONE* **2015**, *10*, e0140566. [CrossRef] [PubMed]

45. Nash, K.R.; Lee, D.C.; Hunt, J.B.; Morganti, J.M.; Selenica, M.-L.L.; Moran, P.; Reid, P.; Brownlow, M.; Yang, C.G.; Savalia, M.; et al. Fractalkine overexpression suppresses tau pathology in a mouse model of tauopathy. *Neurobiol. Aging* **2013**, *34*, 1540–1548. [CrossRef] [PubMed]
46. Lee, S.; Xu, G.; Jay, T.R.; Bhatta, S.; Kim, K.-W.W.; Jung, S.; Landreth, G.E.; Ransohoff, R.M.; Lamb, B.T. Opposing effects of membrane-anchored CX3CL1 on amyloid and tau pathologies via the p38 MAPK pathway. *J. Neurosci.* **2014**, *34*, 12538–12546. [CrossRef] [PubMed]
47. Norden, D.M.; Godbout, J.P. Review: Microglia of the aged brain: Primed to be activated and resistant to regulation. *Neuropathol. Appl. Neurobiol.* **2013**, *39*, 19–34. [CrossRef] [PubMed]
48. Bachstetter, A.D.; Morganti, J.M.; Jernberg, J.; Schlunk, A.; Mitchell, S.H.; Brewster, K.W.; Hudson, C.E.; Cole, M.J.; Harrison, J.K.; Bickford, P.C.; et al. Fractalkine and CX 3 CR1 regulate hippocampal neurogenesis in adult and aged rats. *Neurobiol. Aging* **2011**, *32*, 2030–2044. [CrossRef] [PubMed]
49. Wynne, A.M.; Henry, C.J.; Huang, Y.; Cleland, A.; Godbout, J.P. Protracted downregulation of CX3CR1 on microglia of aged mice after lipopolysaccharide challenge. *Brain Behav. Immun.* **2010**, *24*, 1190–1201. [CrossRef] [PubMed]
50. Surmeier, D.J.; Guzman, J.N.; Sanchez-Padilla, J. Calcium, cellular aging, and selective neuronal vulnerability in Parkinson's disease. *Cell Calcium* **2010**, *47*, 175–182. [CrossRef] [PubMed]
51. Surmeier, D.; Guzman, J.; Sanchez-Padilla, J.; Goldberg, J. What causes the death of dopaminergic neurons in Parkinson's Disease? *Prog. Brain Res.* **2010**, *183*, 59–77. [PubMed]
52. Kim, Y.H.; Koh, H.-K.K.; Kim, D.-S.S. Down-regulation of IL-6 production by astaxanthin via ERK-, MSK-, and NF-κB-mediated signals in activated microglia. *Int. Immunopharmacol.* **2010**, *10*, 1560–1572. [CrossRef] [PubMed]
53. Liu, X.; Shibata, T.; Hisaka, S.; Osawa, T. Astaxanthin inhibits reactive oxygen species-mediated cellular toxicity in dopaminergic SH-SY5Y cells via mitochondria-targeted protective mechanism. *Brain Res.* **2009**, *1254*, 18–27. [CrossRef] [PubMed]
54. Lee, D.-H.H.; Kim, C.-S.S.; Lee, Y.J. Astaxanthin protects against MPTP/MPP+-induced mitochondrial dysfunction and ROS production in vivo and in vitro. *Food Chem. Toxicol.* **2011**, *49*, 271–280. [CrossRef] [PubMed]
55. Kidd, P. Astaxanthin, a cell membrane nutrient with diverse clinical benefits and anti aging potential. *Am. Med. Rev.* **2011**, *16*, 355–364.
56. Park, J.; Mathison, B.; Hayek, M.; Zhang, J.; Reinhart, G.; Chew, B. Astaxanthin modulates age-associated mitochondrial dysfunction in healthy dogs. *J. Anim. Sci.* **2012**, *91*, 268275. [CrossRef] [PubMed]
57. Otton, R.; Marin, D.P.; Bolin, A.P.; Santos, R.C.; Polotow, T.G.; Sampaio, S.C.; de Barros, M.P. Astaxanthin ameliorates the redox imbalance in lymphocytes of experimental diabetic rats. *Chem. Biol. Interact.* **2010**, *186*, 306–315. [CrossRef] [PubMed]
58. Augusti, P.R.; Quatrin, A.; Somacal, S.; Conterato, G.M.; Sobieski, R.; Ruviaro, A.R.; Maurer, L.H.; Duarte, M.M.; Roehrs, M.; Emanuelli, T. Astaxanthin prevents changes in the activities of thioredoxin reductase and paraoxonase in hypercholesterolemic rabbits. *J. Clin. Biochem. Nutr.* **2012**, *51*, 42–49. [CrossRef] [PubMed]
59. Li, Z.; Dong, X.; Liu, H.; Chen, X.; Shi, H.; Fan, Y.; Hou, D.; Zhang, X. Astaxanthin protects ARPE-19 cells from oxidative stress via upregulation of Nrf2-regulated phase II enzymes through activation of PI3K/Akt. *Mol. Vis.* **2013**, *19*, 1656–1666. [PubMed]
60. Wang, H.-Q.Q.; Sun, X.-B.B.; Xu, Y.-X.X.; Zhao, H.; Zhu, Q.-Y.Y.; Zhu, C.-Q.Q. Astaxanthin upregulates heme oxygenase-1 expression through ERK1/2 pathway and its protective effect against beta-amyloid-induced cytotoxicity in SH-SY5Y cells. *Brain Res.* **2010**, *1360*, 159–167. [CrossRef] [PubMed]
61. Brunk, U.T.; Terman, A. The mitochondrial-lysosomal axis theory of aging: Accumulation of damaged mitochondria as a result of imperfect autophagocytosis. *Eur. J. Biochem.* **2002**, *269*, 1996–2002. [CrossRef] [PubMed]
62. Collier, T.J.; Kanaan, N.M.; Kordower, J.H. Ageing as a primary risk factor for Parkinson's disease: Evidence from studies of non-human primates. *Nat. Rev. Neurosci.* **2011**, *12*, 359–366. [CrossRef] [PubMed]
63. Qin, Y.; Sun, X.; Shao, X.; Cheng, C.; Feng, J.; Sun, W.; Gu, D.; Liu, W.; Xu, F.; Duan, Y. Macrophage-microglia networks drive M1 microglia polarization after mycobacterium infection. *Inflammation* **2015**, *38*, 1609–1616. [CrossRef] [PubMed]

64. Minogue, A.M.; Jones, R.S.; Kelly, R.J.; McDonald, C.L.; Connor, T.J.; Lynch, M.A. Age-associated dysregulation of microglial activation is coupled with enhanced blood-brain barrier permeability and pathology in APP/PS1 mice. *Neurobiol. Aging* **2014**, *35*, 1442–1452. [CrossRef] [PubMed]
65. Choi, S.-K.K.; Park, Y.-S.S.; Choi, D.-K.K.; Chang, H.-I.I. Effects of astaxanthin on the production of NO and the expression of COX-2 and iNOS in LPS-stimulated BV2 microglial cells. *J. Microbiol. Biotechnol.* **2008**, *18*, 1990–1996. [PubMed]
66. Sanchez-Padilla, J.; Guzman, J.N.; Ilijic, E.; Kondapalli, J.; Galtieri, D.J.; Yang, B.; Schieber, S.; Oertel, W.; Wokosin, D.; Schumacker, P.T.; et al. Mitochondrial oxidant stress in locus coeruleus is regulated by activity and nitric oxide synthase. *Nat. Neurosci.* **2014**, *17*, 832–840. [CrossRef] [PubMed]
67. Dryanovski, D.I.; Guzman, J.N.; Xie, Z.; Galteri, D.J.; Volpicelli-Daley, L.A.; Lee, V.M.; Miller, R.J.; Schumacker, P.T.; Surmeier, D.J. Calcium entry and α-synuclein inclusions elevate dendritic mitochondrial oxidant stress in dopaminergic neurons. *J. Neurosci.* **2013**, *33*, 10154–10164. [CrossRef] [PubMed]
68. Surmeier, D.J.; Guzman, J.N.; Sanchez-Padilla, J.; Schumacker, P.T. The role of calcium and mitochondrial oxidant stress in the loss of substantia nigra pars compacta dopaminergic neurons in Parkinson's disease. *Neuroscience* **2011**, *198*, 221–231. [CrossRef] [PubMed]
69. Parkinson Study Group. Phase II safety, tolerability, and dose selection study of isradipine as a potential disease-modifying intervention in early Parkinson's disease (STEADY-PD). *Mov. Disord.* **2013**, *28*, 1823–1831.
70. Wolf, A.M.; Asoh, S.; Hiranuma, H.; Ohsawa, I.; Iio, K.; Satou, A.; Ishikura, M.; Ohta, S. Astaxanthin protects mitochondrial redox state and functional integrity against oxidative stress. *J. Nutr. Biochem.* **2010**, *21*, 381–389. [CrossRef] [PubMed]
71. Ye, Q.; Huang, B.; Zhang, X.; Zhu, Y.; Chen, X. Astaxanthin protects against MPP(+)-induced oxidative stress in PC12 cells via the HO-1/NOX2 axis. *BMC Neurosci.* **2012**, *13*, 156. [CrossRef] [PubMed]

Permissions

All chapters in this book were first published by MDPI; hereby published with permission under the Creative Commons Attribution License or equivalent. Every chapter published in this book has been scrutinized by our experts. Their significance has been extensively debated. The topics covered herein carry significant findings which will fuel the growth of the discipline. They may even be implemented as practical applications or may be referred to as a beginning point for another development.

The contributors of this book come from diverse backgrounds, making this book a truly international effort. This book will bring forth new frontiers with its revolutionizing research information and detailed analysis of the nascent developments around the world.

We would like to thank all the contributing authors for lending their expertise to make the book truly unique. They have played a crucial role in the development of this book. Without their invaluable contributions this book wouldn't have been possible. They have made vital efforts to compile up to date information on the varied aspects of this subject to make this book a valuable addition to the collection of many professionals and students.

This book was conceptualized with the vision of imparting up-to-date information and advanced data in this field. To ensure the same, a matchless editorial board was set up. Every individual on the board went through rigorous rounds of assessment to prove their worth. After which they invested a large part of their time researching and compiling the most relevant data for our readers.

The editorial board has been involved in producing this book since its inception. They have spent rigorous hours researching and exploring the diverse topics which have resulted in the successful publishing of this book. They have passed on their knowledge of decades through this book. To expedite this challenging task, the publisher supported the team at every step. A small team of assistant editors was also appointed to further simplify the editing procedure and attain best results for the readers.

Apart from the editorial board, the designing team has also invested a significant amount of their time in understanding the subject and creating the most relevant covers. They scrutinized every image to scout for the most suitable representation of the subject and create an appropriate cover for the book.

The publishing team has been an ardent support to the editorial, designing and production team. Their endless efforts to recruit the best for this project, has resulted in the accomplishment of this book. They are a veteran in the field of academics and their pool of knowledge is as vast as their experience in printing. Their expertise and guidance has proved useful at every step. Their uncompromising quality standards have made this book an exceptional effort. Their encouragement from time to time has been an inspiration for everyone.

The publisher and the editorial board hope that this book will prove to be a valuable piece of knowledge for researchers, students, practitioners and scholars across the globe.

List of Contributors

Damir Nizamutdinov and Lee A. Shapiro
Department of Surgery, Texas A & M University Health Science Center, College of Medicine, Temple, TX 76504, USA
Department of Neurosurgery, Neuroscience Research Institute, Baylor Scott & White Health, Temple, TX 76504, USA

Maria Elena González-Fraguela and Teresa Serrano Sanchez
Immunochemical Department, International Center for Neurological Restoration, 25th Ave, Playa, 15805, PC 11300 Havana, Cuba

Lourdes Lorigados Pedre and María de los Angeles Robinson-Agramonte
Neuroimmunology Laboratory, Immunochemical Department, International Center for Neurological Restoration, Ave 25 # 15805 b/w 158 and 160, Playa, Havana 11300, Cuba
Immunochemical Department, International Center for Neurological Restoration, 25th Ave, Playa, 15805, Havana PC 11300, Cuba

Orlando Ramón Serrano-Barrera
Las Tunas General Hospital, Las Tunas 75100, Cuba

Han Liu, Enquan Xu, Jianuo Liu and Huangui Xiong
Department of Pharmacology and Experimental Neuroscience, University of Nebraska Medical Center, Omaha, NE 68198-5880, USA

Donna Gruol
Molecular and Cellular Neuroscience Department, The Scripps Research Institute, La Jolla, CA 92037, USA

Lázaro Gómez
Non Invasive Brain Stimulation Unit, International Center for Neurological Restoration, 25th Ave, Playa, Havana 15805, Cuba
Clinical Neurophysiology Lab., International Center for Neurological Restoration, 25th Ave. Playa, Havana 15805, Cuba

Belkis Vidal and Maribel Selguera
Child and Adolescent Mental Health Service, Borrás-Marfán Hospital, G and 27 Street, Vedado, Havana 10400, Cuba

Carlos Maragoto, Héctor Vera Cuesta, Marlén Denis, Tairí Marín and Yaumara Cabrera
Non Invasive Brain Stimulation Unit, International Center for Neurological Restoration, 25th Ave, Playa, Havana 15805, Cuba
Neuropediatric Clinic, International Center for Neurological Restoration, 25th Ave. Playa, Havana 15805, Cuba

Lilia Maria Morales, Sheyla Berrillo, Margarita Baez, Celia Alarcón and Lucila Dieguez
Clinical Neurophysiology Lab., International Center for Neurological Restoration, 25th Ave. Playa, Havana 15805, Cuba

Abel Sánchez
Non Invasive Brain Stimulation Unit, International Center for Neurological Restoration, 25th Ave, Playa, Havana 15805, Cuba

Yaima Llanez
Neuropediatric Clinic, International Center for Neurological Restoration, 25th Ave. Playa, Havana 15805, Cuba

María Robinson
Clinical Immunology Lab., International Center for Neurological Restoration, 25th Ave. Playa, Havana 15805, Cuba

Gatambwa Mukandala, Ronan Tynan, Sinead Lanigan and John J. O'Connor
UCD School of Biomolecular and Biomedical Science, UCD Conway Institute of Biomolecular and Biomedical Research, Belfield, Dublin 4, Ireland

Simon Alex Marshall
Department of Psychology & Neuroscience, University of North Carolina-Chapel Hill, Chapel Hill, NC 27599, USA

Chelsea Rhea Geil and Kimberly Nixon
Department of Pharmaceutical Sciences, College of Pharmacy, University of Kentucky, Lexington, KY 40536, USA

Estate M. Sokhadze, Emily L. Casanova, Desmond P. Kelly and Manuel F. Casanova
Department of Biomedical Sciences, University of South Carolina School of Medicine-Greenville, 200 Patewood Dr., Ste A200, Greenville, SC 29615, USA
Developmental Behavioral Unit, Department of Pediatrics, Children's Hospital, Greenville Health System, Greenville, SC 29615, USA

Eva V. Lamina
Department of Biomedical Sciences, University of South Carolina School of Medicine-Greenville, 200 Patewood Dr., Ste A200, Greenville, SC 29615, USA

Ioan Opris
School of Medicine, University of Miami, Miami, FL 33136, USA

Irma Khachidze
Centre of Experimental Biomedicine, 14 Gotya Str., Tbilisi 0160, Georgia

Sulie L. Chang
Institute of NeuroImmune Pharmacology, Seton Hall University, 400 South Orange Avenue, South Orange, NJ 07079, USA
Department of Biological Sciences, Seton Hall University, 400 South Orange Avenue, South Orange, NJ 07079, USA

Wenfei Huang, Xin Mao and Sabroni Sarkar
Institute of NeuroImmune Pharmacology, Seton Hall University, 400 South Orange Avenue, South Orange, NJ 07079, USA

Lisette Blanco Lezcano and Jorge A Bergado Rosado
Immunochemical Department, International Center for Neurological Restoration, 25th Ave, Playa, 15805, Havana PC 11300, Cuba

Esteban Alberti Amador
Molecular Biology Department, International Center of Neurological Restoration (CIREN) Ave. 25 No. 15805 e/158 and 160, Playa, Havana 11300, Cuba

Beatriz Caballero Fernández
Policlínico 26 de Julio, Calle 72 #1313. A. Almendares, Playa, Havana 11300, Cuba

Maria Erta, Mercedes Giralt, Amalia Molinero, Gemma Comes and Juan Hidalgo
Department of Cellular Biology, Physiology and Immunology, Animal Physiology Unit, Faculty of Biosciences, Universitat Autònoma de Barcelona, Bellaterra 08193, Spain
Institute of Neurosciences, Universitat Autònoma de Barcelona, Bellaterra 08193, Spain

Silvia Jiménez
Department of Cellular Biology, Physiology and Immunology, Animal Physiology Unit, Faculty of Biosciences, Universitat Autònoma de Barcelona, Bellaterra 08193, Spain

Lisette Blanco-Lezcano and Caridad Ivette Fernandez-Verdecia
Experimental Neurophysiology Department, International Center of Neurological Restoration (CIREN) Ave. 25 No. 15805 e/158 and 160, Playa, Havana 11300, Cuba

Lidia Leonor Cardellá Rosales
Physiologic Sciences Department, Latin American Medicine School, Carretera Panamericana, Kilómetro 3 1/2 Municipio Playa, Habana 19148, Cuba

Darin J. Knapp
Bowles Center for Alcohol Studies, The University of North Carolina at Chapel Hill, CB7178, Chapel Hill, NC 27599-7178, USA
Department of Psychiatry, The University of North Carolina at Chapel Hill, CB7178, Chapel Hill, NC 27599-7178, USA

Kathryn M. Harper and Zachary Zimomra
Bowles Center for Alcohol Studies, The University of North Carolina at Chapel Hill, CB7178, Chapel Hill, NC 27599-7178, USA

Buddy A. Whitman
Bowles Center for Alcohol Studies, The University of North Carolina at Chapel Hill, CB7178, Chapel Hill, NC 27599-7178, USA
Curriculum in Neurobiology, The University of North Carolina at Chapel Hill, CB7178, Chapel Hill, NC 27599-7178, USA

George R. Breese
Bowles Center for Alcohol Studies, The University of North Carolina at Chapel Hill, CB7178, Chapel Hill, NC 27599-7178, USA
Department of Psychiatry, The University of North Carolina at Chapel Hill, CB7178, Chapel Hill, NC 27599-7178, USA
Curriculum in Neurobiology, The University of North Carolina at Chapel Hill, CB7178, Chapel Hill, NC 27599-7178, USA
Department of Pharmacology, The University of North Carolina at Chapel Hill, CB7178, Chapel Hill, NC 27599-7178, USA
UNC Neuroscience Center, The University of North Carolina at Chapel Hill, CB7178, Chapel Hill, NC 27599-7178, USA

Simone Mori and Bruno Conti
Department of Chemical Physiology, The Scripps Research Institute, 10550 North Torrey Pines Road, La Jolla, CA 92037, USA

Pamela Maher
Cellular Neurobiology Laboratory, Salk Research Institute, La Jolla, CA 92037, USA

Bethany Grimmig
Center of Excellence for Aging and Brain Repair, Department of Neurosurgery and Brain Repair, Morsani College of Medicine, University of South Florida, Tampa, FL 33612, USA

Josh Morganti
Sanders-Brown Center on Aging, Department of Anatomy and Neurobiology, University of Kentucky, Lexington, KY 40508, USA

Kevin Nash
Byrd Alzheimer's Institute, Department of Molecular Pharmacology and Physiology, Morsani College of Medicine, University of South Florida, Tampa, FL 33613, USA

Paula C. Bickford
Center of Excellence for Aging and Brain Repair, Department of Neurosurgery and Brain Repair, Morsani College of Medicine, University of South Florida, Tampa, FL 33612, USA

Index

www.ingramcontent.com/pod-product-compliance
Lightning Source LLC
LaVergne TN
LVHW060552210926
848485LV00005B/1302